THE MENTAL HEALTH OF REFUGEES

Ecological Approaches
to Healing and Adaptation

THE MENTAL HEALTH OF REFUGEES

Ecological Approaches to Healing and Adaptation

Edited by

Kenneth E. Miller
San Francisco State University

Lisa M. Rasco
University of California, Berkeley

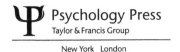
Psychology Press
Taylor & Francis Group

New York   London

Camera ready copy for this book was provided by the editors.

First published by Lawrence Erlbaum Associates, Inc., Publishers
10 Industrial Avenue
Mahwah, New Jersey 07430

Reprinted 2008 by Psychology Press

Psychology Press
Taylor & Francis Group
27 Church Road
Hove, East Sussex BN3 2FA

Cover design by Kathryn Houghtaling Lacey

Library of Congress Cataloging-in-Publication Data

The mental health of refugees: ecological approaches to healing and adaptation / edited by Kenneth E. Miller, Lisa M. Rasco.
    p. cm.

Includes bibliographical references and index.

ISBN 0-8058-4172-5 (cloth : alk. paper)
ISBN 0-8058-4173-3 (pbk. : alk. paper)
1. Refugees—Mental health. 2. Refugees—Mental health services.
   3. Cultural psychiatry. I. Miller, Kenneth E., 1963–   II. Rasco,
   Lisa M., 1970– .
RC451.4.R43F765 2004
362.2'086'914—dc22   2003064154
                                           CIP

Printed in the United States of America
10 9 8 7 6 5 4 3 2 1

To Don Mateo, Doña Maria, Emilio, and Alonzo,
Who taught me about community and the meaning of resilience;
And to my parents: George Miller, a friend and colleague whose support
has been invaluable and without limit,
and Nina Miller, whose commitment to creating a more socially just world
Continues to be an inspiration for the work I do.

—Ken Miller

To Semir and Sonja,
Who opened my eyes to the incredible strength
And healing power of family amidst great loss and transition;
And to my own family: Mom, Dad, Laura, Darren, and Jamie;
Rema, Josh, Ray, and Trish;
Ben, Cara, and Niko—
You sustain me.

—Lisa Rasco

vii

About the Editors

Kenneth E. Miller is an assistant professor of psychology at San Francisco State University. He received a doctorate in clinical psychology from the University of Michigan, and completed two years of postdoctoral training in community and prevention research at Arizona State University and the University of Illinois at Chicago. His research is focused on the impact of war experiences and exile-related stressors on refugee wellbeing, and on the effectiveness of ecological mental health interventions with refugee communities. He has worked with and studied Guatemalan refugee families in southern Mexico, Bosnian refugees in Chicago and the San Francisco Bay Area, and most recently Afghan refugees in the San Francisco Bay Area.

Lisa M. Rasco is a doctoral candidate in clinical psychology and fellow of the Center for the Development of Peace and Well-being at the University of California, Berkeley. Her research has focused on the psychophysiological effects of war-related trauma and currently concerns the impact of trauma and stress on family functioning and the socioemotional development of children. She has consulted on the design of a Bosnian community center and, with Ken Miller, on the development of an ecological mental health intervention for Afghan refugees that integrates mental health concepts and practices into the English as a Second Language classroom.

List of Contributors

Sanela Besic, Department of Psychiatry, University of Illinois at Chicago, Chicago, IL, USA

Jorge Enrique Buitrago Cuéllar, Corporación AVRE, Bogotá, Colombia

Maurice Eisenbruch, University of New South Wales, New South Wales, Australia

The Family Rehabilitation Centre Staff, Sri Lanka

Suzanne Feetham, Department of Psychiatry, University of Illinois at Chicago, Chicago, IL, USA

Jessica Goodkind, California State University Hayward, Hayward, CA, USA

Panfua Hang, Michigan State University, East Lansing, MI, USA

Jon Hubbard, Center for Victims of Torture, Minneapolis, MN, USA

Kathleen Kostelny, Erikson Institute, Chicago, IL, USA, and Christian Children's Fund, Richmond, VA, USA

Yasmina Kulauzovic, Department of Psychiatry, University of Illinois at Chicago, Chicago, IL, USA

Alma Lezic, Department of Psychiatry, University of Illinois at Chicago, Chicago, IL, USA

Kenneth E. Miller, San Francisco State University, San Francisco, CA, USA

Carlinda Monteiro, Christian Children's Fund, Luanda, Angola

Aida Mujagic, Department of Psychiatry, University of Illinois at Chicago, Chicago, IL, USA

Jasmina Muzurovic, Department of Psychiatry, University of Illinois at Chicago, Chicago, IL, USA

Ivan Pavkovic, Department of Psychiatry, University of Illinois at Chicago, Chicago, IL, USA

Nancy Pearson, Center for Victims of Torture, Minneapolis, MN, USA

Lisa M. Rasco, University of California Berkeley, Berkeley, CA, USA

John Rolland, Department of Psychiatry, University of Illinois at Chicago, Chicago, IL, USA

Dzemila Spahovic, Department of Psychiatry, University of Illinois at Chicago, Chicago, IL, USA

Rachel Tribe, University of East London, London, England

Willem A. C. M. van de Put, HealthNet International, Amsterdam, The Netherlands

Stevan M. Weine, Department of Psychiatry, University of Illinois at Chicaco, Chicago, IL USA

Michael Wessells, Christian Children's Fund, Richmond, VA, USA, and Randolph Macon College, Ashland, VA USA

Mee Yang, Michigan State University, East Lansing, MI, USA

Merita Zhubi, Department of Psychiatry, University of Illinois at Chicaco, Chicago, IL USA

PREFACE

At the dawn of the 21st century, we are living in a time of remarkable technological achievement, of extraordinary advancements in our ability to treat and prevent an ever-widening range of disease, and of an expanding global economy that links together the most geographically distant communities. Against this backdrop of impressive development, it is disheartening to observe how little distance we have traveled toward the creation of a more socially, economically, and environmentally just world community. Repressive regimes flourish, often with the covert aid of industrialized nations who profess a deep commitment to democratic ideals. The disparity in wealth between nations of the southern and northern hemispheres continues to worsen, with hundreds of millions of people in developing countries living on the equivalent of a dollar a day, and millions dying of preventable and treatable diseases. Multinational corporate profit is frequently prioritized over the basic human and civil rights of impoverished communities that provide inexpensive labor under conditions of exploitation and stark repression; and extreme ethnic violence, at times reaching the level of genocide, is allowed to proceed essentially unopposed while politicians offer moving speeches honoring the victims of the Nazi Holocaust and promise that such horrors will never again be allowed to occur.

Violent conflict, ethnic and political persecution, and state sanctioned repression continue to drive millions of people into exile or internal displacement, forcing them to leave behind their homes, their communities, and for many, their homelands. Many are forced to flee with little time to prepare for the journey of exile, and carry with them only their most essential and portable possessions. They leave behind houses, plots of land passed down through generations, family members and friends unable or unwilling to go into exile; proximity to the graves of ancestors; and the sense of belonging that comes with living in one's own culture, as a member of one's own community, a citizen of one's own country. They flee after having witnessed the death of loved ones, the destruction of their property, and the humiliation of family members, friends, and neighbors at the hands of sadistic armed combatants; and they flee after enduring their own experiences of physical and sexual violence, arbitrary detention, and prolonged fear and vulnerability. They leave not in search of a better life, but simply to survive, because survival in their own homes and communities has become tenuous if not altogether impossible. They seek safe haven, and many hold tightly to the dream of an eventual return home. History has demonstrated repeatedly, however, that the dreamt of return is often elusive, due to prolonged conflict that makes a safe repatriation impossible.

Psychologists, psychiatrists, and other mental health professionals have begun to recognize and document the high levels of psychological distress experienced by refugees and displaced persons worldwide. There is a rapidly growing body of research documenting patterns of widespread psychological trauma and depression within these communities, a pattern that holds across diverse methodologies and samples. Paralleling this emphasis on research, mental health professionals have begun offering clinical services such as psychotherapy and psychiatric medication to refugees, with the goal of alleviating symptoms of distress and facilitating adjustment to life in exile. Refugee mental health clinics have been established in major cities throughout the industrialized (i.e., "developed") world, as well as in some of the developing countries where the majority of the world's refugees and displaced people reside. The response of the mental health community has been well intentioned, and although empirical data are lacking, it seems reasonable to suggest that clinic-based services have provided much needed assistance to those refugees who have had access to and were willing to utilize them.

This book, which brings together the writings of leading experts in the field of refugee mental health, reflects a growing concern that clinic-based psychological and psychiatric services developed primarily in Western Europe and the United States may be limited in some very fundamental ways in their capacity to address the mental health needs of refugee communities. Rooted in Western conceptions of wellness, distress, and healing, such services are culturally alien to most refugees, who generally come from non-Western societies with very different models of mental health and the mechanisms by which distress should be alleviated. Such services are also limited because they are largely inaccessible to the majority of the world's displaced people, who live in developing countries where Western mental health services are often scarce or non-existent; and they are limited because they are poorly suited to addressing the diverse range of psychosocial stressors that affect refugees on a daily basis (e.g., the loss social support networks, the loss of social roles and of meaningful role-related activity, a lack of access to key resources, difficulties navigating the new setting).

In short, there is a gradual recognition occurring among mental health professionals who work with refugees and internally displaced people that the old paradigm of clinical intervention, though certainly useful, cannot be the cornerstone of our response to the mental health needs of these communities. The authors in this book share a common vision, a commitment to an alternative conceptual framework within which culturally appropriate refugee mental health programs can be developed. As the various chapters illustrate, such programs empower communities to take greater control over their own mental health and the conditions that affect it. Guided by an ecological model that combines elements of public health, empowerment theory, community psychology, clinical psychology, psychiatry, and anthropology, ecological mental health programs have been developed for refugees in highly diverse settings, from Sierra Leonean refugees in Guinean refugee camps, to internally displaced women widowed by the civil war in Sri Lanka, to Bosnian refugees in a large urban center the United States. While the programs differ in their populations, foci, and specific methods, they share a guiding framework that recognizes the inherent strengths and sources of resilience that all refugee communities possess. The diverse projects described in this book are innovative, empowering, and far-reaching in their impact.

Importantly, the contributing authors have not been asked to present models of fully polished, flawless intervention strategies. Instead, the goal has been for this group of creative, resourceful individuals to share a wealth of innovative and impactful intervention experiences that illustrate a new way of thinking about how we can best support the healing and adaptation of communities displaced by violence—communities that are struggling to heal from the wounds of the past, to adapt successfully to the challenges of the present, and to create futures that hold the promise of new life projects, new social roles, and new social networks that provide meaning and value to life.

1

An Ecological Framework for Addressing the Mental Health Needs of Refugee Communities

Kenneth E. Miller and Lisa M. Rasco[1]

This book offers a unique angle of vision from which to consider how mental health professionals can respond effectively to the psychological needs of communities displaced by war and other forms of political violence. The view represents a departure from the medical model that has guided most mental health research and intervention with refugees. That model emphasizes the provision by highly trained professionals of clinic-based services such as psychotherapy and psychiatric medication. The focus is on healing or ameliorating symptoms of psychological distress within individuals, with little attention paid to mending damaged social relations within communities, or to strengthening naturally occurring resources within families and communities that could facilitate healing and adaptation.

In allowing the medical model to so fundamentally shape our response to the mental health needs of refugees, we have—perhaps inadvertently—followed what Kaplan (1964) termed "the law of the instru-

---

[1]The authors wish to thank Rhona Weinstein and Jim Kelly for their invaluable feedback on this chapter.

ment," which dictates that when the only tool in one's possession is a hammer, there is a tendency to see everything as a nail in need of hammering. Having seen the devastating effects of war and displacement on people's mental health, and believing that what we have to offer in response is an array of professionally staffed, clinic-based services, we have opened the doors of our clinics to refugee clients. Specialized treatment centers have been created to serve refugees who have been tortured, and population-specific clinics have been funded to serve the mental health needs of specific refugee groups. With the very best of intentions, we have made available those services with which we are familiar, and which have historically defined the scope of our professional activities.

The extent to which clinic-based services for refugees are effective is largely unknown. Although several case studies and clinical reports have been published, few refugee treatment centers have published systematic evaluations of the services they provide. Despite the lack of empirical data, however, new clinics continue to be developed, guidelines and treatment strategies for clinical work with refugees continue to be published, and clinic-based services continue to represent the cornerstone of the mental health community's response to the mental health needs of refugee communities.

A primary aim of this chapter is to highlight three critical factors that have been overlooked in the process of investing so much time and energy into the development of clinic-based interventions. These factors are:

1. Most refugees have little or no access to the services of mental health professionals, because such services are scarce or nonexistent in those areas where the majority of the world's refugees live, and are often difficult to access for refugees in developed countries, as well;

2. Western mental health services, when they are available, are often underutilized because they are culturally alien to most refugees, the majority of whom come from non-Western societies and bring with them culturally specific ways of understanding and responding to psychological distress;

3. Clinic-based services are of limited value in addressing the constellation of displacement-related stressors that confront refugees on a daily basis, and that represent a significant threat to their psychological well-being. Examples of displacement-related stressors include the loss of social networks and a corresponding sense of isolation and lack of social support, unemployment, the loss of previously valued social roles and role-related activities, a lack of environmental mastery (i.e., possessing the knowledge and skills needed to negotiate the local environment), and the various stressors associated with living in poverty (Beiser, Johnson, & Turner, 1993; Gorst-Unsworth & Goldenberg, 1998; Lavik, Hauff, Skrondal, & Solberg, 1996; Miller, Worthington, Muzurovic, Goldman, & Tipping, 2002; Omidian, 1996; Pernice & Brook, 1996; Silove, 1999; Silove, Sinnerbrink, Field, & Manicavasagar, 1997).[2] As we discuss below, these three factors, when taken together, raise serious questions about the value of our nearly exclusive reliance on Western, clinic-based models of mental health intervention with refugees.

Fortunately, far from holding only a metaphorical hammer in our hands, we have a great many tools available to us that we can use to promote healing and adaptation in communities displaced by political violence. All the world is not a nail, nor need it appear to be so. If we are willing to venture out of our clinics and into the communities in which refugees live; if we are willing to broaden the range of roles we play and the types of activities in which we engage; and if we are willing to learn from colleagues in other disciplines such as public health, community psychology, prevention science, and anthropology, we can have a much farther reaching impact on lowering distress and promoting well-being within refugee communities than was ever possible working exclusively under the medical model and its corresponding set of clinical services.

In short, we believe it is time for a paradigm shift for those who seek to understand and respond effectively to the mental health needs of refugee communities. The good news is that we needn't look far to find a

---

[2]Although refugees often come from highly impoverished countries, refugee camps and other settings of resettlement usually involve a marked reduction of their standard of living (Hitchcox, 1990; UNHCR, 2002).

promising alternative to a primary or sole reliance on the medical model. The ecological paradigm of community psychology, with its roots in public health and its emphasis on collaboration and community empowerment, holds great promise as an alternative framework within which culturally appropriate mental health interventions for refugees can be developed, implemented, and evaluated. In fact, ecological interventions with refugee communities are already being conducted in various regions of the world. Such programs are still quite scarce, however, and program staff work in relative isolation, with little by way of shared experience upon which to draw. They are essentially pioneers, charting new territory as they proceed, drawing on theories and methods that have rarely been implemented in work with refugees. Psychologists, psychiatrists, and others involved in such projects have left the clinic and entered the community, and in so doing, both the rules and the roles have changed. Expert-driven services have been replaced by collaborative endeavors in which community members contribute their expertise and play essential roles in the intervention process; individual treatment has been supplemented or replaced by communal rituals and activities; and the conventional emphasis on treating psychopathology has been complemented by a new focus on identifying and developing community strengths and resources that can promote healing and adaptation.

This book represents a "taking stock" of sorts. It is a pause in the action, a chance for reflection and the sharing of experiences, both successful and problematic. It is an opportunity for those with considerable experience in the field to communicate their experiences and ideas to individuals and groups just getting started. And it is a time for serious consideration of both the possibilities and the potential limitations of ecological interventions with refugee communities. We have asked the authors of each chapter to reflect critically on the projects in which they have been involved, and to address a common set of points regarding the context, design, implementation, and evaluation of their work. There are significant differences among the projects in terms of sociopolitical and cultural contexts, populations of focus, and specific intervention goals and methods. What they have in common is an emphasis on ecological intervention strategies that maximize community participation and involve community members as respected and effective collaborators in the various phases of the intervention process.

In this chapter, we first briefly describe the scope of the world refugee situation. We then provide a short summary of research findings regarding patterns of psychological distress among refugees, and construct an empirical foundation for suggesting that clinic-based intervention strategies are fundamentally limited in their capacity to address these high rates of distress. We then turn to a discussion of the ecological model, and offer a rationale for its adoption as an alternative framework to guide mental health interventions with refugee communities. Finally, we consider some of the key issues and critical challenges inherent in doing community-based mental health work with refugees. The chapter concludes with some brief introductory comments regarding each of the projects described in the book.

THE WORLD REFUGEE SITUATION

This book makes its appearance at the start of the 21st century, a time of profound sociopolitical change and upheaval, of ultra-nationalism and widespread ethno-political violence that has resulted in the forced migration of millions of people. The majority of these are civilians whose only crime was that of living in regions of violent conflict, or belonging to a particular ethno-cultural group subjected to oppression and persecution, extending in some cases to the extremity of genocide. At the time of this writing, there are an estimated 35-38 million people displaced from their homes by civil and interstate war, as well as various forms of state sanctioned repression and persecution (Global IDP Project, 2002; UNHCR, 2002). This figure, which likely underestimates the actual total, includes approximately 13 million individuals formally recognized as refugees or asylum seekers according to the 1951 UN Convention Relating to the Status of Refugees (UNHCR, 1951). The UN Convention defines as a refugee anyone who

> owing to a well-founded fear of being persecuted for reasons of race, religion, nationality, or membership of a particular social group or political opinion, is outside the country of his nationality and is unable, or, owing to such fear, is unwilling to avail himself of the protection of that country.

Critical to this definition is the emphasis on finding oneself *outside the country of one's nationality*. In fact, however, it has become abundantly clear over the past few decades that the majority of people displaced by violence do *not* seek safe haven in other countries; instead, they become "internal refugees," remaining within the boundaries of their homeland either because they cannot or will not avail themselves of protection elsewhere. Their numbers are difficult to assess accurately, for unlike "official" refugees, internally displaced persons (IDPs) do not fall under the protection or jurisdiction of any particular international organization. Outsiders often have limited access to internally displaced communities, making accurate estimates of their numbers particularly difficult. This is especially true in contexts in which repressive governments have a vested interest in denying the existence of communities displaced by the state's own violent practices and human rights violations. Thus, the current estimate of 20-25 million internally displaced people (Global IDP Project, 2002) should be viewed as a crude approximation, with the actual number of IDP's possibly being higher.

Throughout this introductory chapter, we break with tradition and use the term *refugees* to refer collectively to all people forced by political violence to flee their homes and communities, regardless of whether they enter another country or remain within the borders of their homeland. We do this partly out of semantic convenience, and partly out of a belief that the term *internally displaced persons*, although technically accurate, fails to capture the harsh reality experienced by the majority of people who are displaced by political violence. This reality includes a preflight period of exposure to various types of violent experiences, which may include the abduction, murder, or "disappearance" of family members or friends, witnessing or experiencing physical assault, rape and other forms of sexual violence, the destruction of one's home and property, forced participation in acts of violence, and a persistent state of fear and vulnerability. Once the decision to flee is made, a series of profound losses and disruptions is set in motion. These include separation from family members unable or unwilling to flee, the abandonment of one's home and other material possessions, the loss of social networks and of social and occupational roles, and the reality of leaving behind a range of familiar and deeply valued settings, such as a parcel of land attained after years of labor, or an ancestral burial ground that represents continuity with one's ancestors. Although we recognize that internally displaced people and "official" refugees (i.e., those outside of their homeland) often face significantly different sets of resources and challenges as they adapt to their new settings, we believe that their forced migration involves a shared set of core experiences of violence, disruption, and loss. For this reason, as well as the convenience of a somewhat simpler nomenclature, we have opted to use the term *refugees* inclusively, referring to all people forced by political violence to flee their homes and communities.

RESEARCH ON THE MENTAL HEALTH OF REFUGEES

The primary focus of research on the mental health of refugees has been on documenting patterns of psychiatric symptomatology, using questionnaires or structured clinical interviews designed to identify psychiatric syndromes such as post-traumatic stress disorder (PTSD) and major depressive disorder (MDD). Although we believe that there are significant limitations to the nearly exclusive reliance on this approach (e.g., an inattention to indigenous idioms of distress, an exclusive focus on psychopathology that fails to consider the numerous strengths and forms of resiliency within refugee communities, and an underutilization of qualitative methods that would allow refugees to identify, in their own words, critical determinants of their psychological well-being), the psychiatric/symptom-focused approach to documenting refugee distress has nonetheless yielded some compelling findings. With more than 1,000 articles and book chapters on the topic now in print, including studies using clinical and community samples, children as well as adults, and refugees living in a diverse array of settings (internal displacement near zones of ongoing conflict, refugee camps, and resettlement countries), it is now possible to draw some reasonably solid conclusions regarding the impact of political violence and displacement on people's mental health. The following brief review first considers the psychological impact of exposure to political violence, then examines the effects ongoing stressors related to the experience of displacement.

The Traumatic Impact of Political Violence

Exposure to political violence is associated with an increased risk of both acute and chronic post-traumatic stress reactions (Arroyo & Eth, 1986; Fox & Tang, 2000; Hubbard, Realmoto, Northwood, & Masten, 1995; Kinzie, Sack, Angell, Manson, & Rath, 1986; Kinzie, Sack, Angell, Clark, & Ben, 1989; McSharry & Kinney, 1992; Michultka, Blanchard, & Kalous, 1998; Miller, Weine et al., 2002; Mollica et al., 1993, 1998; Shresta et al., 1998; Thabet & Vostanis, 2000; Weine et al., 1998). Most commonly, symptoms of traumatic stress among refugees have been assessed using the diagnostic criteria of post-traumatic stress disorder (PTSD). Although the cross-cultural validity of the PTSD construct and its appropriateness in situations of ongoing violence represent sources of ongoing controversy (a point to which we return later), the constellation of symptoms that comprise the PTSD syndrome have been documented in numerous studies of refugees representing diverse national and ethnic backgrounds. This does *not* mean that the PTSD construct adequately captures the totality of the trauma experience, nor does it negate the possibility that culturally specific expressions of trauma may exist that bear little resemblance to the three symptom cluster model of PTSD. Nor for that matter does it imply that psychological trauma should be understood only or primarily as an individual phenomenon. As we discuss shortly, acknowledging the presence of trauma within individuals in no ways contradicts the idea that trauma may also occur as a *psychosocial* phenomenon that affects entire communities and their underlying fabric of social relationships (Martín Baró, 1989; Summerfield, 1995; Wessells & Monteiro, 2001). Rather, the salience of the PTSD syndrome in a wide spectrum of refugee studies merely suggests that there exists across diverse cultures a set of highly intercorrelated symptoms of distress that develop in the wake of exposure to terrifying experiences over which people have little or no control.

To give the reader an idea of the prevalence of PTSD among diverse refugee groups, we offer a brief summary of research findings. This review is intended to be illustrative rather than comprehensive; readers interested in a more extensive review are referred to an excellent chapter by de Jong (2002).

Perhaps the most oft-cited research on the effects of political violence and exile is a set of studies conducted by David Kinzie and his colleagues with Cambodian refugees in the United States (Kinzie et al., 1986, 1989). Kinzie's group used the Diagnostic Interview Schedule, a structured clinical interview, to assess the prevalence of PTSD in their community study of 46 Cambodian youth. The participants in these studies had endured internment in Khmer Rouge "re-education" camps, been subjected to forced labor, beatings, and starvation, and each had lost an average of three family members under the Pol Pot regime. It is perhaps not surprising, given the severity and chronicity of the violence to which these young people had been exposed, that 50% of the study participants met DSM criteria for PTSD at the time of the initial study, 4 years after their departure from Cambodia. More striking is the fact that in their follow-up study 3 years later, Kinzie et al. (1989) found a nearly identical prevalence of PTSD, although we are not told whether those participants who met criteria for PTSD in the follow-up study were the same youth diagnosed with PTSD in the original assessment.

Richard Mollica and his colleagues (Mollica et al., 1993) have published several studies examining the mental health of Cambodian and Vietnamese refugees in diverse settings, including refugee camps in Southeast Asia and in a major urban center of the United States (Mollica et al., 1998). In a recent study of Vietnamese male torture survivors now living in the United States, Mollica et al. (1998) found that a striking 90% of the study's participants met diagnostic criteria for PTSD on the Harvard Trauma Questionnaire, a measure developed by Mollica, Caspi-Yavin, Bollini, & Truong (1992) specifically for use with Southeast Asians. The authors also noted that there was a direct relationship between the intensity of the torture experience and the severity of subsequent PTSD symptomatology, implying what they termed a "dose-dependent" relationship between degree of exposure to traumatic experiences and the severity of subsequent trauma symptoms. Such a dose-dependent relationship between trauma exposure and PTSD symptoms has been well established in research with non-refugee trauma survivors (Norris, 2002; Pynoos, Steinberg, & Wraith, 1995). In another study, Mollica et al. (1993), conducted a community survey with 993 Cambodian adults in a Thai refugee camp. The majority of participants had experienced multiple acts of violence, loss, and deprivation, and while the prevalence of major depressive disorder was 55%, PTSD was diagnosed in only 15% of study participants — a comparatively low rate given their traumatic life histories.

Other studies, with diverse refugee populations, also have found elevated levels of PTSD, which though variable, are still of an alarming magnitude relative to non-refugee populations (including non-refugee immigrant populations). For example, Michultka, Blanchard, and Kalous (1998) found a 68% prevalence of PTSD in their study of Central American refugee adults, while Fox and Tang (2000) found that 49% of the Sierra Leonian refugees they studied in the Gambia were in the clinical range for PTSD on their measure of trauma, the Harvard Trauma Questionnaire (Mollica et al., 1992).[3] In one of the few randomized community samples involving refugees, McSharry and Kinney (1992) used the DIS to assess the prevalence of psychiatric disorder in 124 Cambodian refugee adults in the United States. Most notable was their finding that 12 to 14 years after resettling in the United States, nearly 43% their sample met diagnostic criteria for PTSD. This finding, like those of the Kinzie et al. studies, highlights the potential of psychological trauma to persist over considerable periods of time.

Finally, in a recent study of Bosnian refugees in Chicago, Miller, Worthington et al. (2002) examined levels of psychological distress among two groups — one attending a mental health clinic and the other a community comparison group. Members of both groups had lived through at least some of the recent war in Bosnia, which exposed them to multiple acts of violence ranging from repeated shelling of their homes and communities to detention, beatings, and witnessing the violent deaths of loved ones. Trauma symptoms were assessed using the self-report version of the PTSD Symptom Scale (PSS; Foa, Riggs, Dancu, & Rothbaum, 1993). The mean PTSD symptom level of the clinic group (i.e., those seeking mental health treatment) was extremely high, in the upper

---

[3]A notable caveat: In this and a great many mental health studies with refugees, assessment instruments have been utilized without adequate standardization for the populations being studied; consequently, results should be viewed cautiously, particularly when clinical cut-offs have been used to determine the presence of PTSD. Unless clinical cut-off levels have been developed and validated using data gathered from the population being studied, it is preferable to report *levels* of trauma symptoms and their relationship to other variables of interest, rather than speak of diagnostic "cases" of psychological trauma when culturally valid criteria for defining "caseness" are not yet established.

quartile of the range of possible scores. For the community group, the mean trauma symptom level also was elevated, although variance in scores suggested a diversity of experience, with some members of the community group experiencing few trauma symptoms, and others experiencing considerable trauma-related distress for which they had not sought treatment.

Studies of refugee children have revealed a greater variability in levels of PTSD, with a critical factor appearing to be the degree to which children were exposed to acts of violence before becoming displaced (Smith, Perrin, Yule, Hacam, & Stuvland, 2002; Thabet & Vostanis, 2000)—essentially the "dose relationship" phenomenon described by Mollica and his colleagues. Thabet and Vostanis (2000), for example, in their study of Palestinian children in the Gaza Strip, found a positive relationship between the number of traumatic events children had experienced and the severity of their PTSD symptomatology. Forty-one percent of the children in their study met diagnostic criteria for PTSD at the time of their initial assessment.[4] The Kinzie et al. studies discussed earlier, in which children's level of exposure to violence was extremely high (i.e., multiple acts of violence over an extended period of time), also illustrate the traumatic impact of high "doses" of war-related violence. The traumatogenic nature of war-related violence was also documented in a recent study by Smith et al. (2002), who examined the mental health of Bosnian children in the devastated city of Mostar in southern Bosnia-Hercegovinia. Using the Revised Impact of Events Scale (RIES; Dyregov & Yule, 1995) in their community sample of nearly 3,000 children, the estimated prevalence of PTSD was 52%. Further, degree of exposure to war-related violence was the strongest predictor of trauma symptoms (while the loss of a loved one was highly associated with level of self-reported grief). The impact of war-related violence was also evident in a small study of Salvadoran children living in Los Angeles, in which 33%

---

[4]It is interesting to note that within a year of the initial assessment, following the formal (if temporary) cessation of hostilities between the Palestinians and Israelis, the prevalence of PTSD in this sample dropped to approximately 10%. This finding underscores the value of using longitudinal research designs, since cross sectional assessments may capture reactive symptoms of distress that are likely to diminish with the passing of time and the normalization of the environment.

of the 30 children studied were diagnosed with PTSD (Arroyo & Eth, 1986).

Other studies of refugee children have found lower rates of psychological trauma, generally reflecting comparatively lower rates of exposure to war-related violence. In their community sample of 61 Tibetan refugee children living in India, Servan-Schreiber, Lin, and Birmaher (1998) found an 11.5% prevalence of PTSD, whereas Miller (1996) found little evidence of post-traumatic stress symptoms in his study of 58 Guatemalan children living in refugee camps in southern Mexico. He attributed the absence of trauma primarily to the fact that most of the children had spent their childhoods in the relative safety of the camps and thus had not been witness to the genocidal violence that drove their families into exile 10 years earlier. In contrast to the children, however, their mothers experienced persistent symptoms of trauma that reflected the violence they had lived through. The intergenerational impact of this maternal trauma was suggested by a significant inverse relation between girls' mental health and the level of distress reported by their mothers. This relationship was not found for boys, who generally spent much more time than girls outside of the home, working with their fathers, gathering firewood, attending school, or playing with peers.

Future Directions for Research on the Effects of Political Violence

A critically important focus for further research is the identification of factors that mediate and/or moderate the impact of exposure to political violence on refugees' mental health. Although there is clear evidence of a strong, positive association between exposure to violence and the development of trauma symptoms, the fact that many people exposed to violence do not develop enduring psychological trauma suggests the presence of protective factors that may buffer the effects of potentially traumatic experiences. The handful of studies that have examined variables that appear to mediate or moderate the impact of violence have yielded findings consistent with those of research on other forms of traumatic stress. Variables such as the nature of the violent events to which people are exposed, the availability of social support following exposure to violence, the meaning which survivors of violence make of their experiences, and the range of coping strategies and resources available to people, all appear to play a critical role in determining the long-term impact of violence on mental health (Dawes, 1990; Gibson, 1989; Punamäki & Suleiman, 1990). For children, gender and age moderate to some extent the type of violent experiences to which they are likely to be exposed (e.g., adolescent girls are more likely to be targets of sexual violence, while adolescent boys are often at high risk of being forcibly recruited into armed conflict or detained for suspicion of guerrilla activity; Aron, Corne, Fursland, & Zelwer, 1991; Dawes, 1990; Garbarino, Kostelny, & Dubray, 1991; Gibson, 1989). Also, several authors have noted that a critical factor mediating the impact of violence on children, particularly infants and younger children, is the extent to which acts of violence result in the loss or psychological incapacitation of their primary caretakers (Boothby, 1988; Frazer, 1973; Garbarino et al., 1991).

Finally, it is clear that political violence and displacement exact a terrible toll on the well-being of communities, as well as individuals and families. To date, however, very few empirical studies have used the community as a unit of analysis; in fact, as illustrated by our brief review, the unit of analysis rarely transcends the individual and his or her psychiatric status, although a small number of studies have examined the impact of violence and displacement on the structure and functioning of families (e.g., Bottinelli, Maldonado, Troya, Herrera, & Rodriguez, 1990).

It is essential that researchers studying the impact of political violence examine its effects at multiple levels. A handful of researchers have begun to move the field in this direction. Writers such as Martín Baró (1985, 1989), Summerfeld (1995), and Wessells and Monteiro (2001) have written poignantly about the destructive impact of political violence on the social fabric of communities. Violent conflict, particularly when accompanied by the propagation of ethnic or religious stereotypes, often fosters attitudes of distrust and hostility, and can destroy previously supportive social relations and undermine faith in social institutions and organizations. In addition, violence can negatively impact communities in other ways: through the widespread use of sexual violence against women and girls (Aron et al., 1991; Landesman, 2002; McKay, 1998), a phenomenon that not only traumatizes victims and but also causes massive disruption to community life (e.g., through the birth of unwanted "children of rape," and the stigmatization of rape survivors who may be viewed as undesirable marriage partners; Landesman, 2002); through the forced recruitment of a community's young people, including children, for participation in armed conflict (Boothby, 1991; Machel, 1996); the destruction of people's limbs resulting from the widespread use of landmines and the corresponding loss of earning capacity and social desirability (Machel, 1996); the widespread creation of orphans who have lost one or both parents to violent conflict, and who must then be cared for by the community (Boothby, 1988; Machel, 1996; Wessells & Monteiro, chapter 2, this volume); and the normalization of violence in which violent approaches to conflict resolution become routine (Martín Baró, 1989; Wessells & Monteiro, chapter 2, this volume).

Putting a Human Face to the Research Findings on Trauma

To give a human face to these numbers regarding the prevalence of trauma among refugees, we offer a few quotations, taken from research done by the first author and his colleagues, with refugees from Guatemala (Miller & Billings, unpublished raw data), Bosnia (Miller, Worthington et al., 2002b), and Afghanistan (Zahir, Kakar, & Miller, 2001).

The first quotation, which illustrates the salience of recurrent nightmares related to previous experiences of violence, is from a Guatemalan woman who fled with her family into Mexico in the wake of a massacre in a village nearby to her own village in Guatemala. As part of an assessment of women's health in the refugee camp, participants were asked whether they were experiencing symptoms of trauma, including nightmares. This woman's response was similar to that of many of the women in the camp:

> I dream that I am being pursued by the army. I see the army burning our home and the soldiers have grabbed us. I see that they're killing my children, and sometimes they're killing me as well.

Recurrent nightmares were also reported by participants in a study examining psychosocial challenges facing Afghan women refugees brought to the United States from Pakistan through arranged marriages to Afghan men already in the United States. In the following quote, a young Afghan woman described her highly distressing symptoms of trauma, which included not only recurrent nightmares, but also persistent hyperarousal, and difficulties with intimacy:

> I still have nightmares about the war. I get up screaming in the middle of the night as I dream of the people I witnessed with their body parts blown up by the rockets and my best friend's death. I get scared when I hear the slightest loud noise and want to duck for cover. I remember the girls that were raped and therefore I have intimacy issues with my current so-called husband.

Another Afghan woman, who had lived through the Soviet invasion and subsequent civil war in her homeland, describes the re-experiencing of unresolved traumatic memories and feelings:

> My head hurts sometimes. Especially when I think back to the war and how there were rockets everywhere. I become really stressed and want to hit myself. I feel so much pressure that I want to hit myself. I often have these attacks when I have difficulty breathing.

In the next quotation, which comes from a narrative study of exile-related stressors facing Bosnian refugees in Chicago, a Bosnian woman who survived "ethnic cleansing" described her experience of insomnia, chronic hyperarousal, impaired concentration, and irritability:

> I didn't have any problems before. But now I am very nervous. Sometimes I start arguing with the people with whom I live. . . . I don't sleep for five nights sometimes. . . . If I fall asleep I have dreams about the war that make no sense . . . almost every time I sleep. If I remember something, I usually forget it within five minutes.

A Bosnian man who survived the horrors of a Serb concentration camp, described his experience of intrusive war-related imagery, and his avoidance of social interactions that might stimulate the distressing images:

> I know I'm not able to stop that, those pictures, but I tried to avoid them. But they come. If someone talks about the war, about those things, I have dreams about that, so I try to avoid company. I try to avoid places where people have been talking about the war. So that's why I want and like to be alone.

Living through the horrors of war and other forms of political violence clearly takes its toll on people's psychological well-being. However, in emphasizing the potentially traumatic nature of exposure to political violence, we do not mean to imply that all refugees who have been exposed to violent events will subsequently develop trauma symptoms. Nor is it the case that symptoms of trauma which appear in the immediate wake of violent events will necessarily persist and develop into full blown PTSD. Many survivors of violent experiences eventually return to normal functioning despite initially experiencing elevated levels of post-traumatic stress symptomatology (Foa & Rothbaum, 1998; Norris, 2001). In addition, although researchers generally direct our attention to the significant number of individuals in their studies who do show evidence of persistent trauma, in the majority of studies we just as easily could focus on the significant number of participants who do *not* show enduring patterns of distress. Finally, we agree with writers such as Summerfield (1995) who caution that we should not assume that elevated levels of traumatic stress necessarily imply impaired psychosocial functioning; on the contrary, we believe that many refugees experience elevated levels of traumatic stress, yet still manage to function well in various domains of their lives. Our point is simply that painful post-traumatic stress reactions do appear to be highly prevalent within refugee communities, and that for a significant number of these trauma survivors, time alone does not appear to lessen their distress.

The Salience of Displacement-Related Stressors

What happens to people after they go into exile or become internally displaced is at least as important to their mental health as their prior exposure to experiences of violence. Numerous studies, both quantitative and qualitative, as well as several clinical reports, have found that displacement-related stressors exert a profound impact on refugees' psychological and physical well-being (Beiser, Johnson, & Turner, 1993; Bennett & Detzner, 1997; Gonsalves, 1990; Gorst-Unsworth & Goldenberg, 1998; Lavik, Hauff, Skrondal, & Solberg, 1996; Miller, Weine et al., 2002, Miller, Worthington et al., 2002; Omidian, 1996; Pernice & Brook, 1996; Silove, 1999; Silove, Sinnerbrink, Field, & Manicavasagar, 1997).

Although early research with refugees focused primarily on understanding the impact of war-related violence on people's mental health, it soon became clear that refugees encountered a set of profound psychosocial stressors *after* they were displaced—stressors related to the multiple losses and changes resulting from the reality of displacement and the challenges of adapting to life in new and unfamiliar settings. Examples of such stressors include social isolation and a loss of traditional social support networks, uncertainty regarding the well-being of loved ones unable or unwilling to make the journey, a lack of income-generation opportunities and a corresponding lack of economic self-sufficiency, discrimination by members of the host society, the loss of valued social roles and a corresponding loss of meaningful role-related activities, and a lack of access to essential health, educational, and economic resources. The available data—again framed primarily within the psychiatric/symptom-based research paradigm—clearly show a strong link between this constellation of ongoing stressors and the development of depression as well as various forms of anxiety. In fact, displacement-related stressors appear to be a primary explanatory factor underlying the high levels of depression found in numerous refugee studies.[5]

We offer here a brief synopsis of research findings on the salience of displacement-related stressors and their relation to mental health status.[6]

---

[5]Although much of the research examining the relationship of displacement-related stressors to mental health is correlational and does not permit causal inference, several ethnographic studies lend strong support to the etiological role of displacement-related stressors in the high rates of depression documented in numerous refugee studies.

[6]The interested reader is referred not only to the original studies cited in this section, but also to the work of Hitchcox (1990) on the experience of Vietnamese refugees in Hong Kong refugee camps, Lundgren and Lang (1989) on the experience of internally displaced Salvadorans, Dybdahl (2001) on internally displaced Bosnians, Boothby (1988) on the impact of displacement on children, Doña and Berry (1999) on the stressors asso-

Pernice and Brook (1996) studied Southeast Asian refugees in New Zealand, and found that post-migration or displacement-related variables such as unemployment, discrimination, and social isolation were all significantly associated with levels of self-reported depression and anxiety. Lavik et al. (1996), who studied a nationally diverse group of refugees attending a mental health clinic in Norway, examined the relation of unemployment and a lack of participation in educational activities to levels of emotional and behavioral difficulties. Both displacement-related variables were positively related to levels of anxiety, depression, and aggressive behavior in their sample. Gorst-Unsworth and Goldenberg (1998), who examined predictors of distress among 84 Iraqi refugee men, found that perceived level of affective social support in exile was associated significantly with levels of PTSD and depression; in fact, perceived level of affective social support was a stronger predictor of depression in this sample than was level of exposure to war-related events. These findings are consistent with those of a recent study of Bosnian refugees by Miller, Weine et al. (2002), in which social isolation and a lack of involvement in meaningful activities were significantly related to levels of depression, while trauma symptoms were accounted for primarily by exposure to war-related violence.

The impact of displacement-related stressors on refugees' mental health has also been documented in several ethnographic studies, including Omidian's (1996) ethnographic study of Afghan refugees in the United States, Englund's (1998) research with Mozambican refugees in Malawi, and Salvado's (1988) study of undocumented Guatemalan refugees in southern Mexico. Omidian (1996) observed high levels of depression within the Afghan community in which she worked, particularly among older Afghans, who had lost many of their social networks, as well as the various social roles they had filled and the corresponding status conferred by those roles. Also lost was the environmental mastery they had experienced in Afghanistan; now, in their new setting in the San Francisco Bay Area, they had to learn new cultural mores, develop proficiency in a new language, and develop other setting-specific skills

ciated with adaptation and acculturation in resettlement countries, von Buchwald (1998) on psychosocial stressors facing residents of refugee camps, and Silove (1999) and Miller (1999) for conceptual/review articles examining the nature of displacement-related stressors and their impact on refugee well-being.

that had not been relevant in their homeland In Englund's (1998) study of Mozambican refugees, a primary source of distress was the lack of opportunities in exile for people to properly observe traditional burial rituals following the loss of loved ones to the violence in Mozambique. In fact, Englund suggests that the refugees were less distressed by their experience of war-related trauma than by their lack of opportunity to bury their dead appropriately and exorcise the vengeful spirits of the deceased. Finally, in his study of undocumented Guatemalan refugees living in southern Mexico, Salvado (1988) noted the pervasive fear of identification, capture, and deportation that characterized people's daily lives, as well as the difficulty they experienced accessing basic health and educational resources due to their undocumented status.

Illustrative Comments Regarding Displacement-Related Stressors

To illustrate the nature and salience of displacement-related stressors, we again present illustrative quotations from two ethnographic studies conducted by Miller and his colleagues with Guatemalan refugees in southern Mexico (Miller & Billings, unpublished raw data), and Bosnian refugees in Chicago (Miller, 1999; Miller, Worthington et al., 2002).

One set of stressors concerns the loss of traditional social networks and the resulting experiences of isolation and a lack of social support. A Bosnian woman who enjoyed a rich social life in Bosnia before her husband was killed and she was forced into exile with her sons, had this to say when asked about her experience of isolation:

> Always. It's always in my soul. I don't have any family members here but my sons. Maybe if there were someone else, I would feel better. I have one neighbor here from Bosnia. Sometimes I eat by myself, sometimes with the children, and sometimes with someone who comes to visit with us . . . but people usually work, and they don't have time.

Another Bosnian, a soft-spoken man who was raising his children alone, talked about the isolation and lack of social support he experienced:

I really don't have anyone here. I am alone with my two children. I'm not able to work and earn anything. I have to cook for my children, to do the laundry. I don't have any friends or cousins who can take care of my children. I am not in contact with anyone else, so no one can help me.

A Guatemalan woman had voiced a similar experience, despite the very different setting in which she was living (a refugee camp in southern Mexico):

I cry when I think about my husband (who died). It's difficult as a widow, having to raise my children without the support of a man to bring the wood, help with the work, and to be generally supportive. The kids were young when he died, and they couldn't help, though now they can and do.

Another Guatemalan woman also described feelings of isolation, despite the insular nature of refugee camp and the opportunities for social interaction outside of the home that it provided:

I have difficulty doing my work in the home because of desperation. I have no-one to talk with. . . . I am lonely. I cry when I am alone in my house. I don't have parents or siblings who help me and visit me.

We recognize, of course, that within refugee communities strong social ties develop, and new social support mechanisms often are created to replace those left behind as a result of being forcibly displaced. There is also considerable variance in the extent to which refugees are able to go into exile together with other family members and friends. To the extent that previous social networks can be maintained in exile or internal displacement, we can expect to find lower levels of social isolation and its negative mental health correlates. Despite the at least partial availability of new or previous social ties and sources of social support within refugee communities, however, isolation and a lack of social support have emerged consistently as among the most salient displacement-related stressors affecting refugees.

Another source of ongoing stress is the loss of life projects and meaningful social roles left behind upon going into exile, coupled with a sense of doubt regarding the possibility of creating new and meaningful projects and roles in the new setting.

> The most difficult thing is that we tried to build something all our lives, and then we lost everything. When we should have been enjoying our lives, when our children got married, we had to leave. When my son got married, and my daughter got married, that was the time when we had everything we needed to enjoy our lives. And that was the best time to live there, and we had to leave that. (Bosnian man in Chicago)

> I feel like my life is interrupted somewhere in the middle, and I'm at the age when I'm not ready for a new beginning, so it's hard. It's too late for a new beginning actually. (Bosnian woman in Chicago)

Poverty and a lack of access to employment-related resources that could help move people out of poverty were sources of ongoing frustration for many participants in both studies. For Guatemalans, this usually meant a lack of land on which to grow corn, beans, and other staples:

> I cry because of what we suffer *here*. We feel very sad, we had all our lands there. Sometimes we run out of food and our land is so far away. (Guatemalan woman in Chiapas)

> I want to work and plant crops and we can't. How are we going to eat? I feel sad because of our poverty. Sometimes I'd rather die because I can't work. I can't buy medicine, I can't earn money to buy medicine. (Guatemalan woman in Chiapas)

For Bosnians, poverty was expressed in terms of poor housing conditions, and a lack of money to meet basic needs:

My daughter is almost 15, and she goes to school, and I live on Social Security Benefits of about $500. My children get $200 in food stamps and $200 in cash, and we all live together in one studio apartment. My daughter is almost an adult, and it's not nice to be all in one room. I know I am eligible for public housing, and I applied, but there is nothing. My daughter needs a coat, and they both need books, notebooks, pencils, and bags, and I'm not able to afford that . . . that is distressing to me. (Bosnian man in Chicago)

I had problems with very high rent, that's why I changed my apartment, and I took a very bad apartment because it was less expensive and I was supposed to pay almost all my income for an apartment, for the rent. My apartment is so bad that the rain comes in when it's raining. And I live on the third floor, so it's too many stairs for me because I'm not able to go up stairs. I have difficulty. I would like to have a nice apartment with nice things inside. Now when I enter my apartment and see the garbage, and I see my broken walls, I really—I just feel very bad. (Bosnian woman in Chicago)

Although Bosnians in Chicago had comparatively greater access to work opportunities than did rural Guatemalans in the camps of Chiapas, the lack of environmental mastery—the knowledge and skills relevant to the new setting—made the process of attaining meaningful employment quite challenging.

It is very difficult. It's very difficult when you go out and you are not able to communicate—when you go to the doctor or when you go shopping, and you are not able to communicate. Life was very hard. We got just a little help—social support for just two months, and after that we were on our own. My husband worked, and I worked too for a while, until I burned my hand. I was supposed to work in one hotel, but in order to reach there, I was supposed to take three buses, and I didn't know how to do that. So, I used to sit down and cry. (Bosnian woman in Chicago)

> I'm not able to speak English. I'm not able to express my feelings
> For me, everything is harder. When I go out, I'm scared of some-
> thing, though nothing is there. When I was in Bosnia and went
> out, I got all the news, I knew what was going on, but here it's
> like I'm blind and deaf. I don't know if you experienced this
> when I went to Sarajevo—people are talking. . . . I don't un-
> derstand what they're talking about. (Bosnian woman in Chi-
> cago)

It is important, of course, to underscore the significant variation among refugees in the degree to which they are affected by, and able to cope with, these and other displacement-related stressors. Refugees often possess remarkable resilience, including a determination to adapt as well as possible to the most challenging of circumstances. This resilience is evident in the development of community organizations and structures that permit some degree of re-establishment of normality and collective coping. It is also evident in the remarkable adaptation of some individuals who, despite significant hardships, master the many challenges facing them and become leaders in their communities.

It is also important to note that experiences of displacement may create opportunities or provide access to resources that were not available in the homeland. For example, Guatemalan refugees in the refugee camps of southern Mexico often had greater access to healthcare and education than they had experienced in Guatemala. For women in particular, nongovernmental organizations working in the camps often were able to provide new opportunities for formal training in midwifery, lay health care, and pedagogy (Billings, 1996); in addition, free from the omnipresence of the Guatemalan army and its network of spies, the camps provided rich opportunities for the development of a political consciousness and the creation of a powerful political organization designed to represent the refugees' interests in negotiations with the Guatemalan government regarding a return to Guatemala (Miller, 1994).

Additional Sources of Distress

This brief review of research findings has identified two key sets of stressors that endanger the mental health of refugees. The first set of stressors

stressors is the violent events that people may have experienced prior to being displaced; the second set is the numerous losses and adaptational demands, referred to here as displacement-related stressors,[7] that confront refugees in their new settings. Taken together, prior exposure to violence and ongoing exposure to displacement-related stressors account for a great deal of the psychological distress that has been documented in so many studies of refugee communities.

There are two additional sets of factors that may contribute to psychological distress within refugee communities. One set includes *pre-displacement* experiences of trauma, loss, and deprivation that are not directly to political violence. It is interesting to note that in most refugee studies, assessments of traumatic stressors rarely inquire about events— such as child abuse, spouse abuse, physical injuries and illnesses, traumatic losses, etc.—that occurred prior to or independent of exposure to political violence. Unfortunately, this approach limits the amount of variance in levels of distress that can be explained by our research, since war-related experiences of violence and loss and displacement-related stressors are unlikely to be the only sources of psychological distress in any population. In addition, it limits our understanding of the ways in which prior exposure to other life stressors may influence people's capacity to cope effectively with traumatic stressors that *are* related directly to political violence.

The other set of factors are psychosocial stressors that occur *following* the move into exile or internal displacement, but that are not directly related to the experience of displacement *per se*. Examples of such factors include spouse abuse, sexual assault (i.e., outside the context of spouse abuse), physical illness and injuries, and interpersonal losses. As previously noted, most refugee studies have limited their assessments of psychosocial stressors to war-related experiences of violence and loss and the constellation of displacement-related stressors discussed above. Un-

---

[7]Although several of the displacement-related stressors discussed in this chapter have also been referred to by some authors as acculturative or resettlement stressors, we prefer the term *displacement-related stressors* because (1) not all displacement-related stressors are associated with the acculturation process (indeed, for refugees living in the insular environment of refugee camps, acculturation to the host society may be quite minimal (Miller, 1996); and (2), the term *resettlement* has come to be associated with permanent resettlement in host societies, while in fact most refugees either return home or remain in situations of temporary safe haven.

fortunately, the failure to consider the impact of other ongoing stressors not directly related to the experience of displacement may lead us to underestimate the importance of factors that have a significant impact on refugee well-being. Domestic violence is a good example. Although most service providers and frontline staff readily acknowledge the problem of spouse abuse in refugee communities, only a handful of the hundreds of published articles and chapters on refugee mental health have examined this phenomenon and its impact on the mental health of refugee women and children(e.g., Walter, 2001). Figure 1.1 depicts the four sets of risk factors discussed earlier and their relation to the well-being of individuals, families, and communities. In the model, political violence exerts a direct effect on individual mental health, and on the well-being of families and communities. Political violence also results in the experience of displacement, which, in turn, confronts people with a constellation of displacement-related stressors. These stressors represent risk factors for the development of individual mental health problems as well as heightened family tensions and difficulties establishing supportive community relations and institutions. In addition, many refugees must also contend with the persistent effects of prewar stressors, or with current stressors not directly related to experiences of war-related violence and displacement. The representation of individual, family, and community well-being as different sides of the same three dimensional cube is meant to reflect the mutually influential relationships among these three levels.

Implications for Mental Health Interventions With Refugees

As we have suggested, not all refugees show evidence of acute or persistent mental health problems, and among those who do, many individuals manage to function effectively despite their experience of internal distress (Summerfield, 1995). It is important to acknowledge this resilience, both for what it tells us about the human spirit in the face of profound crisis, and for the lessons it may offer regarding pathways to adaptive functioning despite exposure to high levels of stress. It is also important, however, that we remain mindful of the darker story told by the research data. These data tell a story of large numbers of refugees who continue to experience symptoms of trauma that have not abated

Figure 1.1. The Adverse Effects of Political Violence and Displacement on Individuals, Families, and Communities

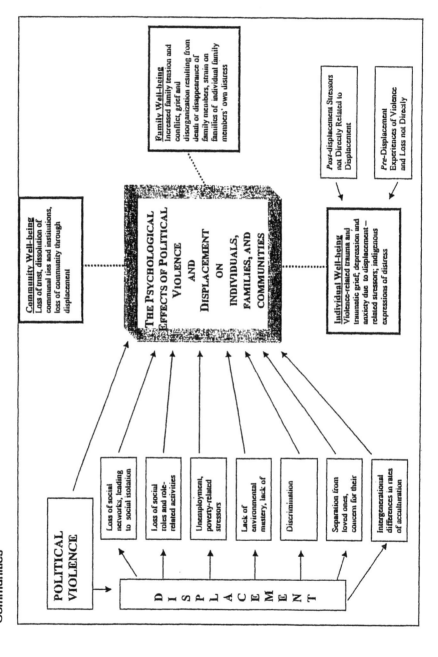

with the passing of time, and of refugee communities struggling to develop new social networks, navigate unfamiliar environments, discover new and meaningful social roles, find ways out of poverty and into self-sufficiency, and manage the day to day sadness of being separated from loved ones unable or unwilling to make the journey out.

What are the implications of these research findings for mental health professionals? Most fundamentally, mental health interventions are needed that alleviate psychological distress and promote effective coping and adaptation within refugee communities. More specifically, the data suggest that refugee mental health programs should have, at minimum, two broad aims. First, they should help traumatized refugees resolve, or at least manage effectively, their symptoms of trauma and traumatic loss, and second, they should enhance the capacity of refugee communities to cope effectively with the numerous displacement-related stressors that confront them on a daily basis and regain adaptive functioning. Although we are accustomed to thinking of coping in individual terms, it may be helpful to broaden that view to include the capacity of *communities* to respond effectively to the mental health and psychosocial needs of community members. For example, a critical displacement-related challenge involves facilitating the development of social networks that can provide much needed social support and a sharing of resources. Because political violence so often divides communities by generating suspicion and hostility among community members, the task of creating supportive social networks may entail an initial process of healing damaged relations within communities so that basic conditions of trust and openness are present. Another approach to enhancing the adaptive capacity of communities could involve the identification or creation of settings within which community members can discover meaningful roles and role-related activities, and carve out new life projects to take the place of those left behind.

Against the backdrop of these two aims (helping refugees manage and resolve traumatic stress reactions, and helping refugee communities cope with displacement-related stressors), we now consider the utility of clinic-based mental health services, which, thus far, have been the cornerstone of the mental health community's response to the psychological needs of refugee communities. In the opening of this chapter, we briefly mentioned three factors that limit the utility of clinic-based services such as psychotherapy and the prescription of psychiatric medication. These are (1) the lack of access that most refugees have to such services; (2) the fact that Western mental health services, even when they are available, are often underutilized because they are culturally alien to refugees from non-Western societies (i.e., the majority of the world's refugees); and (3) the limited capacity of clinic-based services to address the constellation of displacement-related stressors that affect refugees on a daily basis, and that are strongly associated with adverse mental health outcomes such as depression and anxiety. In this section, we briefly consider each of these factors.

Lack of Access to Professional Mental Health Services

Mental health professionals are generally quite scarce in or near regions of violent political conflict, where the majority of the world's refugees live (Boothby, 1996; de Jong, 2002; Lundgren & Lang, 1989). In fact, most mental health professionals are trained and reside in developed nations, geographically distant from the majority of the world's "hot spots" (almost all of them in developing countries) that have given rise to refugee movements during the past 50 years. Those mental health professionals who do live in regions of violent conflict tend to reside in urban centers, where violence is often less pronounced, the standard of living is somewhat higher, and people are more likely to be familiar with Western notions of psychological distress and healing (de Jong, 2002; Lundgren & Lang, 1989). Venturing out into rural areas to provide services to those communities most severely affected by political violence can be hazardous, particularly in settings where local military or paramilitary forces regard mental health work as threatening because it is likely to reveal systematic human rights abuses. Numerous mental health workers have been subjected to harassment, persecution, and even assassinated for their work with communities affected by violence. Examples include Sister Barbara Ford, who was recently murdered in Guatemala by paramilitary forces opposed to her work on the development and implementation of a mental health project for rural Guatemalans affected by the military's repressive practices,[8] and Ignacio Martín Baró, a Salvadoran psychologist and Jesuit priest killed in 1989 by a Salvadoran death squad. Dr. Martín Baró spent much of his career examining the psychosocial effects of state terror and civil war on Salvadoran society (see Martín Baró, 1985, 1989, 1990).

Although the paucity of mental health professionals in or near regions of ongoing conflict helps explain the lack of access to professional mental health services that refugees in developing countries experience, one might reasonably ask whether issues of access are really germane to the experience of refugees in the developed nations, where mental health professionals are plentiful, and mental health clinics for refugees have been developed in many metropolitan areas. In fact, the question of access to mental health services is salient even in the developed nations, since the majority of mental health professionals do not offer their services to refugees, who are often impoverished and unable to pay more than a small fee for such services (Quesada, 1988). In addition, refugees often lack adequate proficiency in the language of the host country, and professional therapists rarely have access to language interpreters; consequently, communication is a formidable obstacle that further limits refugees' access to mental health services (Miller, Silber, Pzdirek, Caruth, & Lopez, 2003; Tribe, 1999). Finally, mental health clinics for refugees typically have small staffs and operate on shoestring budgets; consequently, they typically can reach only a small proportion of individuals in need of mental health assistance (Miller, 1999).[9]

---

[8]Ford, Cabrera, and Searing (2000) have published a wonderful manual entitled *Buscando una buena vida: Tres experiencias de salud mental comunitaria* (*Searching for a better life: Three experiences of community mental health*), which describes the context, rationale, theory, and methods of this project.

[9]To illustrate this point, we offer a quote from Miller (1999):

While psychotherapy may be an effective form of intervention at the individual or small group level, its capacity to reach large numbers of people is limited in part by the number of professionally trained therapists and interpreters available to work with refugees. An example might be helpful in illustrating the problem. The Bosnian Mental Health Program in Chicago, in conjunction with its sister Refugee Mental Health Program, represents one of the largest mental health services in the United States specifically designed to serve Bosnian refugees. With a staff of several psychologists and psychiatrists, 5-6 graduate student trainees, an art therapist, 2 volunteer massage therapists, an interpreter, and 4 mental health counselors/case managers who also provide interpreting for individual and group psychotherapy, the pro-

In sum, most refugees simply do not have access to the services of mental health professionals. Although this is readily evident in or near most regions of violent conflict, where mental health professionals are scarce, issues of access are also salient in developed nations despite the large number of highly trained mental health professionals in those countries.

A Lack of Cultural Fit

Psychotherapy and psychopharmacology are primarily European and American phenomena, and reflect a specifically Western set of beliefs regarding the nature of psychological distress and the range of appropriate methods for addressing it. However, the majority of displaced people come from non-Western societies, and have ways of understanding and responding to emotional distress that differ from the explanatory and treatment models that guide the work of Western-trained mental health professionals (Eisenbruch, 1991, 1988; Farias, 1994; Rosenblatt, 2001; Somasundaram & Jamunanantha, 2002; Torrey, 1972; van de Put & Eisenbruch, 2002). Although it is difficult to generalize across diverse cultures, some major areas of difference between Western and non-Western approaches to mental health include the use of traditional healers in non-Western cultures versus professionals with high levels of formal education in the West; an emphasis on religious and supernatural explanations for psychological distress in many non-Western cultures (Somasundaram & Jamunanantha, 2002; van de Put & Eisenbruch, 2002; Torrey, 1972), versus a focus in the West on intra-individual, natural/scientific explanations (e.g., psychodynamic, cognitive-behavioral, or psychobiological models; Todd & Bohard, 1999); and a view in many non-Western cultures of the self, and of individual well-being, as inseparably embedded within a matrix of social roles and interpersonal rela-

---

gram provides a fairly comprehensive range of services. Caseloads are consistently full, and the program is able to serve a maximum of between 200 and 250 individuals per year. To put this in context, consider that there are an estimated 22,000 Bosnian refugees living in the Chicagoland area (Smajkic, 1999). Given the available data regarding the prevalence of psychological distress among refugees generally, and among Bosnian refugees specifically, it seems reasonable to conclude that the program is serving only a small percentage of those Bosnians who could benefit from some form of psychological intervention. (p. 287)

tions (e.g., Englund, 1998), in contrast to the emphasis on individualism and autonomy that is predominant in Western societies (Triandis, 2001). These cultural differences have important implications for mental health interventions, since Western models of treatment focus on healing dysfunctional psychological or biological processes within individuals, whereas non-Western approaches to healing often involve spiritual and communal rituals meant to restore healthy relations among people and between people and "supernatural" entities, including deceased ancestors or specific deities.

Numerous authors have observed that refugees from non-Western societies tend to underutilize professional mental health services despite their experience of considerable distress (e.g., Ensign, 1995; Omidian, 1996). A primary reason for this pattern of underutilization appears to be the perception among many refugees of such services as culturally alien, and in some cases highly stigmatized. In the West, for example, seeking professional treatment for symptoms of psychological trauma is a widely accepted and commonly recommended course of action. Among Cambodians, however, symptoms of trauma are far more likely to result in a visit to a traditional healer than a mental health professional, even when professional mental health services are readily available (van de Put & Eisenbruch, 2002). Among Afghan refugees, psychological distress is rarely revealed to strangers, and the suggestion that mental health treatment may be indicated is often met with powerful resistance (Shorish-Shamely, 1991).

Refugees from rural Guatemala and El Salvador may frame their experience of psychological distress not in the Western language of trauma, but rather in terms of *susto* or *nervios*, expressions of distress that have no precise equivalent in Western psychiatry, but which are well known to any Central American *curandero* or traditional healer (Farias, 1994; Rubel, O'Neill, & Collado Ardón, 1989). And among Sri Lankans, the psychological devastation caused by the disappearance (i.e., abduction and usually death) of a loved one is often ameliorated with the assistance not of mental health professionals, but of religious healers who offer a set of shared beliefs and culturally familiar rituals that provide some degree of meaning and resolution to the experience of uncertainty and loss (Perera, 2001).

Taken together, these two factors—the lack of access to mental health services and the lack of cultural fit between such services and the cultural belief systems of refugees from non-Western societies—suggest that clinic-based mental health services are neither especially efficient for reaching large numbers of distressed refugees, nor culturally well-matched to the worldviews of those they are intended to serve. This does not mean that therapy and medication have no role to play in the healing process of refugees experiencing distress. On the contrary, we believe that clinical services may play an important role in ameliorating distress, particularly psychological trauma, among those refugees who have access to and are willing to utilize such services. Our point is simply that clinic-based services, by themselves, should not form the cornerstone of our response to the mental health needs of refugee communities.

The Limited Capacity of Clinic-Based Services to Address Displacement-Related Stressors

Earlier, we examined research findings concerning the salience of displacement-related stressors in the lives of refugees and their powerful relation to adverse mental health outcomes such as depression and anxiety. In our view, it is simply outside of the scope of clinic-based mental health services to address these stressors effectively. At issue here is a constellation of core tasks: the development of new social networks that can reduce isolation and increase the availability social support; the identification and/or creation of new social roles and new life projects that can lend meaning and structure to people's lives; the enhancement of knowledge and skills needed to access key resources related to health, education, employment, and legal status; and the mending of social ties within communities devastated by years of living with fear, mutual suspicion, and violence.

Although some might argue that tasks such as these fall outside the scope of mental health professionals, we believe that the strong link between people's mental health and their capacity to effectively manage these displacement-related challenges clearly argues for viewing such work as falling very much within the domain of mental health. It is, however, a different sort of mental health work that is called for—an approach that is rooted in community settings rather than mental health clinics; that is based on collaborative rather than hierarchical relationships with community members; and that is grounded in a thorough and respectful understanding of local values and beliefs regarding psychological well-being and distress. It is here that we face an interesting challenge, for the medical model of psychiatry and clinical psychology that has guided our clinic-based work with refugees cannot adequately guide our work once we leave the clinic and enter the communities in which refugees live. The transition from clinic to community creates the need for a new model, an alternative framework that reflects the complex realities of refugee communities and the altered relationships we will need to develop as we shift from relations of hierarchical expertise to authentic collaboration.

THE ECOLOGICAL MODEL OF COMMUNITY PSYCHOLOGY

Although community psychology in the United States has its roots in social movements and historical developments that date back at least to the settlement houses of the early 1900s (Dalton, Elias, & Wandersman, 2001; Heller, Price, Reinharz, Riger, Wandersman, & D'Aunno 1984), the field itself was organized formally in May of 1965, at a gathering of psychologists in the town of Swampscott, Massachusetts (Bennett et al., 1966). The Swampscott conference took place in the wake of the passage of the Community Mental Health Centers Act (CMHCA) in 1963. The CMHCA had greatly extended the reach of mental health services by funding the development of some 750 community mental health centers throughout the country. The centers offered a diversity of mental health services, which were available to community residents regardless of their ability to pay (Bloom, 1984; Levine & Perkins, 1997). The development of the centers was especially significant in low-income communities, where residents traditionally had limited access to the services of mental health professionals. In addition, studies at the time had documented significantly higher rates of mental health problems in low income communities than those found in more affluent neighborhoods (e.g., Hollingshead & Redlich, 1958), suggesting the need for improved access to high quality mental health services for poor and working class Americans.

Although it is true that the passage of the CMHCA greatly expanded the reach of clinic-based mental health services, particularly in previously underserved communities, critics of the Community Mental Health Movement argued that it was ultimately conservative in nature and limited in scope (Bloom, 1984; Heller et al., 1984). For while the development of the community mental health centers greatly increased the availability of mental health services in low income communities, the centers failed to address the underlying social inequities that gave rise to the very kinds of distress that clinicians were treating in the centers. Although all community mental health centers were supposed to provide services aimed at the *prevention* as well as treatment of mental health problems, less than 5% of center budgets were actually allocated to prevention activities (Heller et al., 1984). Thus, the emphasis remained almost exclusively on treatment rather than prevention, with minimal attention to altering the contextual factors that generated distress in people (e.g., domestic violence, discrimination, unemployment, poor housing conditions, lack of access to community resources, social isolation and a lack of social support systems). Finally, there were few efforts by center administrators to develop collaborative relationships with community members, so that the latter could have an active role in shaping the services that were to be provided (Bloom, 1984). The lack of local input limited the extent to which services could be tailored to the specific needs of different communities.

In response to these and other perceived limitations of the community mental health centers (and of traditional clinical services generally), participants at the Swampscott conference opted to lay the groundwork for a new field, community psychology, that would be guided by a set of principles and priorities quite different from those of clinical psychology and psychiatry. Drawing on parallels between human communities and natural ecosystems, and borrowing from such diverse fields as public health, anthropology, clinical and social psychology, organizational behavior, and sociology, writers such as Jim Kelly (1966, 1970, 1986, 1987), Ed Trickett (1984; Trickett, Kelly, & Vincent, 1985), and others developed an *ecological model* that entailed the following set of core principles to guide the development and implementation of community interventions:[10]

ECOLOGICAL PRINCIPLE #1

Psychological problems often reflect a poor fit between the demands of the settings in which people live and work and the adaptive resources to which they have access. Therefore, ecological interventions seek to alter problematic settings, create alternative settings that are better suited to people's needs and capacities, or enhance people's capacity to adapt effectively to existing sett..gs.

Various writers have noted that how we define problems determines to a great extent how we go about trying to solve them (Caplan & Nelson, 1996). Inherent in most Western mental health interventions are definitions of mental health problems as reflections of damaged or dysfunctional processes *within* people. Naturally, this person-centered approach leads to an emphasis on healing or correcting the internal damage or dysfunction. This framework unquestionably makes sense for certain types of psychological disorders, including those with a strong biological component, as well as other types of distress such as severe trauma that persists long after the traumatic situation has passed and a healthy environment has been established.

From an ecological perspective, however, many types of mental health problems, including most of the displacement-related distress experienced by refugees, are best understood as reflecting problems in the relationship between the demands of the settings in which people live and the adaptive or coping resources at their disposal. This conceptualization leads to a fundamentally different set of intervention strategies, all of which focus on changing the problematic person-setting relationship rather than "fixing" something inside the person experiencing the problem. As suggested earlier, this can happen by altering problematic settings, by creating settings better suited to people's needs and abilities, or

---

[10]The set of ecological principles listed here is only partial. Readers interested in a more thorough discussion of the ecological model, including its implications for community-based research, are referred to Kelly (1966, 1970), Levine and Perkins (1997), Rappaport (1981), and Trickett, Kelly, and Vincent (1985).

by strengthening people's capacity to cope with existing settings. In practice, there is often considerable overlap between these three strategies.

For refugees, all three approaches are viable. Existing settings can be altered in numerous ways. At the macro level, individuals seeking asylum, many of whom experience high levels of trauma and depression, can be treated humanely rather than being detained as criminals while they await their asylum hearings (Postero, 1992). For example, unless asylum applicants pose a clear danger to the community, they could be released pending their hearing, and appropriate referrals could be made to legal, psychosocial, health, and housing resources. Media campaigns can be used to promote tolerance and discourage discrimination against refugees. Resettlement policies can aim at preserving rather than dispersing refugee families and communities, in order to maintain existing sources of social support and minimize painful separations. And pressure can be brought to bear to ensure that refugees are treated fairly under international law and treaties. For example, greater international monitoring of host governments could help ensure that refugees and asylum seekers are not forcibly repatriated, especially when conditions in their countries of origin remain dangerous.

At the local level, refugee camps can be made safer, in order to reduce the occurrence of rape and other forms of sexual violence and exploitation. And instead of refugee assistance strategies that foster dependency, programs can be implemented that promote economic self-sufficiency and thereby enhance self-esteem and a sense of efficacy (Harrell Bond, 1999; von Buchwald, 1998). An excellent example of this approach is the micro-enterprise approach, in which funding is provided to refugees to start small businesses that lead to income generation and diminish the need for outside aid (Forbes Martin, 1992). Local community settings also can be enhanced to more effectively meet specific community needs. For example, in a collaborative project with indigenous Guatemalan refugees in southern Mexico, Miller and Billings (1994) worked with local school teachers in the refugee camps to enhance their capacity to address children's psychosocial development within the school setting. Another approach to changing a local setting involves adapting local language classes to respond more effectively to the unique mental health needs and challenges experienced by many refugees (Cohon et al., 1986), who sometimes experience difficulty with learning a new language due to impairments in concentration, attention, and memory associated with trauma and/or depression (Miller, Worthington et al., 2002). By integrating mental health concepts and strategies into the English as a Second Language (ESL) classroom with refugees in the United States, Cohon et al. (1986) sought to enhance language mastery, develop skills and strategies for coping with psychological distress, and transform the classroom community itself into a source of social support for its members.

New settings also can be created that promote psychological wellness in refugees. In the Bosnian Community Center in Chicago, a setting developed and run by the local Bosnian community, Bosnian refugees have access to companionship, English and computer classes, cultural celebrations, and media resources (T. Robb & A. Smajkic, personal communications). Similar community centers and mutual assistance organizations—most of which function to enhance social support, promote environmental mastery, provide spaces for cultural and religious celebrations, and help community members gain access to important social, economic, educational, and health-related resources—have been developed in many other refugee communities. Numerous other strategies for developing new settings are described in the projects in this book. An example is the development of *learning circles* with Hmong refugees in the United States (Goodkind, Hang, & Yang, chapter 9, this volume). In the learning circles, Hmong community members and students from Michigan State University met regularly to address problems facing the Hmong community (the group approach reflected the strong collectivism in Hmong culture), and participants from the two cultures exchanged knowledge and experiences. Another example is the development of "coffee gatherings" for Bosnian refugee families, in which participants come together as families (reflecting the centrality of the family as a social unit in Bosnia) to share experiences, problem-solve common difficulties, and gain knowledge and access to important community resources, while also strengthening their social networks (Weine et al., chapter 8, this volume).

Finally, ecological interventions with refugees can enhance the capacity of refugee communities to adapt more effectively to existing settings. Tribe and DeSilva (1999; see also Tribe et al., chapter 5, this volume) illustrate this approach nicely in their description of the Women's Empowerment Program, a psychosocial program for women widowed by the violent conflict in Sri Lanka. Among the various components of the program, women gained access to knowledge, social support, and material resources designed to help them cope more effectively with the multiple challenges confronting them as single mothers living in refugee camps. The ESL/Mental Health approach (Cohon et al., 1986) described earlier also has a strong emphasis on strengthening the capacity of refugee communities to adapt to the demands of local settings, for example by helping program participants learn how to access key resources in their new environment, while also helping them master the skills needed to take advantage of those resources (e.g., language skills, mastery of the local transportation system, knowledge of tenants' rights, etc.). All of the projects in this volume describe innovative approaches to helping refugee communities adapt to settings that often are highly challenging.

The ecological emphasis on changing the person/setting relationship as a way of addressing mental health problems in no way negates the value of other more intrapersonally-focused interventions aimed at restoring psychological equilibrium among severely distressed individuals. As we discuss shortly, and as several of the chapters in this volume illustrate, an ecological framework encourages interventions at multiple levels, including the individual, the family, the community, and society as a whole. Whether they are delivered by shamans, *curanderos*, or psychotherapists, individually focused treatments that promote the healing of damaged intrapersonal processes will always have their place in addressing the mental health needs of refugee communities. Our point is simply that such treatments should never become the cornerstone of our response to the mental health needs of refugee communities; instead, they should always represent just one of several intervention strategies in a richly diverse psychological toolbox.

ECOLOGICAL PRINCIPLE #2

Ecological interventions should address problems that are of concern to community members. Intervention priorities should reflect the priorities of the community.

As our earlier review indicates, researchers concerned with the mental health of refugees have focused primarily on assessing the prevalence of psychological trauma. This would seem to imply that trauma represents the most pressing mental health concern within refugee communities. It is not clear how this assumption came to be so widely accepted, nor is it clear that it is necessarily warranted. Certainly, as summarized in our earlier review, the data do show an elevated prevalence of psychological trauma among a diversity of refugee populations. However, this does not mean that refugees themselves perceive psychological trauma as among their most pressing concerns. In fact, there is some evidence suggesting that refugees may actually be more concerned about other stressors affecting their mental health than they are about psychological trauma; examples include unemployment (Hubbard & Pearson, chapter 3, this volume); physical health problems, mood disturbances, and family discord (de Jong, 2002); the lack of opportunity to engage in culturally appropriate burial and mourning rituals for loved ones killed by violence (Englund, 1998); domestic violence (Zahir, Kakar, & Miller, 2001); and poverty-related stressors, such as inadequate housing or the threat of eviction when there is insufficient money to pay the rent (Miller, Worthington et al., 2002).

This is not to suggest that trauma is not a widespread problem among refugees, nor do we mean to suggest that refugees experiencing symptoms of trauma do not find their symptoms distressing. Our point is simply that an exclusive or primary focus on PTSD may be somewhat at odds with the perceived needs and priorities of local community members.

The fact that refugee communities may not prioritize the treatment of trauma symptoms relative to other pressing concerns, including those we have referred to in this chapter as displacement-related stressors, does not mean we should abandon our efforts to help people manage or resolve their experiences of psychological trauma. It *does* mean that we may need to broaden the focus of our interventions to reflect the range of concerns that are salient within the communities in which we work. To know what those concerns are, we simply need to ask community members in ways that allow them to tell us what is most important to them. In practical terms, this means complementing traditional psychiatric as assessment methods with qualitative strategies such as semistructured interviews, focus groups, and participant observation. In contrast to *deductive* methods which are designed to confirm or disprove our own *a priori* hypotheses, inductive methods such as these allow respondents to articulate their own concerns unrestricted by our assumptions about what matters most to them or what aspects of their experience are most in need of attention. Gathering such information is not simply a good idea, it is *essential* to the design of contextually appropriate ecological interventions.

Some readers may understandably object that mental health interventions should not be expected to address all of the problems and challenges that confront communities displaced by political violence. After all, mental health is simply one domain of experience, and other types of organizations may be better suited to addressing concerns related to physical health, employment, housing, and so forth. On the one hand, we believe there is merit to this perspective, and are strong advocates of coordinated, multidisciplinary approaches to addressing the challenges faced by refugee communities. On the other hand, we also believe that mental health interventions are most likely to be successful when they address those stressors that participants identify as most significantly affecting their psychological well-being. For example, to the extent that unemployment is a major stressor affecting the well-being of individuals and families in a refugee community, it may be necessary to help community members increase their access to employment-related opportunities before they are prepared to focus on ameliorating their symptoms of psychological trauma. When family discord is a primary concern, family-focused strategies that reduce stress and enhance functioning may be most appropriate initially, before engaging in trauma-focused interventions that target traumatized individuals. The projects in this book share an emphasis on addressing those mental health-related stressors that are of greatest concern to community members. They have retained their focus on mental health, yet their intervention foci often extend beyond the healing of trauma or the amelioration of psychiatric symptomatology.

ECOLOGICAL PRINCIPLE #3

Whenever possible, prevention should be prioritized over treatment, as preventive interventions are generally more effective, more cost-efficient, and more humane than an exclusive reliance on the treatment of problems once they have developed. This does not negate an important role for treatment; it simply regards individual treatment as one tool in the arsenal of intervention responses.

One might draw a parallel to the problem of smoking and its relation to lung cancer. From a public health perspective, it makes a great deal of sense to prioritize the *prevention* of lung cancer through smoking prevention and cessation programs. At the same time, as long as there are people in need of treatment for lung cancer that has already developed (whether from smoking or other causes), there will continue to be a need for hospital-based treatment services as well as prevention programs.

How does the concept of prevention apply to refugees, many of whom are already experiencing high levels of distress by the time they are resettled? In considering this question, it may be helpful to distinguish between primary and secondary preventive interventions. Primary prevention programs are implemented with whole communities or sub-communities prior to the onset of psychological difficulties, the goal being the prevention of problems before they arise. Secondary prevention programs, in contrast, are aimed at individuals or groups already showing signs of distress, with the aims of restoring psychological equilibrium and preventing the development of enduring psychological difficulties (Goldston, 1977; Kaplan, 1964).

Recall now our earlier suggestion that effective refugee mental health programs should have two primary aims: helping people manage or resolve experiences of psychological trauma and traumatic loss, and assisting communities to cope effectively with ongoing displacement-related stressors. With regard to psychological trauma, there is a growing body of research showing the secondary preventive effects of social support on incipient symptoms of post-traumatic stress reactions (Gist, Lubin, & Redburn, 1999; Kaniasty & Norris, 1999). In the wake of traumatic events, naturally occurring social support systems can be effective buffers against the development of enduring symptoms of trauma. Family members, friends, and community leaders are well positioned to provide affective and instrumental social support to trauma survivors, and can help them identify alternative ways of framing their experiences of victimization (e.g., helping transform their identities from victims to survivors, and offering sociopolitical or religious perspectives that provide some degree of meaning to their experiences). Although severely traumatized individuals may require the assistance of traditional healers or mental health professionals trained in the treatment of psychological trauma, the availability of socially supportive networks, together with the passing of time, is often sufficient to help people exposed to traumatic events recover psychologically (Foa & Rothbaum, 1998; Kaniasty & Norris, 1999). *From an intervention standpoint, this suggests that the secondary prevention of PTSD among refugees should focus on re-establishing or strengthening social support networks within refugee communities.* Indeed, this approach is central to the interventions described in this volume.

There is also some evidence that community narratives may function to transform the meaning of traumatic experiences so as to make them less pathogenic (Dawes, 1990; Punamäki, 1989). To the extent that this is so, another preventive strategy could entail helping communities traumatized by experiences of violence develop communal narratives that provide some degree of shared meaning and eventual resolution to their experiences. This approach is illustrated by Ford, Cabrerra, and Searing (2000), who developed an innovative mental health intervention with Guatemalan Indian communities displaced by the genocidal violence that swept through the largely Indian highlands in the early 1980s (Handy, 1984; Manz, 1988). In that project, the authors collaborated with community members to integrate traditional Mayan and Western mental health beliefs and healing strategies that might help people recover from their experiences of trauma and displacement. They elaborated a communal approach to healing that involved, among other things, culturally familiar activities designed to help people articulate, tolerate, and transform their experiences of trauma. In the narratives that emerged, traumatic events were reframed as acts of unjust social control by a repressive state, rather than as reflections of weakness or failure in the survivors. In a related vein, religious leaders in several Bosnian Muslim communities in which many of the women were raped have sought to minimize the women's sense of shame by publicly declaring them heroines of resistance, thereby reframing their experience in terms devoid of shame (Petevi, 1996). Although it is unlikely that this intervention eliminated the women's suffering, it does represent an innovative community-level approach to ameliorating the effects of war-related trauma, and to creating the conditions under which further healing might occur.

Both primary and secondary preventive interventions are well suited to helping refugee communities cope effectively with exile-related stressors, our other proposed aim of mental health interventions with refugees. To the extent that much of the depression and anxiety experienced by refugees is related to the multiple challenges they encounter as a result of being displaced, enhancing their capacity to cope effectively with displacement-related stressors should exert significant preventive mental health effects. For example, by facilitating the development of social networks, we can reduce isolation and increase the availability of social support (Petevi, 1996). And by helping refugees develop the knowledge and skills needed to negotiate their new settings, we can broaden their social, educational, and employment-related options, which in turn can lead to the discovery of new social and occupational roles, the generation of much needed income, and the identification of new life projects. An example of the latter approach is found in the experience of Guatemalan refugee women in southern Mexico who received formal training in midwifery at a nearby Mexican hospital (Billings, 1996). Because of the advanced training they received, the women were able to play a highly visible and much needed role in the community, helping to ensure safe and healthy deliveries in the camp and assisting new mothers with early childcare practices. For several of the men in the community who had been farmers in Guatemala but who were now without land and thus lacked the capacity to provide for their families, training in pedagogy led to meaningful employment as camp school teachers. Consequently, the men discovered new occupational roles, and were able to once again provide, at least minimally, for their families.

ECOLOGICAL PRINCIPLE #4

Local values and beliefs regarding psychological well-being and distress should be incorporated into the design, implementation, and evaluation of community-based interventions. This increases the likelihood that interventions will be culturally appropriate and therefore enhances the odds of program utilization and effectiveness.

A central theme in the projects included in this volume concerns the importance of understanding and integrating local mental health-related beliefs and practices into the design and implementation of community interventions. In his anthropological study of healers in diverse cultures, Torrey (1972) found that a shared worldview was an essential ingredient in effective helping relationships. A natural extension of Torrey's observation is the idea that people are more likely to utilize mental health and psychosocial programs that embody their own cultural beliefs and include culturally familiar rituals of healing.

This does not mean that Western mental health practices have no place in ecological interventions with refugee communities. Few cultures have evolved systems of healing adequate to address the effects of war-related trauma or the psychosocial impact of mass displacement. Just as importantly, cultures are rarely static, nor do they exist in isolation from other cultural values and practices. Within refugee communities, there may be considerable variation in the extent to which people continue to practice or believe in traditional methods of healing. For example, exposure to Western medicine and the lack of access to traditional *curanderos* has left many Guatemalan refugees in Mexico as likely to seek help from physicians as from traditional healers (Miller & Billings, unpublished raw data). There may also be multiple belief systems and related rituals of healing coexisting within any given refugee community, since people of different ethnic and religious backgrounds may be jointly displaced by the same experience of violent conflict. In such cases, no single "traditional" set of beliefs and practices is likely to adequately represent the community's range of responses to psychological distress.

Taken together, these factors suggest that there is a need for the integration of multiple perspectives and approaches to healing distress within refugee communities. Our concern is with the avoidance of "psychological imperialism" (Dawes, 1997), the reflexive application of Western mental health constructs and practices to non-Western contexts, without regard or respect for local values, beliefs, and rituals of healing. The authors in this volume have been careful to avoid such imperialism, and their projects illustrate a variety of innovative approaches to blending Western and local approaches to understanding and healing psychological distress and promoting positive adaptation among refugees. Examples include the use of local religious ceremonies together with the enhancement of social support and the training of community members in Western counseling methods to help Sierra Leonian refugees heal from experiences of trauma and displacement (Hubbard & Pearson, chapter 3, this volume); and the building of a *jango*, a circular hut that serves as a traditional community center, to enhance the sense of community among displaced Angolans, together with training in various expressive arts and play activities designed to promote healthy psychosocial development among children in the community (Wessells & Monteiro, chapter 2, this volume).

ECOLOGICAL PRINCIPLE #5

Whenever possible, ecological interventions should be integrated into existing community settings and activities, in order to enhance participation in and long-term sustainability of the interventions.

A colleague of ours related an interesting story about trying to provide mental health services to Ethiopian Jewish women who had recently arrived in Israel. The women and their families had faced considerable hardship before coming to Israel, yet they were highly reluctant to take advantage of the mental health services available at a nearby mental health clinic. Eventually, a therapist at the clinic decided to try a different tack. Having noticed that the women did their laundry at a common washing area, she brought her own laundry in and gradually became a regular presence in the group. Over time, she was able to generate discussion about the difficulties the women had faced in Ethiopia as well as those challenges they continued to face in Israel. The washing area had become a *de facto* mental health setting.

Earlier, we discussed the reluctance of many refugees to utilize mental health services located in formal mental health settings such as psychiatric clinics or hospitals because of the social stigma attached to receiving mental health care in such settings. By integrating mental health services into familiar, nonstigmatized community settings, it is possible to enhance program utilization among people who might be disinclined to participate in programs located in formal mental health settings. Ideal community settings include schools, community centers, recreation areas, people's homes, the offices of community organizations, primary care centers, in fact, any setting in which people routinely come together for community-based activities. This point is illustrated in the diversity of community settings in which the programs described in this book are housed.

There are additional advantages to working within existing community settings beyond the avoidance of stigma. For example, in contrast to clinic settings in which hierarchical relationships between patients and helpers are quite pronounced, community settings are more conducive to authentic collaboration and a greater sense of equality among project staff and participants. In our view, this has two benefits. First, egalitarian settings may exert a restraining influence on outside professionals' tendency to assume the role of authority figure vis à vis community members, who may be all too ready to grant such authority to highly educated professionals at the cost of recognizing and valuing their own experiences, abilities, knowledge, and skills. Second, working in nonclinical community settings minimizes the likelihood of program participants falling into the role of "sick patient", a pull that can be quite strong in highly medicalized clinical settings (Goffman, 1961). Although the role of sick patient may be appropriate under certain circumstances, we would suggest that it is not a role that pulls for people's strengths and adaptive resources, nor is it one that promotes active coping in the face of ongoing psychosocial stressors.

ECOLOGICAL PRINCIPLE #6

Capacity building, rather than the direct provision of services by mental health professionals, should be an intervention priority in all communities. This is especially important in communities that either underutilize, or have limited access to, professional mental health services. Capacity building reflects the ecological focus on empowerment, *defined here as helping people achieve greater control over the resources that affect their lives.*

Capacity building within refugee communities means identifying and building upon the strengths that community members possess. It means collaborating with community members in all phases of the intervention process, from the conceptualization and development of community interventions to their implementation and evaluation. The goal of capacity building in refugee communities is to maximize the capacity of communities to address the mental health needs of their members, through prevention as well as treatment, thereby lessening their dependence on scarce outside professionals. Capacity building is also about helping communities enhance the capacity of existing social structures (or develop new structures) to better meet needs of community members.

Capacity building approaches are ultimately more efficient, more effective, and more empowering than expert driven models of community intervention. They are more efficient because they greatly expand the reach of mental health programs that have few professional staff to provide services. They are more effective because ecologically oriented capacity building entails genuine collaboration with community members, which in turn increases the likelihood that interventions will be designed and implemented in ways that reflect and respect local cultural values and norms. And they are more empowering because they enable communities to respond effectively to mental health problems that were previously difficult to address.

A common thread in the projects described in this volume is their emphasis on active collaboration with members of local refugee communities. Although this collaboration takes different forms in the various projects, its most common and perhaps most critical feature involves a shift on the part of mental health professionals from the role of direct service provider to collaborative, capacity building roles such as consultant, trainer, and co-evaluator. The direct service providers in the interventions are generally members of the community, ranging from traditional healers, religious leaders, and community elders, to community members trained as lay mental health staff, competent to engage in a wide variety of mental health-related activities.

We realize that some mental health professionals may have concerns about the use of trained community members (paraprofessionals) doing mental health work with refugees who may be experiencing high levels of distress. We certainly recognize the value of referring severely traumatized individuals for specialized care with traditional healers or mental health professionals trained in the treatment of trauma. More generally, however, we are mindful of the extensive literature documenting the effectiveness of trained paraprofessionals (see Christenson & Jacobson, 1994 for an excellent review). In fact, findings have shown consistently that well trained paraprofessionals are at least as effective as mental health professionals in reducing symptoms of distress and enhancing psychological well-being (Christenson & Jacobson, 1994). The findings from several of the projects in this book, although still preliminary, are consistent with this literature, and support the use of paraprofessionals in refugee settings.

ORGANIZATION AND STRUCTURE OF THE BOOK

In the past 10 years, there has been a remarkable increase in the number of ecological mental health interventions that have been developed with internally displaced and exiled communities. Mental health professionals have begun to recognize the need for a broader conceptual framework for addressing the mental health needs of communities displaced by political violence. We are confronted almost daily with images of the terror and despair faced by survivors of interstate and civil war, political repression, and the systematic persecution of religious and ethnic communities. For those working on the front line, the limitations of an exclusive reliance on clinic-based services have become increasingly clear. For mental health professionals working with refugees in the comparative safety and stability of the developed nations, those same limitations are likewise becoming more evident. There is a new openness to thinking outside the box, to considering alternative ways of defining mental health work and the types of activities it may entail.

It is in the context of this openness to innovation and new ways of seeing familiar problems that this book is presented. Although ecological interventions have now been developed in numerous regions of the world, few opportunities exist for discussion of shared experiences, unique challenges, and innovative solutions. The unifying framework proposed here—the ecological model of community psychology—is our way of giving some conceptual and methodological organization to the array of interventions presented in the book. Some of the authors have developed their work within an explicitly ecological framework; others have used the language of public health and other conceptual frameworks to describe ideas and strategies that are fundamentally consistent (and often synonymous) with the language of the ecological model. Regardless of their language and organizing framework, the interventions described in this book have a common set of emphases, including: (1) collaboration with community members in the development and implementation of culturally appropriate interventions that blend local and Western ideas and practices; (2) the integration of mental health and psychosocial interventions into familiar and nonstigmatized community settings; and (3) a focus on enhancing the capacity of communities to cope effectively with displacement-related stressors, including the structural violence of poverty and discrimination, coupled with a parallel focus on alleviating distress related to experiences of violence and loss.

There is considerable variation in the specific aims and methods of the different projects, and some fit more neatly into an ecological framework than others. Some of the projects focus primarily on displacement-related stressors; others address displacement related stressors while also paying equal attention to helping people heal from the effects of violence and war-related loss. We have intentionally selected projects that represent a diversity of displaced populations, including internally displaced communities in Columbia, Angola, Sri Lanka, and Cambodia, and refugees (in the formal UN Declaration sense of the term) from Sierra Leone living in Guinea, from West Timor living in East Timor, and from Laos and Bosnia living in the United States. The populations included in the volume are not fully representative of the world's displaced peoples. Unfortunately, we were unable identify ecological mental health projects with several of the world's major refugee populations, including Afghans, Palestinians, or Kurds.[11] This does not mean that important mental health work is not being done with these populations, only that we were unable to locate interventions that fit within the ecological framework around which this volume is organized.

---

[11]For an excellent description of an ecological mental health intervention with Sudanese refugees, see Baron (2002).

We have asked the authors of each chapter to follow a standard outline, in order to maintain some degree of consistency of structure and focus across the chapters and to allow for greater ease of comparison among projects. Briefly, authors were asked to provide a bit of background regarding the sociopolitical context that led to the refugee crisis they have addressed, and to outline the mental health consequences of violence and displacement in the populations with which they have worked. We also asked the authors to be explicit about their model of distress: How did they conceptualize the mental health effects of the violence and displacement? To what extent did they blend Western and local views of mental health and mental health problems? In a related vein, authors were encouraged to reflect on their conceptualization of *trauma* and their views of the PTSD construct. Few issues are as contentious in the refugee mental health field as the question of the appropriateness and applicability of the PTSD diagnosis, especially in situations of ongoing conflict. Among the numerous criticisms that have been leveled at the PTSD diagnosis are the following:

1. The notion of a *post*-traumatic stress disorder implies that exposure to the traumatic situation has ended; however, for displaced communities living in or near zones of violent conflict, exposure to traumatic stress is often *ongoing* rather than past (Mayotte, 1992; Straker, 1988).
2. The diagnosis fails to take into account the diverse post-traumatic effects of different types of traumatic experiences, essentially treating all traumatic events equally (with the one distinction being that between natural and interpersonal trauma).
3. The construct fails to capture the totality of the ways in which traumatic experiences affect people (e.g., its impact on the attachment system, on cognitive schemas, and on spirituality; Wilson, Friedman, & Lindy, 2001).
4. The diagnosis creates a negatively biased view of people's mental health, since some studies suggest that survivors of political violence may function effectively despite experiencing elevated levels of PTSD symptoms (Summerfield, 1995).
5. The diagnosis essentially *medicalizes* a set of normal reactions to profoundly abnormal social conditions (Summerfield, 1995).

6. The use of adult-centered diagnostic criteria overlooks important developmental variations in children's vulnerability to and expression of traumatic stress reactions (e.g., Terr, 1990).
7. Cultural variations in the experience and expression of traumatic stress responses are not included in the supposedly universal PTSD criteria (Kleber, Figley, & Gersons, 1995).
8. The diagnosis *individualizes* the effects of political violence; that is, it reduces the effects of violence to its impact on individual mental health, while ignoring its effects on communities and on society as a whole (Martín Baró, 1989; Buitrago Cuéllar, chapter 7, this volume; Wessells & Monteiro, chapter 2, this volume). If one adopts the perspective that repressive governments intentionally use highly visible trauma-inducing strategies (e.g., torture, massacres, rape) to instill widespread fear and silence popular demands for social change, it becomes apparent that conceptualizing the effects of political violence *solely* in terms of PTSD symptoms fails to capture the totality of how violence affects civil society and the psychosocial well-being of communities.

Despite these criticisms, the PTSD construct continues to be used widely in studies of refugees, and advocates point to a growing literature documenting the existence of the PTSD syndrome in diverse cultures, including those from which many of the world's refugee have come. Our view is that both sides ("approaches" —or something less polarizing than "sides") have valid concerns. On the one hand, as we have already shown, the data clearly indicate that a syndrome comprised of the symptoms of PTSD has been found in a wide range of refugee populations. There does seem to be something universal about *certain aspects* of people's reactions to traumatic events. On the other hand, we strongly agree that the PTSD construct is problematic in situations of *ongoing* violence, that it fails to capture the complexity of the trauma experience, and that an exclusive focus on PTSD diverts our attention from the impact of violence on larger social systems (families, communities, and societies). Our aim here, however, is not to resolve this debate about the PTSD construct; instead, we hope that by encouraging authors to make explicit their model of trauma and its relation to their intervention, we can help generate a constructive dialogue rooted in actual field experiences with refugee communities.

Finally, we have asked the authors to describe their interventions and the process of implementation, to consider the challenges they encountered and the lessons they learned along the way, and to provide a summary of evaluation methods and findings. As Hubbard and Miller discuss in chapter 10 of this volume, evaluation has proved to be the Achilles heel of most community-based interventions with refugees, particularly those living in or near situations of ongoing violence. It is an enormous challenge to conduct systematic evaluations of mental health interventions in the chaotic environment of refugee camps, where renewed violence often leads to recurrent displacements, low literacy rates may complicate the use of questionnaires or other written materials, and the concept of systematic evaluation is itself often alien and at times alienating. This does not minimize the need for effective evaluations; it simply underscores the importance of developing evaluation methods that fit the complex and diverse settings in which refugee mental health interventions take place.

Focus of the Chapters

In chapter 2, Michael Wessells and Carlinda Monteiro describe an innovative intervention with internally displaced communities in Angola. Although the primary focus of the intervention is children, the project worked at multiple levels, training thousands of adults to work with children and improving the response of communities to the mental health and psychosocial needs of children affected by their experiences of violence and displacement. The project is particularly rich in its multilevel intervention approach and its holistic conceptualization of children's mental health and psychosocial needs.

In chapter 3, Jon Hubbard and Nancy Pearson present an ecological intervention with refugees from the civil war in Sierra Leone, now living in refugee camps in neighboring Guinea. The intervention is informed by the extensive cross-cultural clinical experience of the authors and their colleagues at the Center for Victims of Torture in Minneapolis, and by important ethnographic work carried out by the project's staff in Guinea.

The chapter offers a compelling description of how community members can be trained to work effectively as mental health paraprofessionals, and illustrates the value of integrating local and Western beliefs and practices in mental health interventions. The chapter also addresses the complexity of conducting systematic program evaluation in a context of ongoing violence and recurrent displacement.

In chapter 4, Willem van de Put and Maurice Eisenbruch offer a richly detailed account of their ecological trauma-focused intervention with Cambodians who survived the genocide and massive displacement that occurred under the Khmer Rouge. The Cambodian intervention is particularly impressive in the extent to which local mental health-related beliefs and practices are integrated into the project, and by the authors' commitment to integrating their work into existing community settings.

In chapter 5, Rachel Tribe and her colleagues at the Family Rehabilitation Center describe an ecological intervention with internally displaced women widowed by the civil war in Sri Lanka and living in refugee camps. Although the intervention model relied more extensively on outside experts for its implementation than many of the other projects in the book, the authors hoped that by using a "cascade model" of training, the participants might in effect become trainers for other women in the refugee camps and thereby transmit the knowledge and skills they had acquired in the intervention workshops. The project is particularly noteworthy for its holistic emphasis on addressing a broad range of variables affecting the women's well-being, ranging from traditional mental health concerns to legal and economic issues, employment concerns, and health-related topics.

Chapter 6 represents a bit of a departure from the previous chapters. In the context of describing a community-based psychosocial intervention with refugees in East Timor, Kathleen Kostelny and Michael Wessells offer a "behind the scenes" look at the complexity of implementing a large-scale psychosocial intervention under highly challenging circumstances. In our view, there is far too little discussion of the many challenges of carrying out precisely the type of work that is the focus of this volume. One could easily imagine, based on reports in professional journals or book chapters, that ecological interventions with refugees (and other communities) are relatively straightforward and uncomplicated. On the contrary, the challenges are numerous and sometimes daunting, and it is only through open dialogue about these challenges that we will move forward, sharing creative solutions and perhaps learning to avoid some of the pitfalls that have befallen those who came before us. We believe that this chapter represents an important contribution to a much needed discussion.

In chapter 7, Jorge Buitrago describes an innovative ecological intervention developed in Columbia. A consistent hallmark of community-based mental health work in Latin America is its explicitly political framework, a contrast to work done elsewhere in which project staff have intentionally sought to remain politically neutral. For Latin Americans working in contexts of ongoing violence and repression, neutrality is often regarded as an impossibility; either one is aligned with the victims of repressive violence, or one becomes complicit (actively or passively) with those who perpetrate the violence (e.g., Kordon & Edelman, 1987; ODHAG, 2000). This report by Jorge Buitrago and his colleagues in Corporación AVRE poignantly illustrates this perspective by describing their ecological work with Columbians affected by the ongoing civil war and state-sanctioned violence in their country. Many of the communities served by the AVRE project have been displaced by the armed conflict in Columbia; others have not been displaced but have been affected in other ways by the ongoing conditions of violence, impunity, and material deprivation. The chapter provides a compelling argument for viewing the effects of violence and displacement not merely in terms of individual symptoms of distress, but also in terms of damage and dysfunction manifested at multiple levels, including the family, the community, and society as a whole. Consequently, the authors advocate that interventions ideally should adopt a multilevel approach and not limit their focus solely to healing distressed individuals.

Chapter 8 is the first of two chapters focused on ecological interventions with refugee communities in the United States. In this chapter, Stevan Weine and his colleagues describe a creative family-focused intervention implemented initially with Bosnians, and subsequently with Kosovars, in the greater Chicago area. The project was staffed completely by members of the target communities, and was implemented in community settings ranging from a local community center to participants' homes. The authors provide a compelling discussion of the hazards of relying exclusively on clinic-based mental health services with refugees, and provide an excellent illustration of how systematic evaluation methods can be applied to ecological interventions.

In chapter 9, Jessica Goodkind, Panufa Hang, and Mee Yang provide a rich discussion of ecological principles as a backdrop to their intervention with Hmong refugees in Michigan. The project represents a fascinating university/community collaboration, based on an advocacy model, in which local university students and Hmong community members met together regularly to address community concerns and develop supportive relationships. Like Weine et al., the authors used particularly strong evaluation methods to examine both the process and outcome of their intervention. The chapter is also noteworthy for its conceptualization of mental health and well-being in holistic terms that transcend the narrow focus on psychiatric symptomatology found in many refugee studies.

In chapter 10, Jon Hubbard and Kenneth Miller explore the challenges of conducting evaluations of refugee mental health interventions, particularly in or near settings of ongoing violence. While recognizing the complexity of doing evaluation work in such contexts, the authors argue that finding context-appropriate evaluation methods is essential if we are to document effective intervention strategies. Drawing on their diverse field experiences, they offer a number of suggestions that organizational staff can use to evaluate both the process and the outcomes of their interventions.

The book concludes with a summary chapter by the editors. The chapter is both reflective and forward-looking. The strengths of ecological mental health projects with refugee communities are considered, as are current limitations. In particular, we underscore the need for more clearly delineated risk and intervention models to guide our interventions, in order to ensure that we are targeting the most appropriate variables using methods that are likely to be maximally effective. We also consider both the importance and the complexity of integrating Western and local beliefs and practices related well-being and distress, and, (echoing Hubbard and Miller) urge program staff to strengthen their efforts to evaluate both the process and outcome of their interventions.

REFERENCES

Aron, A., Corne, S., Fursland, A., & Zelwer, B. (1991). The gender-specific terror of El Salvador and Guatemala: Post-traumatic stress disorder in Central American women. *Women's Studies International Forum, 14*, 37-47.

Arroyo, W., & Eth, S. (1986). Children traumatized by Central American Warfare. In R. Pynoos & S. Eth (Eds.), *Post-traumatic stress disorder in children* (pp. 101-120). Washington, DC: American Psychiatric Press.

Baron, N. (2002). Community based psychosocial and mental health services for southern Sudanese refugees in long term exile in Uganda. In J. de Jong (Ed.), *Trauma, war, and violence: Public mental health in socio-cultural context* (pp. 157-204). New York: Kluwer Academic/Plenum Publishers.

Beiser, M., Johnson, P., & Turner, J. (1993). Unemployment, underemployment and depressive affect among Southeast Asian refugees. *Psychological Medicine, 23*, 731-743.

Bennett, C., Anderson, L., Cooper, S., Hassol, L., Klein, D., & Rosenblum, G. (1966). *Community Psychology: A report of the Boston Conference on the Education of Psychologists for Community Mental Health.* Boston: Boston University..

Bennett, J., & Detzner, D. (1997). Loneliness in cultural context: A look at the life-history narratives of older Southeast Asian refugee women. In A. Lieblich, & J. Ruthellen (Eds.), *The narrative study of lives* (pp. 113-146). Thousand Oaks, CA: Sage.

Billings, D. (1996). *Identity, consciousness, and organizing in exile: Guatemalan refugee women in the camps of southern Mexico.* Unpublished dissertation, University of Michigan, Ann Arbor, Michigan.

Bloom, B. (1984). *Community mental health: A general introduction (2nd ed.).* Monterey, CA: Brooks/Cole.

Boothby, N. (1988). Unaccompanied children from a psychological perspective. In E. Ressler, N. Boothby, & D. Steinbock (Eds.), *Unaccompanied children* (pp. 133-180). Oxford: Oxford University Press.

Boothby, N. (1991). *Working in the war zone: A look at psychological theory and practice from the field.* Paper presented at the Children in War Conference, Jerusalem.

Boothby, N. (1996). Mobilizing communities to meet the psychosocial needs of children in war and refugee crises. In R. Apfel & B. Simon (Eds.), *Minefields in their hearts: The mental health of children in war and communal violence* (pp. 149-164). New Haven, CT: Yale University Press.

Bottinelli, C., Maldonado, I., Troya, E., Herrera, P., & Rodriguez, C. (1990). *Psychological impacts of exile: Salvadoran and Guatemalan families in Mexico.* Washington, DC: Hemispheric Migration Project, Georgetown University.

Caplan, N., & Nelson, S. (1996). On being useful: The nature and consequences of psychological research on social problems. In R. Lorion, I. Iscoe, P. DeLeon, & G. vandenBos (Eds.), *Psychology and public policy* (pp. 123-144). Washington, DC: American Psychological Association.

Christensen, A., & Jacobson, N. (1994). Who (or what) can do psychotherapy. The status and challenge of non-professional therapies. *Psychological Science, 5,* 8-14.

Cohon, J. D., Lucey, M., Paul, M., & LeMarbre Penning, J. (1986). *Preventive mental health in the ESL classroom: A handbook for teachers.* New York: American Council for Nationalities Service.

Dalton, J., Elias, M., & Wandersman, A. (2001). *Community psychology.* Stamford, CT: Wadsworth.

Dawes, A. (1990). The effects of political violence on children: A consideration of South African and related studies. *International Journal of Psychology, 25,* 13-31.

Dawes, A. (1997, July). *Cultural imperialism in the treatment of children following political violence and war: A Southern African perspective.* Paper presented at the Fifth International Symposium on the Contributions of Psychology to Peace, Melbourne.

De Jong, J. (2002). Public mental health, traumatic stress and human rights violations in low income countries. In J. de Jong (Ed.), *Trauma, war, and violence: Public mental health in socio-cultural context* (pp. 1-92). New York: Kluwer Academic/Plenum Publishers.

Doña, G., & Berry, J. (1999) . Refugee acculturation and re-acculturation. In A. Ager (Ed.), *Refugees: Perspectives on the experience of forced migration* (pp. 169-195). London: Pinter.

Dybdahl, R. (2001). A psychosocial support program for children and mothers in war. *Clinical child Psychology and Psychiatry, 6,* 425-436.

Dyregov, A., & Yule, W. (November, 1995). *Screening measures — the development of the UNICEF screening battery.* Paper presented at the Symposium on War Affected Children in Former Yugoslavia at the Eleventh Annual Meeting of the International Society for Traumatic Stress Studies, Boston.

Eisenbruch, M. (1988). Can homesickness kill? In Abbott, M. (Ed.), *Refugee settlement and wellbeing* (pp. 101-117). Auckland, New Zealand: Mental Health Foundation of New Zealand.

Eisenbruch, M. (1991). Is Western mental health care appropriate for refugees? *Refugee Participation Network, 11,* 25-27.

Englund, H. (1998). Death, trauma and ritual: Mozambican refugees in Malawi. *Social Science and Medicine, 46,* 1165-1174.

Ensign, J. (1995). *Traditional healing in the Hmong refugee community of the California central valley.* Unpublished dissertation, California School of Professional Psychology, Fresno, CA.

Farias, P. (1994). Central and South American refugees: Some mental health challenges. In A. Marsella, T. Bornemann, S. Ekblad, & J. Orley (Eds.), *Amidst peril and pain: The mental health and well-being of the world's refugees* (pp. 101-114). Washington, DC: American Psychological Association.

Foa, E., Riggs, D., Dancu, C., & Rothbaum, B. (1993). Reliability and validity of a brief instrument for assessing post-traumatic stress disorder. *Journal of Traumatic Stress, 6,* 459-474.

Foa, E., & Rothbaum, B. (1998). *Treating the trauma of rape: Cognitive behavioral therapy for PTSD.* New York: Guilford.

Forbes Martin, S. (1992). *Refugee women.* London: Zed Books.

Ford, B., Cabrerra, R., & Searing, V. (2000). *Buscando una buena vida: Tres experiencias de salud mental comunitaria [Looking for a better life: Three experiences of community mental health].* Sta. Cruz el Quiche, Guatemala: Cáritas Quiche.

Fox, S., & Tang, S. (2000). The Sierra Leonean refugee experience: Traumatic events and psychiatric sequelae. *Journal of Nervous and Mental Disease, 188,* 490-495.

Frazer, M. (1973). *Children in conflict.* New York: Basic Books.

Garbarino, J., Kostelny, K., & Dubray, N. (1991). *No place to be a child: Growing up in a war zone.* Lexington, MA: Lexington Books.

Gibson, K. (1989). Children in political violence. *Social Science and Medicine, 7,* 659-667.

Gist, R., Lubin, B., & Redburn, B. (1999). Psychosocial, ecological, and community perspectives on disaster response. In R. Gist & B. Lubin (Eds.), *Response to disaster: Psychosocial, ecological, and community approaches.* Philadelphia: Bruner/Mazel.

Goffman, E. (1961). *Asylums: Essays on the social situation of mental patients and other inmates.* Chicago: Aldine.

Goldston, S. (1977). An overview of primary prevention programming. In D. Klein & S. Goldston (Eds.), *Primary prevention: An idea whose time has come.* DHEW Publication No. (ADM) 77-447. Washington, DC: Government Printing Office.

Gonsalves, C. (1990). The psychological effects of political repression on Chilean exiles in the US. *American Journal of Orthopsychiatry, 60,* 143-153.

Gorst-Unsworth, C., & Goldenberg, E. (1998). Psychological sequelae of torture and organized violence suffered by refugees from Iraq: Trauma-related factors compared with social factors in exile. *British Journal of Psychiatry, 172,* 90-94.

Global IDP Project (2002). http://www.idpproject.org

Handy, J. (1984). *Gift of the devil: A history of Guatemala.* Boston: South End Press.

Harrell Bond, B. (1999). The experiences of refugees as recipients of aid. In A. Ager (Ed.), *Refugees: Perspectives on the experience of forced migration* (pp. 136-168). London: Pinter.

Heller, K., Price, R., Reinharz, S., Riger, S., Wandersman, A., & D'Aunno, T. (1984). *Psychology and community change* (pp. 172-226). Pacific Grove, CA: Brooks/Cole.

Hitchcox, L. (1990). *Vietnamese refugees in Southeast Asian refugee camps.* Hampshire, England: MacMillan Academic and Professional, Ltd.

Hollingshead, A., & Redlich, F. (1958). *Social class and mental illness: A community study.* New York: Wiley.

Hubbard, J., Realmuto, G., Northwood, A., & Masten, A. (1995). Comorbidity of psychiatric diagnosis with posttraumatic stress disorder in survivors of childhood trauma. *Journal of the American Academy of Child & Adolescent Psychiatry, Vol. 34,* 1167-1173.

Kaniasty, K., & Norris, F. (1999). The experience of disaster: Individuals and communities sharing trauma. In R. Gist & B. Lubin (Eds.), *Response to disaster* (pp. 25-55). Philadelphia: Bruner Mazel.

Kaplan, A. (1964). *The conduct of inquiry.* San Francisco: Chandler.

Kelly, J. (1966). Ecological constraints on mental health services. *American Psychologist, 48,* 1023-1034.

Kelly, J. (1970). Antidotes for arrogance: Training for community psychology. *American Psychologist, 25,* 524-531.

Kelly, J. (1986). Context and process: An ecological view of the interdependence of practice and research. *American Journal of Community Psychology, 14,* 581-605.

Kelly, J. (1987). An ecological paradigm: Defining mental health consultation as a preventive service. In J. Kelly & R. Hess (Eds.), *The ecology of prevention* (pp. 1-36). New York: The Hawarth Press.

Kinzie, J., Sack, W., Angell, R., Clark, G., & Ben, R. (1989). A three year follow-up of Cambodian young people traumatized as children. *Journal of the American Academy of Child and Adolescent Psychiatry, 28,* 501-504.

Kinzie, J., Sack, W., Angell, R., Manson, S., & Rath, B. (1986). The psychiatric effects of massive trauma on Cambodian children: I. The children. *Journal of the American Academy of Child and Adolescent Psychiatry, 25,* 370-376.

Kleber, R., Figley, C., & Gersons, B. (1995). *Beyond trauma: Cultural and societal dynamics.* New York: Plenum Press.

Kordon, D., & Edelman, L. (1987). *Efectos psicológicos de la repression política [Psychological effects of political repression].* Bueno Aires: Sudamericana-Planeta.

Landesman, P. (2002). A woman's work. *New York Times,* September 15, p. 82.

Lavik, N., Hauff, E., Skrondal, A., & Solberg, O. (1996). Mental disorder among refugees and the impact of persecution and exile: Some findings from an out-patient population. *British Journal of Psychiatry, 169,* 726-732.

Levine, M., & Perkins, D. (1997). *Principles of community psychology* (2nd ed.). New York: Oxford University Press.

Lundgren, R., & Lang, R. (1989). 'There is no sea, only fish': Effects of United States policy on the health of the displaced in El Salvador. *Social Science and Medicine, 28,* 697-706.

Machel, G. (1996). *The impact of armed conflict on children.* Report of the Expert of the Secretary General Cape. New York: United Nations.

Manz, B. (1988). *Refugees of a hidden war.* Albany: State University of New York Press.

Martín Baró, I. (1985). *Acción e ideología: Psicología social desde Centroamerica* San Salvador: UCA Editores.

Martín Baró, I. (1989). Political violence and war as causes of psychosocial trauma in El Salvador. *International Journal of Mental Health, 18,* 3-20.

Martín Baró, I. (August, 1990). *War and the psychosocial trauma of Salvadoran children.* Paper presented posthumously at the annual meeting of the American Psychological Association, Boston, MA.

Mayotte, J. (1992). *Disposable people? The plight of refugees.* Maryknoll, NY: Orbis Books.

McKay, S. (1998). The effects of armed conflict on girls and women. *Journal of Peace and Conflict, 4,* 381-392.

McSharry, S., & Kinney, R. (1992). Prevalence of psychiatric disorders in Cambodian refugees: A community random sample. Unpublished manuscript, Social Research Institute, Graduate School of Social Work, University of Utah, Salt Lake City, Utah..

Michultka, D., Blanchard, E., & Kalous, T. (1998). Responses to civilian war experiences: Predictors of psychological functioning and coping. *Journal of Traumatic Stress, 11,* 571-577.

Miller, K. (1994). *Growing up in exile: Mental health and meaning-making among indigenous Guatemalan refugee children.* Unpublished dissertation, University of Michigan, Ann Arbor, MI.

Miller, K. (1996). The effects of state terrorism and exile on indigenous Guatemalan refugee children: A mental health assessment and an analysis of children's narratives. *Child Development, 67,* 89-106.

Miller K. (1999). Rethinking a familiar model: Psychotherapy and the mental health of refugees. *Journal of Contemporary Psychotherapy, 29,* 283-306.

Miller, K., & Billings, D. (1994). Playing to grow: A primary mental health intervention with Guatemalan refugee children. *American Journal of Orthopsychiatry, 64,* 346-356.

Miller, K., Silber, Z., Pazdirek, L., Caruth, M., & Lopez, D. (2003). *The use of interpreters in psychotherapy with refugees: An exploratory study.* Manuscript submitted for publication.

Miller, K., Weine, S., Ramic, A., Brkic, N., Djuric Bjedic, Z., Smajkic, A., Boskailo, E., & Worthington, G. (2002). The relative contribution of war experiences and exile-related stressors to levels of psychological distress among Bosnian refugees. *Journal of Traumatic Stress.* 15, 377-387.

Miller, K., Worthington, G., Muzurovic, J. Tipping, S., & Goldman, A. (2002). Bosnian refugees and the stressors of exile: A narrative study. *American Journal of Orthopsychiatry, 72,* 341-354.

Mollica, R., McInnes, K., Pham, T., Fawzi, M., Smith, C., Murphy, E., & Lin, L. (1998). The dose-effect relationships between torture and psychiatric symptoms in Vietnamese ex-political detainees and a comparison group. *Journal of Nervous & Mental Disease, 186,* 543-553.

Mollica, R., Donelan, K., Svang, T., Lavelle, J., Elias, C., Frankel, M., & Blendon, R. (1993). The effect of trauma and confinement on functional health and mental health status of Cambodians living in Thailand-Cambodia border camps. *Journal of the American Medical Association, 27,* 581-586.

Mollica, R., Caspi-Yavin, Y., Bollini, P., Truong, T. (1992). The Harvard Trauma Questionnaire: Validation of a cross-cultural instrument for measuring torture, trauma, and posttraumatic stress disorder in Indochinese refugees. *Journal of Nervous and Mental Disease,180,* 111-116.

Norris, F. (2002). *50,000 disaster victims speak: An empirical review of the empirical literature, 1981-2001.* Hanover, NH: The National Center for PTSD.

Norris, F. (2002). Psychosocial consequences of disasters. *PTSD Research Quarterly, 13,* 1-7.

ODHAG (Oficina de Derechos Humanos del Arzobispo de Guatemala). (2000). *Memoria, verdad, y esperanza.* Guatemala City: ODHAG.

Omidian, P. (1996). *Aging and family in an Afghan refugee community: Transitions and transformations.* New York: Garland.

Pernice, R., & Brook, J. (1996). Refugees' and immigrants' mental health: Association of demographic and post-migration factors. *Journal of Social Psychology, 136,* 511-519.

Perera, S. (2001). Spirit possessions and avenging ghosts. In V. Das, A. Kleinman, M. Lock, M. Ramphele, & P. Reynalda (Eds.), *Remaking a world: Violence, social suffering, and recovery* (pp. 157-200). Berkeley: University of California Berkeley Press.

Petevi, M. (1996). Forced displacement: Refugee trauma, protection and assistance. In Y. Danieli, N. Rodley, & L. Weisaeth (Eds.), *International responses to traumatic stress* (pp. 161-192). Amityville, MY: Bayville.

Postero, N. (1992). On trial in the promised land: Seeking asylum. *Women & Therapy, 13,* 155-172.

Punamäki, R. (1989). Predictors and effectiveness of coping with political violence among Palestinian children. *British Journal of Social Psychology, 29,* 67-77.

Punamäki, R., & Suleiman, R. (1990). Predictors and effectiveness of coping with political violence among Palestinian children. *British Journal of Social Psychology, 29,* 67-77.

Pynoos, R., Steinberg, A., & Wraith, R. (1995). A developmental model of childhood traumatic stress. In D. Cicchetti & D. Cohen (Eds.), *Developmental psychopathology, Vol. 2: Risk, disorder, and adaptation* (pp. 72-95). New York: John Wiley & Sons.

Quesada, J. (1988, May 26). Program trains refugees to counsel their compatriots. *Synaspe,* p. 2.

Rappaport, J. (1981). In praise of paradox: A social policy of empowerment over prevention. *American Journal of Community Psychology, 9,* 1-26.

Rosenblatt, P. (2001). A social constructivist perspective on cultural differences in grief. In M. Stroebe, R. Hansson, W. Stroebe, & Henk Schut (Eds.), *Handbook of bereavement research* (pp. 285-300.). Washington, DC: American Psychological Association.

Rubel, A., O'Nell, C., & Collado Ardón, R. (1989). *Susto: A folk illness.* Berkeley: University of California Press.

Salvado, L. (1988). *The other refugees: A study of non-recognized Guatemalan refugees in Chiapas.* Washington, DC: Hemispheric Migration Project, Center for Immigration Policy and Refugee Assistance.

Servan-Schreiber, D., Lin, B., & Birmaher, B. (1998). Prevalence of post-traumatic stress-disorder and major depressive disorder in Tibetan refugee children. *Journal of the American Academy of Child and Adolescent Psychiatry, 37,* 874-879.

Shorish-Shamely, Z. (1991). *The self and other in Afghan cosmology: Concepts of health and illness among the Afghan refugees.* Unpublished dissertation, The University of Wisconsin, Madison.

Shrestha, N., Sharma, B., Van Ommeren, M., Regmi, S., makaju, R., Komproe, I., Shrestha, G., & de Jong, J. (1998). Impact of torture on refugees within the developing world Symptomatology among Bhutanese refugees in Nepal. *Journal of the American Medical Association, 280,* 443-448.

Silove, D. (1999). The psychosocial effects of torture, mass human rights violations, and refugee trauma. *Journal of Nervous and Mental Disease, 187,* 200-207.

Silove, D., Sinnerbrink, I., Field, A., & Manicavasagar, V. (1997). Anxiety, depression, and PTSD in asylum-seekers: Associations with pre-migration trauma and post-migration stressors. British Journal of Psychiatry, 170, 351-357.

Smajkic, A. (1999). *Relapse of PTSD and depression in a treatment of refugees, survivors of war and genocide.* Paper presented at the 15th Annual Meeting of the International Society for Traumatic Stress Studies, Miami, FL.

Smith, P., Perrin, S., Yule, W., Hacam, B., & Stuvland, R. (2002). War exposure among children from Bosnia-Hercegovina: Psychological adjustment in a community sample. *Journal of Traumatic Stress, 15,* 147-156.

Somasundaram, D., & Jamunanantha, C. (2002). Psychosocial consequences of war. In J. de Jong (Ed.), *Trauma, war, and violence: Public mental health in sociocultural context* (pp. 205-258). New York: Kluwer Academic/Plenum Publishers.

Straker, G. (1988). Post-traumatic stress disorder: A reaction to state-supported child abuse and neglect. *Child Abuse and Neglect, 12,* 383-395.

Summerfield. D. (1995). Addressing human response to war and atrocity: Major challenges in research and practices and the limitations of Western psychiatric models. In R. Kleber, C. Figley, & B. Gersons (Eds.), *Beyond trauma: Cultural and societal dynamics* (pp. 17-29). New York: Plenum Press.

Terr, L. (1990). *Too scared to cry: Psychic trauma in childhood* (pp. 1-51). New York: Harper & Row.

Thabet, A., & Vostanis, P. (2000). Post-traumatic stress disorder reactions in children of war: A longitudinal study. *Child Abuse and Neglect, 24,* 291-298.

Todd, J., & Bohard, A. (1999). *Foundations of clinical and counseling psychology.* New York: Addison Wesley Longman, Inc

Torrey, E. F. (1972). *Witchdoctors and psychiatrists: The common roots of psychotherapy and its future.* New York: Harper & Row.

Triandis, H. (2001). Individualism-collectivism and personality. *Journal of Personality, 69,* 907-924.

Tribe, R. (1999). Bridging the gap or damming the flow? Some observations on using interpreters/bicultural workers when working with refugee clients, many of whom have been tortured. *British Journal of Medical Psychology, 72,* 567-576

Tribe, R., & De Silva, P. (1999). Psychological intervention with displace widows in Sri Lanka. *International Review of Psychiatry, 11,* 184-190.

Trickett, E. (1984). Toward a distinctive community psychology: An ecological metaphor for the conduct of community research and the nature of training. *American Journal of Community Psychology, 12,* 264-279.

Trickett, E., Kelly, J., & Vincent, T. (1985). The spirit of ecological inquiry in community research. In E. Susskind & D. Klein (Eds.), *Community research: Methods, paradigms, and applications* (pp. 283-333). New York: Praeger.

United Nations High Commissioner for Refugees (UNHCR). (1951). Article I, UN Convention relating to the status of refugees. Retrieved on July 28, 2003 from http://www.unhcr.ch/cgi-bin/texis/vtx/basics.

United Nations High Commissioner for Refugees (UNHCR). (2002). *The state of the world's refugees.* Oxford, England: Oxford University Press.

US Committee for Refugees. (2002). *World refugee survey.* Washington, DC.: IRSA.

van de Put, W., & Eisenbruch, M. (2002). The Cambodian experience. In J. de Jong (Ed.), *Trauma, war, and violence: Public mental health in socio-cultural context* (pp. 93-156). New York: Kluwer Academic/Plenum Publishers.

Von Buchwald, U. (1998). Refugee dependency: Origins and consequences. In A. Marsella, T. Bornemann, S. Ekblad, & J. Orley (Eds.), *Amidst pain and peril: The mental health and well-being of the world's refugees* (pp. 229-238). Washington, DC: American Psychological Association.

Walter, J. (2001). Refugees and domestic violence: Model-building as a prelude to services research. *Journal of Social Work Research and Evaluation, 2,* 237-249.

Weine, S., Vojvoda, D., Becker, D., McGlashan, T., Hodzic, E., Laub, D., Hyman, L., Sawyer, M., & Lazrove, S. (1998). PTSD symptoms in Bosnian refugees 1 year after resettlement in the United States. *American Journal of Psychiatry, 155,* 562-564.

Wessells, M. G., & Monteiro, C. (2001). Psychosocial interventions and post-war reconstruction in Angola: Interweaving Western and traditional approaches. In D. Christie, R. V. Wagner, & D. Winter (Eds.), *Peace, conflict, and violence: Peace psychology for the 21st century* (pp. 262-275). Upper Saddle River, NJ: Prentice-Hall.

Wilson, J., Friedman, M., & Lindy, J. (2001). A holistic, organismic approach to healing trauma and PTSD. In J. Wilson, M. Friedman, & J. Lindy (Eds.), *Treating psychological trauma and PTSD* (pp. 22-56). New York: Guilford Press.

Zahir, G., Kakar, K., & Miller, K. (2001, June). *Psychosocial challenges facing Afghan women refugees in the United States.* Presented as part of a symposium on "Qualitative Approaches to Researching Refugee Communities" (K. Miller, Chair), at the biennial meeting of the Society for Community Research and Action (Division 27 of the American Psychological Association), Atlanta, Georgia.

PART I

PROGRAMS IN AFRICA AND ASIA

2

Internally Displaced Angolans: A Child-Focused, Community-Based Intervention

Michael Wessells and Carlinda Monteiro

Approximately half of the world's displaced people are children, defined under international law as individuals younger than 18 years of age. In Angola, large numbers of children have been displaced and affected in other ways by 40 years of armed conflict. This chapter outlines the Angolan context and its implications for children's emotional, social, and spiritual well-being. Arguing that intervention approaches focused on mental health and trauma are too narrow, culturally biased, and impractical in Angola, it describes a five-province, community-based intervention program by Christian Children's Fund (CCF) that aimed to stabilize communities, restore a sense of normalcy, and enable healthy development amidst difficult circumstances. It suggests that effective psychosocial interventions should focus less on clinical approaches, emphasize holistic well-being, and mobilize communities in ways that build tolerance, respect for local culture, and hope.

BACKGROUND

Sociopolitical Context

The Angolan war has occurred in multiple stages (Minter, 1994), the first of which (1961–1975) was a struggle for independence from colonial Portugal. Second was ∴ post-independence fight (1975–1991) between the Angolan government (GOA), which then had a Marxist orientation and received support from the former Soviet Union and Cuba, and the opposition group, UNITA (the National Union for the Total Independence of Angola), which was backed by the United States and South Africa. The end of the Cold War lifted hopes for peace, and the first free elections occurred under the Bicesse Accords in 1991. Unfortunately, Jonas Savimbi, UNITA's leader, lost the election but refused to accept the results, plunging the country into war once again. In stage three of the war (1992–1994) some of the worst fighting occurred, and as a result, UNICEF estimated that nearly 1,000 people died per day during this period. The Lusaka Protocol, signed in 1994, achieved a ceasefire, but demilitarization did not occur, and UNITA retained control over particular regions of the country, making Angola effectively a country inside a country. Failures to implement fully the provisions of the Lusaka Protocol escalated tensions and led to mutual blaming on the part of the GOA and UNITA. As both sides became convinced that the conflict could be settled only through violence, fighting re-erupted in December of 1998, continuing until March of 2002.

The recent fighting has occurred mostly in rural areas and has consisted primarily of guerilla raids and hit-and-run tactics. Since the fighting has occurred in and around communities and is overlain on a base of already severe, chronic poverty, the impact on civilians has been enormous. By 2001, an estimated 3.8 million people—nearly one third of the Angolan population—were internally displaced, and large numbers of people had been affected by war. The toll on children has been particularly severe. The infant mortality rate in Angola is 195 per 1,000 births compared to a sub-Saharan average of 106. Thirty-five percent of Angolan children under the age of 5 show signs of malnutrition, and in some areas, nearly 1 in 3 children die before they have reached the age of 5 years. The war has shattered children's basic rights, including their right

to education, which is a gateway for the development of social, intellectual, and occupational competencies and life options. Fifty-eight percent
of the adult and youth population of 15 years and over is illiterate compared to a 41% regional average. Thirty-four percent of primary school
age children are in school compared to a regional average of 56%. In
1999, UNICEF described Angola as "the country whose children are at
the greatest risk of death, malnutrition, abuse and development failure."
Although hopes run high that the situation will improve following the
ceasefire signed on April 4, 2002, poverty and militarization remain
chronic problems, and the risks of continued struggles over precious resources, such as diamonds, remain strong (Dietrich, 2000).

Mental Health and Psychosocial Implications

For children, who comprise approximately half the population of Angola, the war has imposed heavy emotional and social burdens. Internally displaced children, for example, have suffered the loss of their
homes and the stable routines that provide a sense of security, support,
and continuity. Loss of home and farmland increases already severe
poverty, reduces social and economic status, and creates feelings of
hopelessness. Many children have lost parents or family members, and
experience profound grief, insecurity, and uncertainty about how their
needs will be met. Amidst the daily challenges of survival in Angola,
there may be little space for grieving and coming to terms with what has
happened. Traumatic distress is prevalent, as recent research indicates
70% to 90% rates of post-traumatic stress disorder among Angolan teenagers who have had extensive exposure to war (Eyber, 2002; McIntyre &
Ventura, in press).

When CCF began its work on behalf of war-affected children in 1995,
it used a trauma idiom and measured children's traumatic experiences
and symptoms. It soon became clear, however, that a trauma focus was
inadvisable in Angola. Trauma is a small part of a much wider array of
psychosocial impacts related to loss, displacement, orphaning, sexual
violence, poverty, landmines, and separation from parents (cf. Bracken &
Petty, 1998). Thousands of children, both boys and girls, have been
forced into soldiering, and they face profound difficulties such as stigma-

tization, fear of re-abduction, difficulties earning a living, and internalization of values associated with violence and military identity. Similarly, tens of thousands of child victims of landmines face issues of disfigurement, social isolation, stigma, and difficulties obtaining necessary medical treatment. At many levels, violence has become normalized, and two generations have grown up having war as a constant feature of daily life. Because these broad psychosocial problems extend well beyond trauma and other categories of mental illness, the documentation of trauma prevalence is not very helpful in establishing intervention priorities or methodology.

A related difficulty is that the trauma idiom focuses excessively on psychological sources of suffering, when much distress in a war zone relates to poverty and the inability to meet basic needs (Summerfield, 1999). In local idioms of distress, physical suffering—through the inability to feed or clothe oneself or one's family—is inextricably interwoven with emotional suffering associated with violence and loss (Eyber, 2002). Further, the mental illness idiom pathologizes people and focuses on deficits, when in fact, most children in war zones are remarkably resilient and function rather well. To portray them as damaged goods or as victims overlooks their capacities and their agency and labels them in ways that can become self-fulfilling prophecies. Furthermore, programs should not simply address needs and deficits—to be sustainable they should build on local resources and strengths. Rather than focusing on illness and deficits, programs can be built around local strengths, seeking to bolster and add to the supports that already exist for children's resilience.

Trauma counseling is not an appropriate option for psychosocial intervention in Angola, as it has no basis in Angolan culture and is unsustainable. Particularly in rural areas, people do not naturally talk out their problems, and, as explained shortly, they do not interpret their difficulties at the individual level. In addition, Angola has only a handful of trained psychologists in a population of approximately 11 million people, most of whom are war-affected. Our assessment is that programs often focus on trauma because of the ease of measurement, the standardization of treatment methods, and the availability of funding. In addition, local people may seek the use of instruments and nomenclature that carry the imprimatur of Western science. Whether this approach should be the highest priority in a context saturated with broad psychosocial suffering, including poverty and the failure to meet basic needs, is questionable.

Local Beliefs and Practices

Culturally constructed meanings mediate one's response to potentially traumatic events, making it important to understand local beliefs and to avoid imposing preconceptions about trauma when working with culturally diverse populations (Eyber, 2002; Reynolds, 1996; Wessells, 1999). In addition, local people often cope with death and calamities by conducting rituals and ceremonies referred to collectively as "traditions" or "traditional practices." Contrary to what the name suggests, traditions are not fossilized, unchanging practices handed down directly from the ancestors, but are the product of the dynamic interaction between different cultures and ethnic groups within the various regions of Angola. For this reason, it is more accurate to refer to systems of local beliefs and practices, recognizing that variations exist in different parts of Angola. It is important not to romanticize local beliefs and practices, which, like all cultural practices, exhibit a mixture of strengths and weaknesses. The position taken in this chapter is that local beliefs and practices constitute potentially useful resources for psychosocial support. To avoid harm, however, it is essential to document these practices, assess their efficacy, and examine them critically with respect to issues of ethics and power.

A core belief in rural Angola is that when someone dies, the life of the person continues in the world of the ancestors, the spirit world. The ancestors' spirits protect the living community, which is an extension of the ancestral community. The ancestors must be honored through the teaching of traditions and the practice of appropriate rituals, such as burial rituals. Otherwise, the spirits will cause problems such as poor health, crop failure, social disruption, and even war. Life on earth and beyond are continuous and interdependent (Altuna, 1985; Tempels, 1965), and events in the visible world are attributed to events in the spirit world. Through the practice of traditions, local people achieve the harmony between the living and the ancestors that is needed for communal well-being. In this belief system, spirituality is at the center of life, and local people interpret events in terms of spiritual processes rather than the mechanistic accounts familiar to most Westerners. Furthermore, they understand their well-being or suffering not as individual factors, but as expressions of harmony or tension between the living community and the ancestral world.

When someone dies, the family members must conduct a funeral rite that typically includes washing, dressing, and perfuming the body of the deceased person; the placement of personal objects with the dead person to help meet his or her needs during the "journey" to the realm of the ancestors; the assembly of the entire, extended family to honor the dead person; and ceremonies involving eating, drinking, and dancing to honor the life of the dead person and to enable the dead person's spirit to make the transition to the spirit world. By conducting the funeral rite, the family and community "promote" the deceased to the realm of the ancestors, thereby establishing harmony with the spirit world. Without proper burial, it is believed that the dead person's spirit wanders around lost and disgraced and may wreak vengeance on the living. This problem is viewed as communal since the entire living community is placed at risk.

An elder in Huambo described the psychological consequences of his failure to conduct the burial rituals of a loved one:

> During the war my father was killed. I did not perform a burial because I thought that in times of war there is no need for that. But I dreamed with my father telling me that "I am dead but I haven't reached the place of the dead, you have to perform my *obito* [burial rites] because I can see the way to the place where other dead people are but I have no way to get there." (After this dream) I performed the ritual, and I have never dreamed of my father again. (Honwana, 1998, pp. 26–27)

Similarly, a boy soldier who has killed someone may exhibit trauma symptoms such as nightmares, flashbacks, and hypervigilance. Subjectively, however, the boy may view his biggest problem as one of being haunted by the unavenged spirit of a person he had killed (Honwana, 1998; Wessells, 1997). In the view of local people, the problem is one of spiritual contamination, and it is communal in nature. If a returning soldier who is haunted by an unavenged spirit returns to the village, the haunting spirit causes bad behavior, creating problems such as crime and killing in the community. The members of the living community are obligated to restore spiritual harmony by conducting an appropriate purification ritual (lead by a local healer or *kimbanda*) that avenges the spirits of those who had been killed.

Typically, the purification ritual entails the demarcation of a safe space into which the bad spirit cannot enter; the sacrifice of an animal and the offering of gifts to the bad spirit; the ritual washing of the person who is believed to be contaminated; and the inhalation of fumes of special herbs. At the end of the ceremony, the healer has the contaminated person—such as a former child soldier—step across the threshold of his hut and announces, for example, that the boy's life as a soldier has ended and he is rejoining the life of the village. Following such a ceremony, the belief is that it is inappropriate and dangerous to talk about what had happened, because talking could bring back the spirit that had caused the problem (Honwana, 1999). The conduct of the ceremony is significant for the recipient, who is then able to reenter his community without contaminating it. Equally important, the ritual reestablishes harmony between the living and the ancestral communities.

As both examples indicate, local people are affected by war, loss, and violence in ways that lie outside the boundaries of Western psychology. This situation creates an opportunity for learning about indigenous approaches to healing and for developing ways of interweaving Western and local approaches. In the project described next, which had initially been oriented toward trauma, a key piece of learning occurred when, in one of its early projects, CCF staff interviewed an 11-year-old girl who had lost her parents and home in an attack. She reported that her greatest stress was that she had had to run away before having completed the culturally appropriate burial ritual for her parents. In this case, the conduct of the traditional burial ritual was an important intervention although this kind of intervention approach is very different from Western, clinical approaches that focus on individuals and on grieving through emotional expression and support from loved ones.

Having learned from this and related cases, CCF began documenting local beliefs and practices related to bereavement, healing, and reconciliation. CCF learned that the best assistance for war-affected children came not from Western methods alone, but from the blending of Western and local approaches (Wessells & Monteiro, 2001). Furthermore, local people, who had learned from colonial domination to see their own culture as inferior, often began to regain their sense of cultural pride and self-esteem when their approaches to healing were respected and honored. Participation in the traditions conferred a sense of social meaning and continuity in difficult circumstances, thereby providing a form of familiar psychosocial support. Unfortunately, Western-trained psychologists often enter emergencies with little interest in learning about indigenous concepts of mental health and illness. As Western approaches are imposed, local approaches and voices are marginalized. In this situation, psychology becomes a tool of imperialism that cements Western power and control (Dawes, 1997; Wessells, 1999).

The following project took as its point of departure a holistic conception of children's well-being that interconnects physical, social, emotional, cognitive, and spiritual elements. It aimed to increase the well-being of children and adults in Angolan IDP camps and settlement areas, as these combined a high concentration of individuals in need with a paucity of available services. Because the intervention approach we describe is ecologically grounded, it focused not on trauma reduction, symptom measurement, and clinical intervention, but on social integration and community mobilization around meeting children's needs (Boothby, 1996). As used in this chapter, social integration includes engagement in socially meaningful activities, participation in age-appropriate peer interaction, and support of local networks that build social competencies and provide solidarity among community members.

INTERVENTION

The conceptual frame for the intervention is situated at the intersection of four intersecting theoretical frameworks: an ecological model of child development (Bronfenbrenner, 1979), a psychosocial well-being approach (Ahearn, 2000), an empowerment framework for community action and social change (Friere, 1970), and a systems theoretic perspective (e.g., Lederach, 1997; Wessells & Bretherton, 2000) that links healing, nonviolent conflict transformation, and social justice. These are complemented by use of a critical social perspective that challenges the pre-

sumed universality of Western ideas about mental health and the definition of childhood (Boyden & Mann, 2000). Although space limitations
preclude a detailed delimitation, an integrated, summary framework of
the conceptual model that guided our intervention is presented next.
Referred to as an "ecological systems framework," it emphasizes the systemic nature of violence and the importance of restoring community
processes of empowerment and support for children following the
shocks of war and displacement.

Theory and Rationale

Healthy child development occurs within nested systems of family,
community, and society (Bronfenbrenner, 1979; Dawes & Donald, 2000).
The family, including the extended family in the sub-Saharan context, is
the key microsystem within which children develop and where basic
protections and needs are provided. Outside the family, schools and
houses of religious activity provide the first encounter with social institutions and are important spheres of interaction between children, their
peers, and significant adults, such as teachers. At a wider, macrosystemic
level, children's socialization and development occur within social systems that include norms with respect to children's rights, rules of law,
forms of conflict resolution, cultural bereavement processes, and educational opportunities.

Armed conflict is best conceptualized as producing neither masses of
traumatized individuals nor a traumatized population (Bracken & Petty,
1998; Wessells, 1999). Rather, an ecological systems framework that emphasizes community stabilization, the reduction of risks, and the
strengthening of resilience is more appropriate for understanding and
developing interventions to address the repercussions of conflict. In particular, armed conflict provides an ecological shock or destabilization
that creates a culture of violence that damages child protection and supports at multiple, interacting levels. At the level of the macrosystem, internal war shatters societal peace and social trust, contests legitimacy of
institutions and government-defined laws, amplifies poverty and structural violence, and damages infrastructure and child supportive institutions such as schools and health clinics (Machel, 2001). It also establishes

a societal norm of violence, divides the population, and creates structural violence through denial of access to services to meet basic human needs. In Angola, key macrosytemic effects of chronic conflict are urbanization and erosion of traditional culture. As many people have fled to cities to escape fighting in the rural areas and in hopes of earning a living, their lives are shaped more by globalized, colonial culture than by the rural, traditional culture from their places of origin. Following several decades of fighting, many people have grown up viewing war as a constant feature of their social reality.

Community destabilization and disempowerment have been two major consequences of the war. Amidst mass displacement, family members may become separated from one another, and people may live in refugee or IDP camps and areas where they know few people, have relatively little social support, or may be intermixed with other ethnic groups that marginalize them and with whom they feel little affinity (Andrade, de Carvalho, & Cohen, 2001). War disrupts civic society groups—such as women's, church, and youth groups—that offer support for children. It also undermines familiar routines and social networks that provide a sense of continuity, support, and meaning to people's lives. Even when entire groups relocate together in the crisis of war, they may no longer function as a community. There may be no community meetings, little collective planning and action, disruption of leadership and organization, and a pervasive sense of uncertainty and hopelessness.

Life in settlement areas and camps is typically desperate, isolating, and boring (cf. Ager, 1999). In numerous war zones, the authors have talked with people who report feeling despondent, helpless, and apathetic in situations of displacement. Facing shortages of food, water, shelter, and other necessities, people often fend for themselves and their families, eroding further the communal fabric. Not infrequently, camps and settlement areas are difficult to reach or located in areas that are dangerous, and this isolates displaced people from outside services and supports. Even when basic needs are met, apathy and hopelessness may prevail. With normal social roles and activities suspended and with little opportunity for excitement and development, people often lose their sense of self-efficacy, sink into a pattern of listlessness and dependency on outside agencies, and focus on their losses and despair. In many camps, there is little to do, and children spend large amounts of time idling, thereby putting them at risk for engaging in a variety of destructive activities. In this sense, living in a camp or settlement area can be psychologically debilitating in itself.

Moreover, tension and fighting often occur at the community level. In rural Angola, destructive conflict often occurs when displaced people move into an area beside a relatively stable community, increasing pressure on local resources. Displaced people are often marginalized and denied access to basic services. Within settlement areas, fear and suspicions may arise as people who had been dominated by UNITA and isolated for decades now live beside people who had lived in government-controlled areas and who come from a different ethnic group.

Micro-systemically, war may produce extensive damage and loss of social and economic supports. Parents, family members, and friends may be killed or wounded. The authors' observations in diverse war zones indicates that parents, overwhelmed by their war experiences and current situation, may lapse into ineffective parenting or may be in a poor position to make good decisions about their children's well-being. Not infrequently, children spend large amounts of time without adult supervision or protection. Displacement may tear children away from friends and rob them of the support they had had from a favorite teacher or uncle. War amplifies poverty, increases economic stresses on families, and robs people of productive employment, farming, and social roles. Among displaced people in Angola, we have observed that overcrowding and lack of privacy is a significant source of stress and conflict within and between families.

As stresses accumulate, the risks of family violence increase (Wolfe, 1987). In war zones, the impact of family violence on children may be as severe as that of political violence (Garbarino & Kostelny, 1996). In addition, family violence, which relates to accumulated war stresses and unhealed trauma, can be intergenerational (Widom, 1989)—particularly in a situation in which harsh corporal punishment is normative and viewed as a necessary method for teaching obedience and respect. Detrimental effects of chronic and cumulative war-related stress on peer interactions also occur. Competing in desperate circumstances, older, larger children may use violence as a means of obtaining scarce resources, such as food, from younger children. Play, too, is affected. On streets throughout Angola, we have frequently observed children acting out fighting scenes like those they have witnessed.

In this context, a mental health focus is too narrow, individualistic, and deficits-focused to provide an appropriate point of entry for intervention work (Ahearn, 2000). A stronger approach is to focus on community mobilization and children's well-being, defined in a holistic manner that includes physical, cognitive, emotional, social, and spiritual elements. In particular, a high priority is to support children's resilience by empowering the community to strengthen basic care and supports for children (Boothby, 1996; Gibbs, 1997; Wessells & Monteiro, 2001). Often, engagement around meeting children's needs helps to reestablish a collective focus, build cooperation, and increase hope among community members. As communities take steps to care for their children, they regain the sense of control that traumatic experiences undermine, and this sense of self-reliance provides a platform for longer term development and movement beyond a crisis, reactive mode (Wessells & Monteiro, 2001).

To mobilize communities, it is important to work through local networks of influence and action that are pre-existing and sustainable. Rather than trying to mobilize everyone, a more strategic method is to identify and work through key community members who can function as leverage points for collective action and planning, and who can enable the systemic change that benefits children and strengthens communal and family patterns of nonviolence. Often, it is midlevel leaders who are in the most favorable position to effect social change (Lederach, 1997) and who, in this sense, can serve as key leverage points. At the community level, traditional leaders, councils of elders, groups of influential women, and church leaders are among those who represent key leverage points for helping to stimulate collective planning and action on behalf of children.

Focus of Intervention

The project, which was part of a much larger program focused on youth, used a community-based approach to support displaced people, who are among the most vulnerable in Angola. The project addressed five key

problems: community disruption and destabilization, material deprivation, weak supports for children in camps and settlement areas, destructive conflict between displaced groups and relatively stable communities, and inappropriate supports for orphans.

Community Disruption

To enable displaced groups to get back on their feet and function as
communities, the project sought to empower communities and to enable
collective planning and action on behalf of children. A key strategy was
to valorize and work through traditional leadership, which had been
marginalized during colonial rule, and to demonstrate respect for local
values and resources. Traditional leadership was valorized by holding
initial meetings with the traditional chief (*soba*) and elders of the community. Respect for local values and resources was demonstrated
through meetings with traditional healers and discussions about local
beliefs in which CCF staff affirmed the value of local rituals of healing
and cleansing. This helped to build trust among community participants
and to strengthen the sense of shared cultural identity, which increases
solidarity and provides a foundation for collective meaning and confidence (Honwana, 1999; Volkan, 1997). Consultation with local chiefs and
elders opened the door for subsequent meetings with influential women,
parents, and teachers. These meetings raised awareness about children's
needs, and also began the process of collectively taking stock of how to
support children.

Material Deprivation

For displaced people, psychosocial stress is intimately connected
with material deprivation and living in circumstances of poverty and
destruction (Eyber, 2002). Making material improvements is a key step
toward community empowerment and well-being. In fact, local leaders
said it was difficult to act as a community since they had no appropriate
meeting place. Traditionally, rural Angolan communities meet in a *jango*,
a circular hut built with lodgepoles and a thatched roof, that serves as a
community center and a Court of Justice where local issues are discussed
and disputes heard. Meeting there is itself a way to honor tradition and

draw on the strength of the ancestors. Accordingly, CCF partnered in building the *jangoes,* with the communities supplying the labor and CCF providing the materials. CCF staff also supported the communities in planning regarding children and advising on the development of play spaces and supervision for children's activities. CCF facilitated the construction of community playgrounds for children, and in some areas, the construction of schools.

Weak Supports for Children

The war had pushed children's issues to the margins, and elders and parents showed low levels of awareness about the needs of vulnerable children, creating a need for sensitization about children's issues and means of supporting children. To end the idleness commonly observed in camps and help to restore a sense of normalcy and continuity for children, the project organized structured activities for girls and boys, with an emphasis on school-aged and adolescent children. Although Angolan children typically assist with household tasks and often try to contribute to household income, play is also a significant part of their development. Normalizing activities, which often consisted of traditional songs, dances, and games, were organized for children by Angolan adults who themselves knew and valued the activities. They also included activities such as drawing, which, like singing and dancing, enables emotional expression. The project emphasized social integration and group activities such as soccer and playing games. By building playgrounds, the project sought to enable play, which helps develop physical and social competencies and nourishes positive interactions between children and adults. In addition, because adolescents identified illiteracy as a significant problem, the project provided basic literacy courses for young people which were taught mostly by local teachers or former teachers.

Prevalence of Destructive Conflict

At various levels, conflict has become so normalized in Angola that a strong need exists for the creation of skills and opportunities for nonviolent conflict resolution. To help reduce normalized violence, structured play activities for children and sensitization dialogues with adults emphasized nonviolent methods of handling conflict. Where displaced groups lived near relatively stable communities, and tensions existed between them, the project attempted to reduce conflict by enabling cooperation between the groups—such as, by working together to build a shared playground for children. This approach embodied the psychological method of cooperation on superordinate goals as a means of reducing intergroup conflict (Sherif & Sherif, 1969).

Inappropriate Support for Orphans

Significant numbers of separated and orphaned children in Angola have been placed recently in orphanages and foster homes where crowding, understimulation, and other problems create an environment that does not meet children's needs well. Although few accurate data exist, there are repeated reports of mothers abandoning their children to orphanages in hopes that their children will be better fed. In collaboration with Save the Children/UK, CCF lobbied for child supportive policies, such as intensified efforts to reunite these children with their nuclear families, with the extended families that remain a powerful support network for children in Africa, or with selected foster families. CCF also sought to train orphanage staff on children's psychosocial needs and how to assist children through activities such as drawing, singing, informal education, and enabling a sense of individual identity and self-worth.

Implementation

The project was implemented from March of 1999 through December of 2001, before the achievement of the recent ceasefire. The main project sites were 15 IDP camps and informal settlement areas in Luanda and six war-affected provinces—Benguela, Bie, Huambo, Huila, Moxico, and Uige—where there were large numbers of displaced people. However, the war situation demanded considerable flexibility and willingness to respond to emergent needs. Guerilla attacks in rural areas drove large numbers of people into province capitals such as Kuito (capitol of Bie province) and Huambo (capitol of Huambo province), where there was a secure perimeter of approximately 50 kilometers. As the security of the situation permitted, work was extended to Kuito and Huambo. However, throughout the project, security remained a major concern and limited the placement of permanent staff in some of the highest need areas, such as Huambo.

A second challenge to project implementation concerned the diversity of the social structures and situations of displaced groups. In Kuito, many groups had fled together from the conflict-torn rural areas and retained in the camps and settlement areas some of the traditional leadership structures and sense of solidarity with their neighbors. In Luanda, however, the situation was quite different. Many individuals had fled on their own to Luanda, while others, who had begun their emigration to Luanda in a group, had become separated en route. As a result, the IDP camps and settlement areas in Luanda often included a mosaic of people from different regions and ethnic groups. Few community networks or local groups existed, and those that did exist were typically through the local churches (Robson, 2001). Many people did not know their neighbors well, and there was little sense of cultural solidarity. Desperation and competition between households for scarce resources increased the isolation. The net result was a weak social foundation for community-based work in Luanda.

To achieve scale and sustainability, the project used a dual strategy of mobile training and integration of psychosocial aspects into ongoing program activities. Because the project areas were unstable, geographically dispersed, and difficult to reach, CCF decided to work via a mobile team of two Angolan trainers who had extensive training skills and who were in a good position to bring forward the lessons learned from the previous psychosocial projects. These trainers made 1-week visits to each of 15 IDP camps and settlement areas to build positive community relations, provide training, and enable start-up activities for children. Subsequently, the trainers made regular follow-up visits, security permitting, to provide continuing support for the trainees, to help them consolidate their learning, and to advise them on how to handle problems that arose in implementation. With respect to training, the project used a layering strategy that provided multiple levels of expertise. The mobile trainers had been trained by a five-person Angolan national team (CCF staff), who had received extensive psychosocial training from international and regional consultants. The national team also provided regular support and advice directly to the mobile training team.

High costs and security concerns prohibited the establishment of local CCF teams in each camp to work with children. In addition, the program sought to build local capacities for assisting children. Already in the camps there were a variety of groups—such as local NGOs, international NGOs, church groups, and government agencies—that provided assistance such as food relief, emergency feeding, and health services. Too often, however, such humanitarian groups conduct their work in a manner that promotes dependency and does little to support children. CCF chose to train selected workers in local NGOs, churches, and agencies on children's psychosocial development, the impact of violence on children, and how to assist war-affected children. The trainees were selected through a process of consultation with the local groups and according to their motivation to advance children's emotional and social well-being. Practically, the emphasis was on enabling the local staff to integrate activities for children into their work or to conduct their work in a manner more supportive of children. For example, an agency that provided food might learn how to invite young people to participate in food distribution or to organize expressive or socially integrative games for children as the adults collected the food.

Assistance to IDPs

The implementation process began with a participatory situation assessment that used a funneling strategy. Initially, information was collected on a wide array of geographical areas in Angola, followed by progressive narrowing and focus on areas that had high concentrations of IDPs, high levels of need, and a paucity of psychosocial assistance available. At the grassroots level, the strategy was to use rapid assessments that avoided raising community expectations too high and linked talk with assistance, because groups in difficult circumstances lose faith in outsiders unless they see tangible benefits relatively quickly. Using key informant interviews and focus group discussions, the participatory assessment collected qualitative information about the local community, children's emotional and social situation, people's social networks, and key people and groups who supported children. Although not highly detailed, the assessments provided social maps of the most vulnerable groups, child supportive networks, and local actors in an optimal position to offer sustainable assistance. The latter were selected for subsequent training.

Once key people from local NGOs, churches, government agencies, and the IDP group itself were identified and recruited for participation in the project, project trainers conducted week-long training seminars for groups consisting of approximately 20 trainees. The seminar topics included children's healthy psychosocial development, the impact of war and displacement on children, traditional and Western means of healing and assisting children affected by violence, and nonviolent conflict resolution. The importance of treating people with respect was a central theme because displaced people are often treated in a disrespectful manner. Among the displaced, norms of respect have weakened.

The training seminars used a highly participatory methodology that included dramatizations; group reflections on the past, present, and future; and discussions about traditional healing and the importance of Angolan culture. Because most participants were illiterate, the training methodology employed visual aids and metaphors while avoiding abstract, written material. For example, to illustrate the devastating effects of war, the trainer gave each trainee a large sheet of paper and asked him or her to spend 2 minutes tearing it up, which most trainees did with considerable enthusiasm. Next, the trainer asked the trainees to spend 15 or 20 minutes putting the paper back together, an activity that elicited much frustration. Following the activity, trainees discussed how easy it is to destroy something that has unity and integrity and how difficult it is to rebuild following extensive destruction. Applying this metaphor to Angola, they appreciated the importance of the prevention of further community destruction and of moving beyond crisis and survival modes of operation.

A second example of the training methodology concerned the linkage of past, present, and future in regard to the impact of severe corporal punishment, which is practiced widely in Angola. Rather than lecture on the damage done by beating children, the trainer asked the trainees to close their eyes and think back to a time when they were small children, had done something deemed wrong, and were being punished by their parents. Next, the trainer asked the trainees to describe how they felt. Typically, they answered that they felt small, helpless, afraid, and upset. Using silence to create a space for reflection, the trainer sat quietly. Most often, one of the trainees broke the silence with an excited report reflecting an "aha" type of insight. One trainee, for example, exclaimed, "Oh my God, that's what I'm doing to my children now!" Such reports triggered discussions of how child-rearing practices get transmitted across generations. They also provided a platform for discussing how children's behavior could be managed without use of violence.

Following the seminars, the trainers made follow-up visits twice each month to provide support and advice on handling difficult situations. If, for example, a trainee reported that particular children were fighting, the trainer would help to identify a strategy for preventing and containing the fighting. Similarly, if an NGO worker said that he was unsure how to provide activities for very young children brought by their mother to a feeding center, then the trainer would advise on age-appropriate activities. Not infrequently, the trainers made suggestions regarding how to assist children who exhibited particular problems such as a high level of withdrawal.

The project trained 795 adults, 110 of whom were staff of national or inter-national NGOs. These staff subsequently worked to integrate their learning into their ongoing work and to provide normalizing activities for children. These activities were documented through trainee reports and descriptions, reports from adults in the area, and direct observation during follow-up visits by trainers. For example, an NGO worker, who provided therapeutic feeding for malnourished children, organized play activities for children who accompanied their mothers and sick siblings to the center. Similarly, adult trainees from the IDP group organized, on a volunteer basis, normalizing group activities such as soccer games. In a settlement area where there had been little to do, these games drew huge, animated crowds who cheered on the children. To facilitate emotional expression and reintegration, trainees also organized drawing and drama activities.

Initially, the trainees attempted to count the number of children who participated in the normalizing activities. However, this approach soon proved to be impractical since, amidst the boredom and previous lack of activity in the areas, the initiation of an activity typically brought out all

the area children in the camp who then took turns observing and participating. Because all the children in the targeted age groups participated,
the total number of participating children — which was over 17,000 — was
estimated on the basis of the total number of children in the relevant target groups in the camps. Although the quality of activities and adult–
child interactions could have been higher had there been fewer participants, one should not underestimate the importance of engaging large
numbers of children in play and normalizing activities under such difficult living conditions. In addition, in numerous camps, the project provided basic literacy courses to build life skills for youth and engaged 166
young men and 200 young women in these courses.

As part of the situation assessment, the trainers convened discussions with community leaders, teachers, youth group leaders, and others
to sensitize the local community to the situation and needs of children.
These discussions, coupled with those sparked by the training seminars,
generated ideas about community projects, such as the construction of a
playground, a school, or a *jango* that would benefit children. The mobile
team encouraged planning of these projects and negotiated a partnership
approach wherein the community donated the labor while CCF donated
materials and transportation. By its midpoint, the project had assisted
with more than 25 such community projects. Whenever possible, CCF
enabled dialogues and cooperative activities between displaced groups
and relatively stable communities, which typically had more resources
and often marginalized recently displaced people.

Assistance to Orphans

The mobile training team conducted training seminars for the staff
who worked in orphanages and centers where separated children lived
in groups under adult supervision. Training focused on children's psychosocial needs, such as the need for individual identity, which could be
supported by enabling children to have their own clothing and beds and
to decorate their own personal space. In addition, staff were encouraged
to facilitate and support the interaction of the children, many of whom
had little knowledge of the social world beyond the orphanage, with
community members outside. Staff also learned about how to implement
activities suited to the developmental needs of children in different age

groups. At its midterm, the project had trained 94 staff members of centers for orphaned children. Following the training, the mobile team made periodic visits to the staff to provide follow-up support.

CHALLENGES AND LESSONS LEARNED

This project brought forward numerous lessons that reflect the ecological systems framework and have implications for psychosocial assistance to refugees and displaced people in other settings. First, we found that the use of a mobile team enables provision of support in the broad, flexible manner demanded by a complex emergency. The team's mobility was a powerful asset, since displaced people were spread out geographically over a very wide area. During the project, some areas became too dangerous to access, while others opened and harbored large numbers of displaced people. As these changes occurred, the mobile team adapted accordingly, providing support in a timely manner where it was possible to do so, while avoiding the exposure of staff to excessive security risks.

Second, although stand-alone psychosocial programs can be useful, they are limited by their failure to meet the wider array of needs in a war zone. Understandably, hungry people often seek food before they seek emotional and social support. When psychologists arrive in a camp, they may be greeted by hundreds or thousands of people who eagerly seek food and who are puzzled and frustrated when none is provided. This project addressed this problem by training people from different NGOs that provide material assistance, thereby enabling the integration of psychosocial and material support. This approach also aided sustainability in the sense that the NGO staff who were trained had a long-term presence in camps and settlement areas and a long-term commitment to continuing the activities on behalf of children.

Third, the strengthening of cultural supports increased the efficacy of the project. The engagement of elders, the support for traditional planning processes conducted inside the *jango*, and the respect demonstrated for local culture helped to overcome the helplessness and despair associated with the colonially implanted sense of collective inferiority of local culture and people. Belief and pride in one's own culture can provide a sense of continuity and psychosocial support amidst rapid changes.

The fourth lesson is that emergency and long-term development work can be bridged effectively, thereby avoiding the gap between relief and development that sometimes marks humanitarian efforts. In this project, collective planning and action provided that bridge. Too often, displaced people are treated as victims or beneficiaries who cannot effectively control their own circumstances. In this project, displaced people learned to organize themselves and to restart the processes of collective planning and action that are the foundation of long-term development. By facilitating collective planning, the project helped to bring together groups of people who had been fragmented from each other and to build local linkages, strengthening the social foundation for following the peace agreement signed on April 4, 2002. As large numbers of Angolans resettle or return home, the need for attention to displaced people will remain strong. A central part of this work will be the support of collective planning and action, which is vital to Angola's long-term task of peace-building.

EVALUATION

The training seminars had numerous important effects, which were documented through the administration of pre- and posttests in the appropriate local language. Administered by trainers in one-on-one interviews to a random sample of trainees immediately before and following a week-long training seminar, these tests evaluated the scope and depth of knowledge of topics, such as emotional factors that contribute to children's healthy development and the benefits for children of conducting death ceremonies for the deceased. Trainees showed significant increases in their ability to identify important emotional factors—such as love, respect, communication, and attention—in children's healthy psychosocial development. In addition, training resulted in substantial increases in the ability to identify activities such as music, song, games, and traditional treatments that can help children affected by war. Significant increases also occurred in participants' awareness of the positive benefits to war-affected children of conducting culturally appropriate death ceremonies.

Further, trainees showed increased awareness of the value of apology, forgiveness, and listening as part of the nonviolent management of conflict. One trainee, who had watched children fight over a ball made of stockings (few commercially made balls are available in rural areas), reported:

> . . . children from my area used to fight a lot. I personally used to watch said conflicts prior to the seminar and never bothered myself. Now, after the seminar, I have started to recognize that children were practicing violence, and I resolved the problem very easily. I made another stocking-ball for them and they all now play without problems.

Overall, trainees showed as much learning about traditional methods as about Western methods that emphasized emotional expression. Trainees also reported that they had acquired through the seminars an increased awareness of and respect for local traditions, enhanced awareness of the needs of displaced children, and a better understanding of how to support displaced children.

Numerous challenges made it difficult to conduct a formal evaluation. First, as the numbers of displaced people increased and as word circulated that CCF was providing valuable support, demand for assistance from the mobile team increased, creating the difficult choice of whether to devote project resources to assistance or to evaluation. Conceptually, this is a false dichotomy, since the provision of quality assistance and careful documentation of what works should be complementary endeavors. Practically, however, there are limits on how much a training team can do. In light of the dire needs of displaced people in Angola, the team decided to enlarge the scope of its assistance rather than document fully the impact of its intervention. Second, the Angolan team lacks expertise in the use of qualitative methodologies of the kind that are best suited to documenting the psychosocial impact of this type of program. In the long run, CCF plans to address this situation by expanding the number of staff who work with displaced people and by providing evaluation training and support from members of its global Technical Assistance Group.

Nevertheless, the project has conducted ongoing monitoring of post-training activities, and it has also collected impact information through group discussions with trainees, parents, elders, and community people. In addition, the trainers have observed directly the various activities and behavior of participant children. Although triangulation methods have been used to some extent, the data are best regarded as primarily anecdotal and preliminary.

With regard to children, the project appears to have increased significantly the levels of social activity and integration of children in participant communities. The extensive participation in structured activities reduced the previously widespread idling and apathy that had placed children at risk of engaging in damaging activities such as crime. As children engaged in soccer and other group activities, they learned patterns of cooperation, communication, and nonviolent conflict management. Children who participated in the activities reported feeling more hopeful, supportive of each other, and less inclined to make trouble and disobey adults. Adults reported that through recreation on playgrounds, children fought less with each other and spent more time than they had previously spent in safe environments. Adults also reported that their relations with children had improved significantly through the positive interactions that had occurred on the playground.

The work with orphans increased the awareness of staff and policy leaders about the needs of orphans and the hazards of institutionalization. Staff reported having an increased sense of orphans' individuality and their needs for stimulation and interaction with the outside world. As additional waves of displacement occurred, there were increased pressures to institutionalize children rather than to reunite them with their extended families. Through dialogues with policy leaders, the CCF trainers increased awareness of the importance of family reintegration. Although few hard data are available, most child protection agencies believe that this work with policy leaders has slowed the pace of institutionalization of children.

In both small focus groups and larger, community discussions, adults consistently reported significant increases in their levels of awareness, organization, and empowerment. They reported that the dialogues about children increased their understanding of and attention to meeting children's needs. NGO workers commented that they, as a result of the training, had implemented activities that made their feeding and material assistance activities more participatory, interactive, and supportive of children. Elders among the displaced reported that the planning of the community projects had increased their social organization, reestablished patterns of planning and action, and made them more hopeful. As *jangoes* were constructed, the physical structures were seen as symbolic of the process of collective reconstruction and organization. Elders said that the respect shown for their traditional processes had helped to strengthen their collective identity and to rekindle their belief in their own ability to impact their circumstances. Through the facilitation of collective planning and action, previously fragmented groups became better organized and felt more empowered to govern themselves. Furthermore, many adults said that the construction of playgrounds and schools had made them feel, for the first time, important and equal to people in urban areas who had long enjoyed access to such facilities. The recreational and normalizing activities also helped to kindle a sense of community spirit and engagement. As the public spaces filled with activities, such as soccer games, people interacted more frequently with their neighbors and took pride in participating in group activities. These increased interactions are fundamental to the construction of social networks and the repair of civic society.

The project also had positive impacts in strengthening norms of nonviolence and respect. In Cambila, Uige, the mobile team brought together the leaders of adjacent displaced and relatively stable communities to broker cooperative planning of a shared playground. The leaders of both communities reported that this had been very useful in reducing the tensions that existed and improving intergroup relations. Many displaced people reported that the project had helped them to regain a sense of their own dignity since people from NGOs and other groups treated them with increased respect. In addition, discussions of mutual respect increased awareness that Angolans comprise one people despite the political divisions and ethnic differences. This sense of unity is vital for the tasks of nation building that lie ahead.

REFERENCES

Ager, A. (1999). Perspectives on the refugee experience. In A. Ager (Ed.), *Refugees: Perspectives on the experience of forced migration* (pp. 1-23). London: Pinter.

Ahearn, F. (2000). Psychosocial wellness: Methodological approaches to the study of refugees. In F. Ahearn (Ed.), *Psychosocial wellness of refugees* (pp. 3-23). New York: Berghahn.

Altuna, P. A. (1985). *Cultural tradicional banto*. Luanda: Secretariado Arquidiocesano de Pastoral.

Andrade, F., de Carvalho, P., & Cohen, G. (2001). A life of improvisation: Displaced people in Malanje and Benguela. In P. Robson (Ed.), *Communities and reconstruction in Angola* (pp. 120-161). Guelph, Canada: Development Workshop.

Boothby, N. (1996). Mobilizing communities to meet the psychosocial needs of children in war and refugee crises. In R. J. Apfel & B. Simon (Eds.), *Minefields in their hearts: The mental health of children in war and communal violence* (pp. 149-164). New Haven, CT: Yale University Press.

Boyden, J., & Mann, G. (2000, September). *Children's risk, resilience and coping in extreme situations*. Unpublished background paper for the Consultation on Children in Adversity, Oxford University, England.

Bracken, P., & Petty, C. (1998). *Rethinking the trauma of war*. London: Free Association.

Bronfenbrenner, U. (1979). *The ecology of human development*. Cambridge, MA: Harvard University Press.

Dawes, A. (1997, July). *Cultural imperialism in the treatment of children following political violence and war: A Southern African perspective*. Paper presented at the Fifth International Symposium on the Contributions of Psychology to Peace, Melbourne, Australia.

Dawes, A., & Donald, D. (2000). Improving children's chances: Developmental theory and effective interventions in community contexts. In D. Donald, A. Dawes, & J. Louw (Eds.), *Addressing childhood adversity* (pp. 1-25). Cape Town: David Philip.

Dietrich, C. (2000). Power struggles in the diamond fields. In J. Cilliers & C. Dietrich (Eds.), *Angola's war economy: The role of oil and diamonds* (pp.173-194). Pretoria: Institute for Security Studies.

Eyber, C. (2002). *Alleviating psychosocial suffering: An analysis of approaches to coping with war-related distress in Angola*. Unpublished doctoral dissertation. Edinburgh: Queen Margaret University College.

Freire, P. (1970). *Pedagogy of the oppressed*. New York: Seabury.

Garbarino, J., & Kostelny, K. (1996). The effects of political violence on Palestinian children's behavior problems: A risk accumulation model. *Child Development, 67,* 33-45.

Gibbs, S. (1997). Postwar social reconstruction in Mozambique: Reframing children's experiences of trauma and healing. In K. Kumar (Ed.), *Rebuilding wartorn societies: Critical areas for international assistance* (pp. 227-238). Boulder, CO: Lynne Rienner.

Honwana, A. (1998). *'Okusiakala ondalo yokalye': Let us light a new fire.* Luanda: Christian Children's Fund/Angola.

Honwana, A. (1999). Non-western concepts of mental health. In M. Loughry & A. Ager (Eds.), *The refugee experience* (Vol. 1, pp. 103-119). University of Oxford: Refugee Studies Programme.

Lederach, J. (1997). *Building peace: Sustainable reconciliation in divided societies.* Washington, DC: U.S. Institute of Peace.

Machel, G. (2001). *The impact of war on children.* Cape Town: David Philip.

McIntyre, T., & Ventura, M. (2003). Children of war: Psychosocial sequelae of war trauma in Angolan adolescents. In T. McIntyre & S. Krippner (Eds.), *The psychological impact of war trauma on civilians: An international perspective* (pp. 179-191). New York: Greenwood.

Minter, W. (1994). *Apartheid's contras: An inquiry into the roots of war in Angola and Mozambique.* London: Zed Books.

Reynolds, P. (1996). *Traditional healers and childhood in Zimbabwe.* Athens: University of Ohio Press.

Robson, P. (2001). Communities and community institutions in Luanda. In P. Robson (Ed.), *Communities and reconstruction in Angola* (pp. 166-181). Guelph: Development Workshop.

Sherif, M., & Sherif, C. W. (1969). *Social psychology.* New York: Harper & Row.

Summerfield, D. (1999). The nature of conflict and the implications for appropriate psychosocial responses. In M. Loughry & A. Ager (Eds.), *The refugee experience* (Vol. 1, pp. 28-56). University of Oxford: Refugee Studies Programme.

Tempels, P. (1965). *La philosophie bantoue* [Bantu philosophy]. Paris: Presence Africaine.

Volkan, V. (1997). *Bloodlines.* New York: Farrar, Straus & Giroux.

Wessells, M. (1997). Child soldiers. *Bulletin of the Atomic Scientists, 53*(6), 32-39.

Wessells, M. G. (1999). Culture, power, and community: Intercultural approaches to psychosocial assistance and healing. In K. Nader, N. Dubrow, & B. Stamm (Eds.), *Honoring differences: Cultural issues in the treatment of trauma and loss* (pp. 276-282). New York: Taylor & Francis.

Wessells, M. G., & Bretherton, D. (2000). Psychological reconciliation: National and international perspectives. *Australian Psychologist, 35*(2), 19.

Wessells, M. G., & Monteiro, C. (2001). Psychosocial interventions and post-war reconstruction in Angola: Interweaving Western and traditional approaches. In D. Christie, R. V. Wagner, & D. Winter (Eds.), *Peace, conflict, and violence: Peace psychology for the 21st century* (pp. 262-275). Upper Saddle River, NJ: Prentice-Hall.

Widom, C. (1989). Does violence beget violence? A critical examination of the literature. *Psychological Bulletin, 106,* 3-28.

Wolfe, D. (1987). Child abuse: Implications for child development and psychopathology. Newbury Park, CA: Sage.

3

Sierra Leonean Refugees in Guinea: Addressing the Mental Health Effects of Massive Community Violence

Jon Hubbard and Nancy Pearson

This chapter describes a psychosocial program for Sierra Leonean refugees living in camps in Guinea as it has developed over the past two and a half years. The goal of the project is two-fold: to provide a mental health intervention and to train refugees to become peer-counselors and mental health resources in their own communities. The program is, by design, a work in progress. It represents a collaboration between the Center for Victims of Torture staff and the Sierra Leonean refugee community with whom we work in Guinea. The program may best be viewed as the first step of a process that hopefully will have a lasting impact on the post-war recovery of Sierra Leone.

Since 1985, the Center for Victims of Torture (CVT) in Minneapolis, Minnesota, has been providing rehabilitation services to survivors of politically motivated torture. Aware that most torture survivors in the world are not seeking treatment in Western resettlement countries, but rather remain displaced in their homelands or in refugee camps of neighboring developing countries, the Center has been exploring ways to intervene with this vast and underserved population. In 1999, the U.S. State Department presented the Center with an opportunity to develop a program to address the mental health needs of refugees from Sierra Leone residing in refugee camps in Guinea. This opportunity seemed a good fit for the Center, as the majority of our clients were currently coming from Africa, and we had served a significant number of West African torture survivors during the 1990s.

BACKGROUND

To understand the problems this program was developed to address, it is important to describe briefly the sociopolitical context and conditions that have led nearly a half-million West Africans to seek refuge in Guinea and which continue to impact the lives of the people of Sierra Leone.

Sociopolitical Context

Sierra Leone, a country of approximately 4.5 million people, is comprised of fourteen ethnic groups following a variety of Islamic, Christian and animist traditions (Coomaraswamy, 2002). The country gained independence from Great Britain in 1961. Yet, despite rich mineral and human resources, the country began a process of decline, and "by 1990, 82 percent of the population lived below the poverty line, and Sierra Leone had one of the most skewed income distributions in the world" (World Bank Group, 2002, p. 1).

In his 1998 testimony to the U.S. House of Representatives Subcommittee on Africa, John Earnest Leigh, Sierra Leone's Ambassador to the United States, stated that the roots of the declining situation in Sierra Leone could be found in over three decades of political, social, and economic difficulties. These included "misrule, corruption, military coups, civil war, plunder, carnage, mayhem and the collapse of civil society," and resulted in continuing challenges for national restoration (Leigh, 1998).

The first influx of refugees from Sierra Leone into Guinea began in March of 1991 (Van Damme, 1999) as a result of attempts by the Revolutionary United Front (RUF), backed by Charles Taylor's National Patriotic Front for Liberia (NPFL), to overthrow the ruling party of Sierra Leone, the All People's Congress (APC) regime headed by Major General Joseph Momoh. Although the RUF's stated program was to fight for democracy and fair distribution of resources, they actually conducted systematic and brutal assaults on the civilian population, and used their control over the diamond-producing region to illegally sell diamonds, timber, and other resources to support the on-going conflict (Rice, 1999).

In 1992, the APC was overthrown in a popular military coup led by Captain Valentine Strasser who formed the National Provisional Ruling Council (NPRC) government. This regime was soon fraught with corruption, and when the RUF gained significant territory and was closing in on Freetown in 1995, the NPRC hired the Executive Outcomes (EO), a mercenary firm. The EO successfully pushed the RUF back to their base camps and restored security to most of Sierra Leone (Rice, 1999). Elections were held in 1996, with President Ahmad Tejan Kabbah and a 5-party Parliament elected to power. Subsequently, strides were made towards peace, and a Peace Agreement, known as the Abidjan Accord, was signed with the RUF later that same year (Leigh, 1998).

This was, however, a short-lived peace. In May of 1997, elements within the Sierra Leonean Army (SLA)—called the Armed Forces Revolutionary Council (AFRC)—overthrew the Kabbah government. The leader of the AFRC, Major Johnny Paul Koroma, invited Foday Sankoh, leader of the RUF, and other RUF officials into his government (Berman, 2000).

In June of 1997, the Revolutionary United Front (RUF) made a statement of apology to the nation saying:

> For the past six years or so, we have been living in an environment of hatred and divisiveness. We looked at our brothers and killed them in cold blood, we removed our sisters from their hiding places to undo their femininity, we slaughtered our mothers and butchered our fathers. It was really a gruesome experience which has left a terrible landmark in our history. . . . In the process of cleaning the system, however, we have wronged the great

majority of our countrymen. We have sinned both in the sight of our Sierra Leonean brothers and sisters, for all the terror and the mayhem we unleashed on you in our bid to make Sierra Leone a country that all Sierra Leoneans would be proud of. (RUF, 1997, paragraphs 1-2)

Despite public apologies, however, the AFRC/RUF regime proved to be as brutal as their fighting had been. The Economic Community of West African States (ECOWAS) mobilized in order to oust the AFRC/RUF regime. The ECOWAS Monitoring Group (ECOMOG), first established in 1990 to bring peace in Liberia, was mandated to intervene in Sierra Leone and re-installed President Kabbah in March of 1998, ten months after he had been deposed (Berman, 2000). This horrific period resulted in Sierra Leoneans fleeing into Guinea and Liberia, making up the largest refugee population in the region, with numbers fluctuating from 330,000 to 410,000 (United Nations General Assembly, 1998, March).

The AFRC/RUF forces regrouped once again and attacked Freetown in January of 1999. ECOMOG was able to reverse the takeover of Freetown, but only at great cost to human life and property.

In the month of January 1999 alone, over 4,000 children were abducted during the incursion of the RUF and the Armed Forces Revolutionary Council (AFRC) into Freetown. It is estimated that 60 percent of abducted children were girls, the vast majority of whom are reported to have been sexually abused. . . . Over 3 million Sierra Leoneans—two thirds of the total population— have been displaced by war within and outside their country, more than 60 percent of them children. . . . Many children are suffering from serious psychosocial trauma. (United Nations General Assembly, 1999, 54th Session, Paragraph 13)

Reports regarding the devastation to human life and resulting trauma from the war vary greatly. In 1999, the United Nations High Commissioner for Human Rights reported: "It is estimated that 4,000 people have been hospitalized with amputation wounds, 50 percent of them women. It is estimated that for every person hospitalized, four others suffered severe injuries but did not get hospital treatment. In January 1999, between 5,000 and 7,000 people were killed in Freetown alone" (United Nations General Assembly, 1999, October 1, paragraph 13).

Once again, ceasefire and peace negotiations were undertaken in Togo and eventually resulted in the signing of the Lomé Peace Agreement on July 7, 1999 (Berman, 2000). The Lomé Agreement included provisions for amnesty as well as the disarmament and demobilization of combatants, including child soldiers who were estimated at more than 10,000 among the three main fighting groups: the RUF, AFRC and the Civil Defense Force (CDF) (United Nations General Assembly, 1999, October 1, paragraph 131). However, the conflict resumed yet again in May of 2000 with RUF attacks, detention of UN peacekeepers, and eventually cross-border fighting into Guinea and Liberia. There was an extensive use of child combatants by all sides (RUF, AFRC/ex-SLA, and CDF) of the conflict during this period. At times the rebels controlled up to 70% of the territory, making movement in any direction extremely hazardous. This period culminated in another ceasefire agreement—the Abuja Agreement—which provided a monitoring role for the United Nations Observer Mission to Sierra Leone (UNAMSIL) (UNHCR Global Report 2000, 2001).

Armed border incursions from Sierra Leone into Guinea, during the period from August of 2000 to January of 2001, resulted in ongoing exposure of the refugee population to human rights abuses by rebel forces, as well as local and government forces within Guinea (OHCHR, 2001). Fear resulting from instability at the border and from within Guinea led to the voluntary repatriation of many refugees back to Sierra Leone. At the close of 2000, Guinea was still host to the second largest refugee population on the African continent, which included an estimated 309,100 Sierra Leoneans. In addition, there were 300,000 internally displaced persons (IDPs) within Sierra Leone, along with 40,900 refugees who had returned home (UNHCR Global Report 2000, 2001).

Currently, there are an estimated 95,000 refugees remaining in Guinea. The UNHCR has accounted for 90,000 refugee returnees and estimates that 70,000 individuals spontaneously returned to Sierra Leone without any assistance (OHCHR, 2002). Plans for continuing the repatriation process of the remaining refugees in Guinea and other countries in the region are in motion against the political backdrop of national elections in Sierra Leone having taken place on May 14, 2002. In addition, the process for the establishment of a truth and reconciliation commission (TRC) and the creation of an independent special court for jurisdiction over crimes against humanity, war crimes, and other serious violations of international humanitarian law are underway (OHCHR, 2001).

Mental Health and Psychosocial Implications

In the summer of 1999, at the request of the U.S. State Department, the Center for Victims of Torture conducted an assessment of the mental health needs of refugees living in the camps surrounding Guéckédou, Guinea. The State Department expressed concerns over reports of refugees being too traumatized to take advantage of services or programs being offered by international non-governmental organizations (NGOs), such as Handicapped International and the American Refugee Committee (ARC). Examples were given of people being too depressed to bring in their children to be fitted for prosthetics, to follow-through with medical treatments or to benefit from skills training.

The initial needs-assessment included discussions with NGOs already established and working in the camps, meetings with camp leaders to discuss the problems facing refugees, and spending time in the camps talking directly with people about their needs. NGO staff suggested that, while many refugees were benefiting from social and vocational training programs, a significant number were in need of specific mental health interventions to make use of existing programs. The incidence of mental health problems was never systematically assessed. However, it was clear, based on the observed and expressed needs of the refugees and the sheer number of people (approximately 400,000) in the camps at that time, that there would be a greater need for services than could possibly be addressed by our organization.

Psychological Trauma

Even for staff who work daily with survivors of torture, the scarred bodies and stories of the refugees on such a massive scale was overwhelming. The atrocities that have taken place in Sierra Leone are beyond comprehension (HRW, 2001; Reis, Amowitz, Lyons & Iacopino, 2002). The number of refugees who have suffered trauma is generally understood to be the entire population in varying degrees. As one person expressed to us, "For every person directly victimized, there were 30 others who witnessed the atrocity or were made to actually perpetrate it." Most refugees witnessed atrocities of some sort, including watching as their entire families was brutally executed, seeing dead bodies strewn about, or witnessing family members or friends being raped or mutilated. Direct victims include those who have had their limbs amputated; had the letters RUF or AFRC carved into their chests or arms; been burned, mutilated, raped repeatedly; held captive as sex slaves for groups of military men, or forced to do labor. The rebels abducted thousands of children, and those who were made into child combatants commonly were drugged, indoctrinated, and sometimes made to lead invasions and massacres of their own towns, and in some cases, against their own families. Girls as young as seven or eight were used as sex slaves. Other girls as young as eleven are now pregnant as a result of the massive rapes, or have given birth to babies they reject or for whom they are unable to care. Perhaps one of the most horrific forms of torture inflicted on victims was forced cannibalism.

Clearly, Sierra Leonean refugees have experienced massive trauma and loss, and their resultant suffering is evidenced by common expressions of sadness, flat affect, lethargy, anxiety and social withdrawal, as well as more severe mental health difficulties where symptoms have escalated to full-blown psychosis. Somatic symptoms such as headaches and body pains are common; however, with health care scarce and disease rampant, it is difficult to know whether somatic symptoms have a psychological or physical basis (de Jong, Mulhem, Ford, van der Kam, & Kleber, 2000).

Population of Focus

Due to the massive scope of the traumas experienced by Sierra Leonean refugees, interventions were designed to encompass the entire community. However, the primary focus of the intervention program described in this chapter is refugees whose experiences have resulted in significant mental health consequences that impair their ability to function in important daily activities. This project targets children and adults through community-wide, group, family and individual interventions.

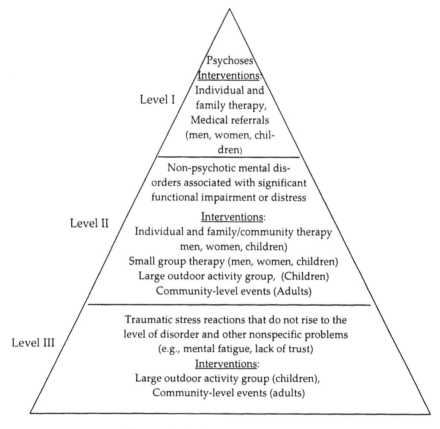

Figure 3.1: Levels of Impairment and Modes of Intervention

Figure 3.1 presents a summary of mental health problems experienced by Sierra Leonean refugees categorized in decreasing order of functional impairment. At each level is a list of interventions we offer to address each domain of problems. Level I of the pyramid represents those refugees with psychotic mental disorders or who present with symptoms requiring medication or hospitalization. We are not staffed to provide psychopharmacological treatment; however, medical referrals are made whenever possible. Other interventions we provide at this level include individual and family therapy designed to educate, support, and facilitate recovery, and community-wide psychoeducation about severe traumatic reactions.Refugees who fall into Level II of the pyramid represent the primary focus of the project described in this chapter. These refugees present with severe depression, anxiety, traumatic stress symptoms, or somatization, and they often exhibit significant decrements in social or occupational functioning or experience severe distress. Small group (10 to 12 individuals), individual, and/or family interventions are used at this level.

Level III of the pyramid, which represents those experiencing the least psychological and functional impairment, comprises the majority of the refugee population. Interventions we utilize at this level include large-group activities (sports and play) for children and community-level events (e.g., psychoeducational dramas or traditional ceremonies). These activities are primarily psychoeducational and/or incorporate traditional healing customs, and they are open to all refugees in the camp.

Specific numbers for each of these populations are not available and are difficult to determine. This is, in part, because self-identification of victims is oftentimes rare, especially in cases where the traumatic event carries a stigma and risk of rejection from the community—such as in the case of child combatants and those who were sexually assaulted (Reis et al., 2002). Others simply are ashamed of what happened to them and develop the coping mechanism of forgetting what happened, or lack adequate levels of trust to reveal their traumas. Part of the work with this population, then, is the development of trust and safety so that their needs can be addressed and they can begin psychological healing. Also, unless there is a compelling reason to provide treatment for a "special population" (such as sexually assaulted girls), we try to treat everyone within their larger peer groups. For example, we have found it useful to treat child ex-combatants among their adolescent peers. Singling them out for special attention only adds to their feelings of isolation and rejection from the larger community and reinforces their status as combatants. As our goal is to reintegrate them with their peers, families and the community, it has been useful to facilitate this process from the beginning. As issues surrounding their status as former soldiers arise, through the ex-combatants themselves or their peers, feelings are shared and processed in a safe and facilitated setting. This process provides the adolescents with a model for the reintegration work that will need to take place when these young men and women return to their villages in Sierra Leone.

INTERVENTION

Theory and Rationale

Our intervention model may best be described as flowing from an ecological perspective—targeting the multiple levels of the individual, family, and the community with appropriate interventions. The ultimate hope is that the program will have a lasting impact on the larger Sierra Leonean society by leaving behind a cadre of individuals with intensive training on how to help individuals and communities recover from the traumas of war.

We knew from the outset that we did not have the staff or resources to meet the needs of all the people in the camps who could benefit from mental health services; therefore, our model became one of capacity building for the community. As such, the training of Psychosocial Agents (PSAs)—peer counselors from the refugee community—became the core component of our program. Should we be forced to leave suddenly, or when the day comes that funding for our program runs out, the PSAs will be the program's legacy.

It is important to note that, while it is likely that the entire Sierra Leonean population has experienced some degree of trauma, the Center does not believe that all, or even most refugees are traumatized to an extent that requires a mental health intervention to help them get on with their lives. The Center agrees with others who have voiced concern over pathologizing refugee populations and deeming everyone in need of 'treatment' (de Jong, 1999; Summerfield, 1998). In our experience, refugees tend to demonstrate remarkable resilience and most—given a supportive environment and an opportunity to be productive—will regain meaning and purpose and rebuild their lives. The Center adheres to the belief that if given a "good enough" environment, people tend to move in a direction of resilience. However, there are individual refugees with significant post-trauma mental health problems who are in need of assistance in regaining their capacity for resilience.[1] Even if this group represents only 5% to 10% of the refugee population around Gueckedou, this could include 20,000 to 40,000 people in need of mental health services. This is the portion of the population on which we are primarily focused, and for whom simply providing social opportunities or skills training is not enough. These are people who can benefit from therapeutic mental health interventions to support and regain life functioning.

In designing the Guinea Program, Center staff considered our own experience treating West African torture survivors in Minnesota, the literature on mental health interventions in refugee camps and for displaced persons (Cairns & Dawes, 1996; Kreitzer, 2002; McCallin, 1999; Swiss & Giller, 1993; and van der Veer, 2000) and discussions with colleagues working in the area. We built the program around several principals.

First, we believed that we needed to make a long-term commitment to the project. We knew from our own work with torture survivors that recovery from the kind of atrocities experienced by the people of Sierra Leone takes considerable time. However, there was no local capacity (e.g., treatment center or staff) to provide ongoing treatment. Refugees were seeking assistance from traditional healers; however, the scope and severity of the post-traumatic symptoms being exhibited appeared outside their treatment expertise. Therefore, to create the capacity within the refugee communities to provide much needed mental health services, we believed it would be necessary to maintain a permanent staff of expatriate mental health professionals working year round on the ground until there was enough *demonstrated* capacity among trained local staff to ensure that they could adequately run the program and provide the needed services. We did this because we had observed that the most predominantly used model for mental health interventions in similar situations was one in which professional expatriate staff (e.g., PhD or MD clinicians or trainers) provided relatively brief training (several weeks to a month)

---

[1] We do not know all the reasons why some refugees are more severely affected by trauma than others, but some risk factors may include previous trauma history, compromised development history, chronic trauma exposure, inadequate personal coping skills, and lack of adequate social supports.

to local staff, and then left the trained paraprofessionals to run the program. Unfortunately, when the professional staff returned after a period of months to check on the program, things were rarely operating as planned.

In addition, our intention was not simply to train Sierra Leonean counselors in a model of "Western" psychotherapy, but rather, to create a program that blended Western knowledge with local wisdom and understanding about trauma and recovery. As such, we would need to find creative ways to join with the community and facilitate their input and participation in all aspects the program from the initial needs assessment and training of staff to the development of the intervention and evaluation components of the program.

Finally, we knew that it would take considerable training and supervision to teach local staff the skills needed to become peer-counselors for their communities. In the West, we require aspiring counselors to pass significant educational and experiential requirements prior to being allowed to provide psychological interventions. However, in refugee camps of the developing world, there appears to be a belief (undoubtedly driven by scarce resources) that several weeks training and a manual is adequate preparation for treating people who have experienced massive trauma and have debilitating post-trauma symptoms. It was this concern that led us to include an intensive and long-term training program for the refugee staff as a central part of the program.

In the end, what was developed was a program to train a cadre of refugee peer-counselors built around a mental health intervention. To address the wide array of identified mental health needs, interventions range from individual casework to community-wide activities. However, for practical reasons (i.e., more need than we can provide individualized services for), a majority of the program's interventions are delivered through small group therapy—which has proven to be an ideal setting for training Psychosocial Agents. Occasionally, clients request or require individual therapy—for example, when they fear rejection from the community should their experiences become known. Family work is included as an adjunct to or in place of group work when appropriate, and Psychosocial Agents regularly visit the families of our clients to build social connections and make links between the work done in group therapy and the family environment. Psychoeducation and ceremonial events—such as cleansing ceremonies—are conducted at a community-wide level.

Implementation

Process

The therapeutic interventions, particularly small group therapy, provide the environment for training the Psychosocial Agents (PSAs) who, in turn, allow us to reach more refugees by expanding our program. When a significant number of PSAs are able to facilitate groups and activities on their own, we recruit and begin training additional staff (once or twice a year). In the end, the Psychosocial Agents are the most important outcome or 'product' of the program. We have currently trained about 80 Sierra Leoneans to be PSAs, with some of the original trainees now having almost three years experience. While there is no certainty as to how many PSAs will pursue counseling as a career when they leave our program, they all will be potential resources to their communities when they return home. While, in practice, the training components and therapeutic interventions are woven together, it is easier to describe them individually.

Recruitment and Training of Refugee Psychosocial Agents. The refugees we train become long-term employees with our program and counselors to their communities, and thus, recruiting the appropriate people is very important. We go to each camp where we plan to set up our program and post notices of job descriptions and requirements for PSAs. Requirements of applicants include a written resume with a cover letter stating their reasons for applying for this position and a description of the level of education completed, including a copy of the certificate of education if available. Applicants are selected on the basis of their resumes and then sit for an examination. The purpose of the examination—which utilizes a case study—is to get a sense of the applicant's ability to be empathic and flexible, and to assess their natural counseling skills. The written examinations are evaluated and rated independently by several staff who then jointly select the top candidates. These candidates are then asked to participate in small group discussions (of 5-6 people per group) during which staff observe their ability to interact, facilitate discussion, present ideas clearly, be respectful, listen to the ideas of others, and work constructively as a team. Each group of candidates is given the same question to be discussed, but the group determines the direction of the discussion. Observers rate candidates on their performance, and the final selection of PSAs is made based upon the results of both the written exam and the small group experience.

Psychosocial Agents are considered to be in training the entire time they work with the program. As they gain skills and take on new responsibilities, PSAs are promoted within the organization but they never "graduate" from the program. We have found "certificates of training," which are granted plentifully in the area, to be difficult to interpret and sometimes misleading. Unless you have direct knowledge of another program's curriculum and standards for participants, it is difficult to know what is implied by having "completed the training." Instead, PSAs who are leaving our program for any reason (e.g., returning to Sierra Leone or looking for a new job) are provided with individualized letters that describe the type of training they have received, their length of employment, their area of specialization (e.g., therapy groups for children), and the level of skill and knowledge they demonstrated through their work. We believe that this approach not only supplies more accurate information about what the PSAs learned in their time with us, but also, because it rewards those who master their training and can demonstrate their skills, it motivates learning in a way that simply awarding certificates does not.

Psychosocial Agents are brought together for their initial training (approximately two weeks) outside of the refugee camps where they have an opportunity to learn together and build group cohesion. The initial training is conducted jointly by the expatriate staff and the training and mental health staff from CVT in Minneapolis. Having staff from the Minnesota program participate brings a broader range of experience to the training, allows for an exchange of knowledge between CVT's U.S.-based and overseas professional staff, and keeps the programs connected as part of one organization. Forty PSAs were trained together when the program first began. As this group increased their skills and required less supervision from the expatriate staff, smaller groups of approximately 15 to 25 new PSAs have been added. The training consists of both experiential and didactic components covering a variety of basic counseling skills and psychoeducation on the effects of war trauma. Topics include basic listening and attending skills, interpreter skills (as Sierra Leonean refugees speak a variety of languages), effects of war trauma, and an introduction to assessment. In addition, time is spent during this initial training exploring with the PSAs their own trauma experiences, the impact of the ongoing conflict and displacement on their communities, and their cultural understandings of the effects of war. As the PSAs are part of the community we are serving, insights into their beliefs around trauma and healing are important to our program. Part of their ongoing responsibility will be to integrate what they are learning from us with their own knowledge and with the traditions and practices of the larger community in an effort to move the program forward.

Throughout the year, PSAs are brought together for additional trainings—lasting from 1 to 3 days—to build on previous skills and learn new skills as they become relevant. The idea behind having multiple trainings spread out over time is to minimize the potential of overwhelming the PSAs with more information than they can absorb at one time, and to allow the PSAs to practice and master basic skills before more advanced techniques are introduced.

The most important training, however, is the day-to-day modeling and the "on-the-job" instruction and supervision the PSAs receive from the professional staff. In the beginning, all the therapy, whether individual or small group, is conducted by the professional expatriate staff. However, PSAs participate in the therapy in a variety of roles. To begin, they participate much as clients would; however, they also act as interpreters between the professional staff and the clients. While English is the official language of Sierra Leone, many refugees are much more fluent in Sierra Leonean Krio or various local languages (e.g., Mende, Kissi, or Kono) than they are in English. As such, groups are generally conducted in English (the primary language of the expatriate staff) and then translated by the PSAs into one (or more) of the local languages. The PSAs continue acting as interpreters for an entire group cycle (approximately 10 to 12 weeks). In the next group cycle, PSAs work as cofacilitators, and finally, in their third cycle, those who have demonstrated the necessary skills, begin to lead their own groups under the guidance and supervision of the professional staff.

The on-going, intensive training of the PSAs during the group therapy sessions takes place during:

1. Pre-session orientation—prior to each session, PSAs meet with the professional staff person to discuss the goals and objectives of the therapy session (approximately 1 hour).

2. In-session modeling—during the session, professional staff model counseling and facilitation skills for the PSAs who observe the interactions of the group (approximately 2 hours).

3. Post-session de-briefing—following the session, the professional staff meet with the PSAs to discuss what happened during the session. An important aspect of the teaching role of the professional staff is to be transparent about their process, discussing what went well and what could have been done differently. This is also an important opportunity for professional staff to elicit valuable feedback from PSAs on the cultural appropriateness of the interventions. PSAs are asked to describe specific ways to make the material or interventions more culturally appropriate (approximately 1 hour).

In our estimation, the use of pre-session orientation, in-session modeling, and post-session de-briefing, as contexts for training and supervision of the PSAs, is an extremely effective method for facilitating the development of counseling skills among local staff.

Professional staff also provide weekly group supervision for PSAs. They discuss general issues that have come up during counseling, discuss case studies, explore the PSAs' personal reactions (e.g., vicarious traumatization or re-traumatization) to what they have heard in their sessions, and address other issues they may be facing in their work or personal lives.

Types of Intervention

The majority of the therapy for adults or children takes place in small groups. Small group therapy is an important method in Western approaches to treating survivors of trauma with similar trauma histories. It is frequently used in Western countries because of its efficacy in treating diverse traumatized populations, such as African torture survivors (Smith, 1998), survivors of sexual abuse (Herman & Schatzow, 1987) and rape (Yassen & Glass, 1984), concentration camp survivors (Danieli, 1985), and war veterans (Parson, 1985). Small group therapy has been used as an effective intervention strategy for assisting young refugees to share their experiences with others, generate ways of affirming a sense of self, increase feelings of self-control, normalize traumatic experiences, and increase their trust in themselves and others (Victorian Foundation for Survivors of Torture, 1996). Also, before our arrival to the area, groups were being used in Guinea by Handicapped International and by the International Rescue Committee (IRC) to provide assistance and support to victims of amputation and rape in the Gueckedou area, and these agencies reported that group work was accepted by the community as a way to come together to solve problems and receive services. Community and group interventions are recommended as the treatment of choice for African populations and other cultures that are collectivist in orientation (Chester, 1992; Drees, 2000; Wessells, 1999). However, a wide variety of clinical situations can necessitate individualized or family-based intervention. These include a reluctance or refusal to participate in groups due to issues of confidentiality (e.g., the presence of perpetrators in the camps, extreme anxiety about sharing histories of abuse with other group members, etc.), extreme withdrawal, and severe levels of psychological impairment that require an individual or family focus.

The primary intervention for children exhibiting psychological distress in response to trauma is to establish a safe and predictable environment, and to allow them developmentally appropriate options for integrating their memories into a clear sense of a valued self in a hopeful universe (Ressler, 1993). In small-group therapy, children have the opportunity to form multiple supportive relationships with therapists, Psychosocial Agents, and other group members to do this work.

A major form of entertainment in Africa is sharing stories and talking about life. For our intervention groups, we have drawn upon the familiarity of group sharing to facilitate the discussion of current life challenges facing group members. Discussion topics may include experiences from the war that continue to bother group participants, recent losses, or experiences in the camps. Groups are often gender-specific or issue-specific, depending on the needs of individuals seeking treatment at any given time. Traditional approaches of helping are incorporated, such as the inclusion in the group of community leaders, elders, rituals, and friends.

Communities often have difficulty acknowledging the psychosocial impacts of atrocities, resulting in collective denial, increased isolation and alienation of community members, and community disintegration. The reversal of this collective denial is thus a crucial component of psychosocial rehabilitation for torture survivors (Fischman, 1998). Community-wide events provide opportunities for collective acknowledgement, elaboration, and validation of the trauma. This type of intervention is critical in addressing the collective or communal aspects of political trauma, and treatment models that have arisen from clinical experience in treating survivors of torture worldwide uniformly stress the importance of addressing trauma at the community level (e.g., Cienfuegos & Monelli, 1983; Fischman, 1998). Several times a year we have helped the community organize cleansing ceremonies. Cleansing ceremonies are beginning to be used with war victims or combatants in a number of post-conflict countries in contemporary Africa (e.g., Wessells, 1999).

What all these techniques have in common is that they involve people coming together in groups to share their experiences and strengths in an effort to process their traumatic experiences, reduce post-trauma suffering (e.g., psychological symptoms and grief), and rebuild social connections and support.

Examples of Techniques. Over time, through an interactive process with the refugee community, we have incorporated a variety of techniques into our programs. Some examples are:

ROLE PLAYS

Role play and dramatic representation are methods commonly used across cultures for telling stories, teaching, or expressing ideas, emotions, and opinions. Our program utilizes these techniques in a variety of ways. They are often used as a method for training Psychosocial Agents and for the professional staff to assess the level of Psychosocial Agents' skills. Role plays also make psychoeducational material meaningful in group activities with children and adults. Sometimes it is easier for clients to share their stories in the form of role plays than it is for them to tell their stories in a direct, verbal way. For example, adolescents who had participated in the therapeutic groups developed role plays which they presented to the wider refugee community. In these role plays, the youth acted out people coming to CVT's program with common war-related symptoms and problems and presented the process of receiving help in therapy. This process appeared to be an active way for the adolescents to translate and express to the larger community their own experiences with our therapeutic interventions. In doing so, they provided valuable psychoeducation—and a good advertisement for the program—helping the community understand what the program has to offer in a way that they could easily understand.

USE OF RITUAL

Adult therapy groups are opened with Christian and Muslim prayers (a common local practice for opening meetings) and frequently the room is blessed with a broom and water. This is followed by several songs. A calabash filled with water is placed in the center of the room and a kola nut—one for each group member—is placed in the calabash. These latter practices were developed by the members of our first intervention groups. As refugees from many different ethnic and religious backgrounds are represented in the therapy groups, it is not always clear that the practices have the same meaning to all participants. But many have expressed that the act of incorporating ritual into the groups makes them feel connected and comfortable and may be more important than the actual content of the ritual.

At times, group members have expressed the belief that some of their problems are related to not having preformed particular traditional ceremonies since arriving in the camps—for example, rituals of death or honoring or appeasing their ancestors. This has been noted by others working with refugees and displaced persons (Englund, 1998; Harrell-Bond & Wilson, 1990; Honwana, 1999). When this happens, our staff works with group members to organize the appropriate ritual or ceremony that will serve their expressed needs or purposes. Frequently, both professional staff and participants report a significant and positive shift in the group following the completion of the ritual. Members may be more relaxed, open, and ready to work together on finding new ways of relieving post-trauma problems.

Incorporating traditional and ceremonial techniques into the therapy process appears to make the intervention more culturally accessible to many in the community. We learned, however, that it is important not to make assumptions about the meaning or appropriateness of particular ceremonies across members of a group (or from one group to the next). For example, Sierra Leoneans represent a variety of spiritual or religious beliefs, and some of the Christian members of our groups expressed serious concern over the inclusion of traditional practices, such as appeasement of ancestors, since they considered these practices to be sacreligious. On the other hand, we have found that it *is* important to include some type of ceremony in the groups. To overcome this contradiction, we encourage group members to come up with their own ceremony — that may or may not be based in past tradition, but that holds meaning for them. For example, one group of men decided to celebrate the end of their 12 weeks of therapy by inviting family and community members to accompany them to the river with a boat one member had carved for the occasion. Each member placed something symbolic to him in the boat (e.g., a leaf, a seed or a note) with a wish for the future. After placing their wishes in the boat, they sent it off toward Sierra Leone while they sang and waved. While the ceremony had no previous meaning for the group members, it was an extremely moving experience for all who attended.

Similar adjustments are required when community-wide activities, such as cleansing ceremonies, are held. Cleansing ceremonies appear to be a common practice across West Africa; however, the specifics of the ceremonies vary from region to region, or even village to village. Most include a community meal and a ritual 'cleansing' of individuals who are seen as somehow contaminated by their experiences (e.g., child soldiers

or rape survivors). The cleansing ceremony brings the community together to acknowledge events that have taken place and to allow them to
move forward (Honwana, 1999; Leslie & Millard, 2000). At the same
time, individual trauma survivors, who may be suffering as much from
feeling "dirty" in the eyes of the community as they are from the trauma
itself, receive a sense of relief from these rituals. Our role has been to
bring together local traditional healers, spiritual leaders, camp leaders,
and group members to organize these ceremonies to serve the needs of
various refugee camp communities and to supply the resources needed
to carry them out.

USE OF SOCIAL SUPPORT

Included in the adult small group experience is the expectation that
group members will take the time to visit each other between sessions.
The incorporation of an expectation of social support relieves each individual member of the burden of having to specifically request visitors if
they feel the need for them, but also acknowledges, reinforces, and
draws upon the capacity of group members to give support to others in
the group who may be in need. The cycle of visiting among the women
of one group resulted in the development of a communal garden which
provided women who had previously been isolated from one another an
opportunity to build a social network, as well as a much needed method
of meeting family food needs. As individuals, they did not have the capacity or the resources to tend a garden; however, together they could
contribute the sufficient resources to till, plant, and harvest a communal
garden. Other "post-therapy" groups have included tie-dying and hair
dressing activities. These supportive group activities provide participants opportunities for reengaging in normal, daily endeavors—such as
meeting socioeconomic concerns—while maintaining and strengthening
new social connections.

CHALLENGES AND LESSONS LEARNED

One could easily devote an entire chapter to describing the challenges
and/or lessons learned in creating and implementing a program like this.
We learned quickly as we began setting up the program that everything

we did had to be seen as part of our intervention and as something that could either facilitate or undermine our efforts—often in unforeseen ways. For example, rather than setting up makeshift quarters in the camps, we started from the ground up. We wanted our program to become an integrated part of the camp communities we were serving. We enlisted community members to help clear the forest for children's play areas and soccer fields. In each camp, volunteers were organized to make over 10,000 mud blocks which were used to build three traditional buildings—a staff office and child and adult therapy buildings. Occasionally, the work would stop and the volunteers would threaten to strike if they were not paid for their time. Over many years in the camps, community members had become accustomed to being paid (with money or food) for participating in any activity organized by an NGO.[2] When the work on the buildings would stop, meetings would be held to discuss how this was going to be *their* community mental health center where members of the community who were suffering from the war could get help. We had frank discussions about how refugee camp life can breed dependence and the important role self-motivation would play in rebuilding after war. It was not an easy process, and it took much longer than expected; however, in the end, the construction of the buildings and the discussions surrounding them connected us with the community in ways we could have never predicted. By the time the site construction was completed, the refugees reported feeling that the program was their own and took great pride in what they had accomplished. In addition to therapy, the buildings' uses have included church services, community meetings, and funerals. The building process was an intervention in and of itself. On one day there were nearly 500 refugees working on buildings in the camps. People expressed satisfaction in the work they were doing and pride that they were creating a setting where their friends and family who were suffering could get the help they needed.

We also learned the importance of having a skilled, full-time professional staff on-site, not only to train and provide services, but to guide the program during times of crisis. One of the most fundamental chal-

---

[2]In one instance, adults who came together for a recreational inter-camp soccer game refused to play unless they were provided food and T-shirts. The game had been organized at the request of the refugees as a way to overcome boredom and enjoy themselves.

lenges facing this sort of intervention is the need to constantly adapt the program as conditions change—often quickly and quite unpredictably. During the 3 years we have been in Guinea, we have had to evacuate our staff numerous times due to rebel attacks and increased volatility in the region. In September of 2000, the town of Gueckedou was destroyed in a rebel attack that left as many as 300 Guineans and refugees dead. Our compound was destroyed. Following this, the UNHCR determined that the refugee camps were too close to the border and began relocating the entire refugee population to camps further into the interior of Guinea. We moved our operations inland to Kissidougou. Overnight the focus of our work had to shift from "recovery therapy" to managing escalating fears and situational distress as the refugee population was re-traumatized. Professional staff met with Psychosocial Agents and developed a plan to address the changing needs of the refugee community. As a consequence, the PSAs—utilizing the status and trust they had fostered working in their communities—began holding groups that allowed people to express their immediate fears, provided the community with information, and organized discussions around issues of repatriation as fearful refugees debated the merits of returning home (rather than move inland to new camps where they heard they would be surrounded by Guinean military and an increasingly hostile Guinean population).

Setting up new camps meant moving thousands of refugees to small Guinean villages that would never be the same. There were strong feelings on both sides—by the refugees who were being told where they had to live, and by the Guineans whose towns were being over-run with refugees. Our staff organized and facilitated meetings between the camp leaders and the Guinean villagers to discuss and share their feelings. As the discussions progressed, our staff observed a reduction in expressed distress and animosity from both the refugees and the Guineans, and participants reported that the dialogues were useful in helping them to understand the stresses and lack of control felt by both sides.

Times like these tested the expectation that the professional staff would continually adapt the program to the actual needs and circumstances encountered; however, their ability to make these adjustments has turned out to be a strength of the program. Without their constant involvement and oversight, the program would have folded at any of a number of junctures.

Another challenge was the recruitment of women in the process of finding "qualified" Psychosocial Agents. The majority of refugees are women and children, yet the method of seeking qualified PSAs placed women at a disadvantage to men as there were far fewer educational opportunities for women than men in Sierra Leone. Therefore, the initial application requirement of having to write, in English, a cover letter stating one's interest and intention for employment, as well as demonstrating educational attainment, prohibited women—who often have natural helping skills and interest, but no formal education—from applying. The written examination presented an additional hurdle for those women who did manage to make the initial selection. To address this issue, we applied affirmative action principles by selecting (without overly scrutinizing their education, spelling or grammar skills) women who were able to get their ideas and experiences across. For women, an emphasis was placed on the second phase of selection where candidates were required to participate in small groups. This provided women an opportunity to demonstrate their interpersonal skills. In addition, the small group interactions provided our staff a method for observing how the men interacted with women (e.g., did they listen to them, show them respect, and facilitate participation of all group members?). Having more women applicants in the small groups was an unforeseen benefit to the selection process, as it helped us identify male candidates who could demonstrate sensitivity and respect to women.

When fully staffed, our Guinea program employs five expatriate staff, including a country director and four mental health professionals. However, it has been a constant challenge, as well as an energy and resource consuming endeavor, to maintain a minimum of three professional staff to provide the training, teaching, modeling, and supervision of the Psychosocial Agents. It has been very difficult to find mental health professionals with sufficient expertise in trauma therapy, experience working with refugee populations, and adequate training skills who also have a desire to work under the difficult conditions presented by the refugee camps of West Africa. In addition to the lack of basic life amenities and danger of contracting tropical diseases, staff have to travel many hours on difficult roads in oppressive weather conditions to reach many of the camps. They must contend with unpredictable and, at times, unstable and dangerous political situations and constant demands to increase the number of small groups in order to reach more refugees. However, we have been able to attract a talented international staff from diverse cultural and linguistic backgrounds (e.g., African, European, Asian, and North American). Bringing together staff with different world-views and professional backgrounds has been an enriching experience for the individuals themselves and, in addition, has benefited the program by providing a unique impetus to continue to explore, clarify, artd develop new ideas and methods.

Challenges related to language and communication affect all groups involved in the program: the Sierra Leonean refugees, the PSAs working with their fellow refugees, as well as the professional staff working with the PSAs and their refugee clients. When the refugee population was moved from the region near Gueckedou to areas further inland, there was a greater mixing of populations from different linguistic backgrounds. At one point, after a small therapy group had been organized, the professional staff realized that there was no common language among the group participants. Interpretation was required in four separate languages for this group. This created so many complications—such as time needed for interpretation and lack of group cohesion—that the group needed to be reconfigured and the process started again.

Another challenge involved balancing our desire to create increased intervention capacity—by quickly passing on the needed skills to our trainees so that they could begin providing services—with the ability of the PSAs to absorb and master the material. Initially, we taught too much too fast. We discovered that our initial two-week training for PSAs covered far too much material and was too in-depth for the PSAs to comprehend and incorporate at the pace we had established. Exploring common ground and teaching new concepts and terms takes a great deal of time, as does modeling basic listening, attending, and communication skills. In addition, the PSAs have their own traumas and life experiences to address, and it is essential that time is allotted for processing this material to prepare them to deal with the problems and issues that their fellow refugees bring to them. We learned to focus the initial training on the most fundamental skills that the PSAs would be using first (e.g., interpreting, listening, and empathizing). The initial training now focuses on providing opportunities to master these basic skills before moving on to more advanced training.

Another continuing challenge is the severe dearth of referral resources for those with major mental disorders or psychotic symptoms
who require psychotropic medication to facilitate their recovery. As
stated earlier, our program in Guinea is not equipped with the personnel
or the medications to provide treatment and pharmacological interventions for individuals with psychotic disorders. This relatively small but
highly needy population remains significantly underserved.

EVALUATION

Methods

Organizations frequently find it difficult to assess the impact of mental
health interventions among refugee populations—particularly when the
interventions are conducted in refugee camp settings. The reasons for
this are numerous and include: cultural differences in symptom expression, the lack of measures validated for use with particular populations
(e.g., Sierra Leoneans) in particular contexts (e.g., a refugee camp in
Guinea), and the difficulty training local paraprofessionals to understand
the constructs being measured (e.g., "flashbacks" or "emotional numbing") and to conduct assessments and evaluations in standardized and
reliable ways. In addition, interventions often target large groups or
communities, making assessment of impact even more difficult. Given
the lack of appropriate assessment tools available, programs often resort
(for many practical reasons) to using translated measures that have been
developed and validated on very different (e.g., Western) and often
unique (e.g., Vietnam Veteran) populations. Very few programs have the
staff expertise, time, or resources to adapt existing measures, or to develop new measures, when they begin a mental health intervention in a
refugee camp. Developing and validating measures and training staff in
their use are time consuming and expensive (both monetarily and in staff
time) endeavors; therefore, the decision to "go with what is available" in
refugee mental health assessment is understandable. Particularly given
that the time and resources used to develop, test, and implement new
assessment and evaluation measures and procedures reduces the
amount of resources available for direct services to refugee populations.

Nonetheless, developing appropriate assessment measures and procedures is extremely important. Refugee mental health interventions are expensive. Not only do we need to know if we are having the impact we intend, but we need to identify the components of our interventions that are having the greatest impact on particular segments of our target populations. We have been attempting to do this in the program evaluation we have undertaken in our Guinea program.

We decided to approach assessment on two separate tracks: (1) using "traditional" indicators of posttraumatic psychological and psychosocial problems (i.e., to begin with what we had), and (2) developing new measures of functional adaptation and post-trauma problems based on the concerns and concepts of the refugees we are serving in the camps around Kissidougou, Guinea.

The Use of Traditional Assessment Measures

Adult and child assessment measures were created based on our experience assessing similar populations at our program in Minnesota, our review of assessments conducted by other refugee camp interventions, discussions with colleagues providing mental health services in West Africa, and our own observations of the difficulties experienced of the local refugee population. Intake measures cover basic demographics (e.g., age, gender, educational attainment), a brief trauma history (e.g., war experiences, losses, separations from family), indicators of social support (e.g., how many people can you go to for help?), the current problems that led to treatment-seeking, and a range of post-trauma symptoms.[3] To assess the post-trauma symptoms, clients were asked to rate the degree to which each symptom had affected them *during the past two week period* using the following 4-point scale: *Never, Rarely, Sometimes,* and *Often*. Clients were taught to use this scale using a diagram of

---

[3]Post-trauma symptoms include the 10 anxiety and 15 depression symptoms from the Hopkins Symptom Checklist 25 (Mollica, Wyshak, de Marneffe, Khuon, & Lavelle, 1987) and the 17 symptoms that comprise Posttraumatic Stress Disorder in the *DSM-IV* (American Psychiatric Association, 1994). West African clients seen at the Center for Victims of Torture in Minnesota report experiencing high rates of symptoms in these domains, so we believed that they should be useful constructs to assess in our program in Guinea. We also included seven somatic symptoms reported frequently during our "war problems" assessment (see next section).

glasses which ranged from empty to full. In addition, we assessed several client-specific problems (e.g., argues with spouse) which are quantified (e.g., twice a day) so that changes can be monitored over time. The assessments have been translated (from English) into four languages: Kissi, Mende, Kono, and the local Krio.[4]

All refugees seeking services from our programs receive an intake assessment. The information gathered in the assessment is used to prepare an appropriate intervention plan for the individual (e.g., individual therapy, group therapy or activity groups) as well as make necessary referrals for other needed services. Follow-up assessments are conducted, on average, at 1.5 months (mid-treatment), 4 months (1 month post-treatment) and at 6 months. The follow-up assessments repeat questions concerning presenting problems, social support, and post-trauma symptoms.

The Development of New Measures

During the setup phase of our program, we conducted a substantial number of brief interviews with refugees to gather information on their views of what constitutes positive adaptation and war-related problems for refugees in the camp. One hundred and sixty adults were asked to think of a man and a woman in the camp who were "doing well." They were then asked to describe the ways in which these people were doing well. One hundred and sixty parents were asked to provide similar information about adolescents and young boys and girls who were doing well. A second round of interviews used the same procedure, but asked the interviewees to think of people who had problems as a result of their war experiences, and then describe the kinds of problems these people had.

The information gathered in this process proved to be immediately useful in informing our staff about how the refugees themselves view positive adaptation and war related problems. For example, staff learned that in parents' descriptions of young boys, getting an education was the

---

[4]The translation process included translation and blind back-translation, as well as translator-back translator consensus of discrepancies. This was followed by group consensus from PSAs who were fluent in English and the second language and who were familiar with the psychological phenomena being measured by the items.

most important factor in judging who was "doing well." However, when describing boys in early adolescence, the emphasis shifted to how well boys were able to help provide for their families. For women to be considered "doing well," it is important for them to be obedient (according to both men's and women's responses). Many of our expatriate staff were dismayed by these findings; however, it was important information for them to understand as they began to intervene in the community.

We are trying to develop a brief and systematic method for sampling community ideas and beliefs that requires relatively little training and can be used by a staff with minimal research skills. While informative in its own right, the data gathered through these interviews has the potential for being used to create new assessment measures based on the constructs of adaptation and war problems that emerged from the responses. The resulting measures would be culture and context specific to the setting in which we are working and could be used along with, or in place of, our original assessment measures (those based on "traditional" Western constructs).

Through this process of creating new assessment measures, we are trying to address the frequently raised concern that measures created based on "outsider" or etic understandings of trauma may not assess adequately the post-trauma problems and/or healing processes of other cultural groups. In addition, allowing our target population to define "well-being" and "war problems" broadly and in their own way gives us a much more holistic picture of their needs and concerns. For example, the loss of jobs and financial or social status are sometimes listed as the greatest post-war problems experienced by refugees—even those who report other significant war-related atrocities. While our program is not designed to address these non-mental health related problems directly, understanding their importance to our clients allows our staff to acknowledge these losses as part of the treatment process (e.g., giving clients the opportunity to talk about material losses) and to make referrals to other programs that are prepared to offer assistance in these areas.

These new assessment measures will also allow us to conduct a more comprehensive program evaluation and to measure changes in refugee health, which we may not be capturing with our traditional Western-based measures. In the long run, it may be the creation of a *procedure for developing new measures* that is most important and useful to us and other organizations providing refugee mental health interventions. The measures we are developing will, after all, be specific to refugees from Sierra Leone living in a refugee camp in Guinea and may not necessarily be appropriate for Ethiopians in a Kenyan refugee camp. However, the *process* of measure development we are creating will be transportable to other settings where new measures based on the ideas and beliefs of those refugees can be created.

Results and Challenges

Developing the assessment component of the program was relatively easy compared to the challenge of obtaining the data needed to carry out the program evaluation. During the first year we collected intake assessments on nearly 1,700 refugees. However, we ended up with follow-up data on only a handful. The same challenges of constant and unpredictable change, that apply to the program in general, make ongoing assessment and data collection difficult, to say the least. When camps are suddenly closed and people move, it is difficult to locate individuals for follow-up assessments. Data is sometimes purposefully destroyed for the safety of the clients when our staff is forced to evacuate on short notice. Also, the constant barrage of situational stressors—like rumors of rebel attacks or "bad news from home"—make it difficult to interpret the symptom data we do get. Data on improved daily functioning would be useful, but with so few opportunities to demonstrate changed performance (e.g., few employment opportunities, long lines for other skill training programs), this is difficult to assess.

Because of these obstacles, it has remained a challenge to collect follow-up assessment data on our clients. Disruptions in activities and disbursement of clients due to rebel hostilities, relocation, and, more recently, repatriation movements have added to the usual difficulties of tracking displaced populations. However, from October of 2001 through the summer of 2002, relative stability allowed our staff to complete ongoing assessments and analyze the data from several cohorts of clients. We are pleased with the results, as it appears that the program is having the desired effect of decreasing post-trauma psychological distress and increasing social connectedness and support.

In general, clients endorsed a wide range of symptoms including high levels of anxiety, depression, and symptoms of posttraumatic stress. Not surprisingly, sadness and frequent crying were particularly common, as were symptoms of panic, sleep problems (including nightmares that are often related to trauma experiences), and avoidance of conversations or reminders of the atrocities that took place. Composites (mean) symptom scores were created by averaging symptom item scores (i.e., summing item scores: *Never* = 1 to *Often* = 4 and dividing by the number of symptoms in the domain) within each domain (somatic, anxiety, depression and PTSS). At intake, composite mean scores ranged from 2.3 for somatic symptoms to 2.9 for depression. It is important to note that these scales have not been normed or validated for use with Sierra Leoneans; however, as a point of reference, average scores >1.75 on the depression and anxiety scales (from the Hopkins Symptom Checklist) are considered to be clinically significant among Southeast Asian refugees (Mollica et al., 1987). We do not use these measures diagnostically but rather as a means of assessing change across time within symptom domains.

In this regard, *all* of the symptom composites showed statistically significant reductions between each successive assessment point. On average, symptom composites dropped nearly a half point between the intake and mid-treatment assessment (1.5 months), showed a similar drop between 1.5 months and 4 months, and dropped just under a quarter point between the 4 month and 6 month post-treatment assessments. Symptom changes of this magnitude across a population of clients are not only highly statistically significant, but more importantly, appear to represent meaningful reductions in distress. Symptoms were reduced by nearly half in those clients who were followed for the full six months. Depression and post-traumatic stress symptoms (PTSS) dropped slightly more than anxiety; however, given the ongoing stress of living in the camps and the uncertainty over repatriation, it is understandable that anxiety might be more resistant to treatment than symptoms of depression and PTSS—which may be more related to past traumatic experiences. Somatic symptoms decreased at about half the rate of the other symptoms. This too would be expected, as many of the somatic symptoms (e.g., headaches or stomachaches) are likely to be related to physical problems that were not addressed by our intervention. When individual symptoms were examined, changes occurred in ways we would expect. For example, symptoms like loneliness, feeling worthless, and helplessness—which are more amenable to psychotherapy—change more than physiologically based post-trauma symptoms, such as increased startle response or hypervigilance.

Measures of social support also indicated significant and meaningful changes in perceived connectedness for our clients. Across assessment periods, there were significant increases in the number of clients who reported feeling that they had people in the camps that they could turn to for help, and there were important increases in the average number of people that clients reported they could turn to for support (from less than 2.5 people at intake to more than 5 people at 6 months post-treatment). We were encouraged that clients continued to report decreased symptoms and increased social support after leaving treatment. We believe this indicates that they are continuing to use the skills they learned in therapy even after they leave the direct support of the group.

It is important to point out that, while we are encouraged by these assessment results, interpretation of them remains limited by the lack of an adequate control group. We are trying to address this in a variety of ways. We have been able to collect data on several additional cohorts of clients as they have moved through our program, and we are finding strikingly similar results (i.e., clients entering the program with similarly high symptom levels and reporting similar symptom reductions at mid- and post-treatment assessments). We are presently analyzing group attendance data to see if clients who are participating to a greater degree are experiencing increased benefits. In addition, we have begun collecting follow-up data on clients who receive intake assessments but who do not return to participate in groups as a comparison sample.

Although we are encouraged by our assessment results, like many clinical interventionists, we also rely heavily on anecdotal data to know if the program is working. Both the expatriate and local staff report numerous stories that suggest that the program is having its intended impact. For example, one of the authors sat in on a women's group shortly after the program began. The women went around the circle talking about their week and reporting about whom they had visited. One woman explained that several nights earlier, she and her husband had talked about witnessing the murder of their daughter several years earlier. She said they had not discussed this since they fled Freetown and came to the camps. She described how they talked and cried well into the night. She paused, and added, "I think I am sleeping better the last few nights." In another instance, an adolescent boy in the program was asked how things were going lately. He looked up from the picture he was drawing and said, "It's better now. Since my mother and father go to CVT, there is less fighting in our house." He then smiled and returned to his project. A woman who had completed a 12-week cycle of groups in our program was asked if she thought it had helped her. She responded, "I laugh now. And I cry. I had not done those things in a long time. I have hope." The "CVT has given me hope" response is one we hear a lot. We are sure it means a lot of different things to different clients, but it sounds positive.

CONCLUSION

This project has been a learning process for everyone involved. We have attempted to translate what we have learned treating torture survivors in the U.S. into something that fits the conditions of Sierra Leonean refugees in the Guinean camps. After 3 years on ground, and with several thousand clients having passed through the program, we are pleased with what has developed. We believed from the beginning that the best approach would be to develop a good starting plan and then send in a group of smart and devoted staff to figure out, in collaboration with the refugee community, how to make it work. The anecdotal feedback we receive from our refugee clients about changes they have experienced, the counseling skills demonstrated by our PSAs, and the program evaluation data we have collected all suggest that the program is working.

Ultimately, the most significant impact we will have will be through those we have trained. The PSAs will have the opportunity to keep alive and growing in their communities ideas about how individuals, families, and communities are affected by and can heal from war trauma and torture experiences. In Fall of 2000, Gueckedou was overrun by rebels, and we were forced to evacuate our professional expatriate staff. Six weeks later, when we were able to return to the camps, we were delighted to see that the PSAs were continuing to provide services to their communities. Therapy groups continued to meet; however, the PSAs had made a conscious decision to focus on problem-solving and psychoeducational material and to avoid the processing of past traumatic experiences in the absence of the supervision and support of expatriate staff. To us, this demonstrated their clinical insight into to the changing needs of their clients and communities and an awareness of their own current strengths and limitations as counselors. The PSAs played instrumental roles in keeping the community calm by providing accurate information about the UNHCR's unfolding plans for relocating them to new camps and organized group discussions to help people process decisions about remaining in Guinea or returning to Sierra Leone.

As noted at the beginning of this chapter, the program in Guinea was conceived as the first step in a long-term, post-war recovery process. In September of 2001, we began setting up services in the camps near Kenema, Sierra Leone, to address the mental health needs of repatriating refugees. Buildings were once again constructed and new PSAs were trained; however, this time segments of the training were led by PSAs from our program in Guinea who returned home to Sierra Leone to help us build the program there. In the spring of 2002, the repatriation camps in Sierra Leone were suddenly closed (or were repopulated with refugees fleeing Liberia), and the Sierra Leonean refugees began returning to their homes in the countryside. As they return home, they are facing new challenges. Many are finding their villages burned, their homes and possessions stolen and destroyed, and loved ones, who they hoped were alive, killed or missing. As the rebel-held areas of the country are opened up and people are allowed to return home to rebuild their communities, we have had to begin to transform our program, once again, in order to provide services in the villages and chiefdoms of Sierra Leone. PSAs continue to take on more responsibilities for the program, as it changes from a model for refugee camp based mental health services to one of community based mental health. If funding continues to be available, we hope to remain in Sierra Leone long enough to leave behind a viable self-sustaining local program of some kind. As PSAs rise to leadership roles in the program over the next several years, we will be able to get by with fewer and fewer expatriate staff and turn over more and more of the control and responsibility for the program to the local staff. How this actually unfolds will depend on a variety of presently unknown factors, such as the ongoing needs of the community, support from the Sierra Leonean government, the desire of PSAs to continue working as counselors, and the ability to develop ongoing funding sources for the program. There remains much to be done and more to learn, but it feels like we have begun to make inroads toward creating a sustainable mental health program for Sierra Leone.

REFERENCES

American Psychiatric Association (1994). *Diagnostic and statistical manual of mental disorders* (4th ed.). Washington, DC: American Psychiatric Association.

Berman, E. G. (2000, December). Re-Armament in Sierra Leone: One year after the Lomé Peace Agreement, *Small Arms Survey*, Occasional Paper No. 1 (p. 11). Retrieved from http://www.smallarmssurvey.org/OccasionalPapers. Html.

Cairns, E., & Dawes, A. (1996). Children: Ethnic and political violence—A commentary, *Child Development, 67*(1), 129-139.

Chester, B. (1992). Women and political torture: Work with refugee survivors in exile. In E. Cole, O. M. Espin, & E. D. Rothblum (Eds.), *Refugee women and their mental health: Shattered societies, shattered lives* (pp. 217-219). New York: Harrington Park Press.

Cienfuegos, A. J., & Monelli, C. (1983). The testimony of political repression as a therapeutic instrument. *American Journal of Orthopsychiatry, 53,* 43-51.

Coomaraswamy, R. (2002, February 11). Commission on Human Rights, 58th Session, Report of the Special Rapporteur on violence against women, its causes and consequences, *Mission to Sierra Leone,* 21-29 2001 (para. 21). UN Economic and Social Council Document: E/CN.4/2002/83/Add.2.

Danieli, Y. (1985). The treatment and prevention of long-term effects and intergenerational transmission of victimization: A lesson from Holocaust survivors and their children. In C. R. Figley (Ed.), *Trauma and its wake* (Vol. 1). New York: Brunner/Mazel.

de Jong, K. (1999). Uses and abuses of the concept of trauma: A response to Summerfield. In A. Ager & M. Loughry (Eds.), *The refugee experience: Psychosocial training module.* Retrieved from the Refugee Studies Centre, University of Oxford website: http://earlybird.qeh.ox.ac.uk/rfgexp/rsp_tre/student/natconf/toc.htm

de Jong, K., Mulhem, M., Ford, N., van der Kam, S., & Kleber, R. (2000). The trauma of war in Sierra Leone. *The Lancet, 355*, 2067-2068.

Drees, A. (2000). Intuitive dialogues in the field of victims of torture. *Torture, 10*(3), 77-80.

Englund, H. (1998). Death, trauma and ritual: Mozambican refugees in Malawi. *Social Science & Medicine, 46*(9), 1165-1174.

Fischman, Y. (1998). Metaclinical issues in the treatment of psychopolitical trauma. *American Journal of Orthopsychiatry, 68*, 27-38.

Harrell-Bond, B., & Wilson, K. (1990). Dealing with dying: Some anthropological reflections on the need for assistance by refugee relief programmes for bereavement and burial. *Journal of Refugee Studies, 3*(3), 228-243.

Herman, J., & Schatzow, E. (1987). Recovery and verification of memories of childhood sexual trauma. *Psychoanalytic Psychology, 4*, 1-14.

Honwana, A. (1999). Non-western concepts of mental health. In A. Ager & M. Loughry (Eds.), *The refugee experience: Psychosocial training module.* Retrieved from the Refugee Studies Centre, University of Oxford website http://earlybird.qeh.ox.ac.uk/rfgexp/rsp_tre/student/natconf/toc.htm

Human Rights Watch (2001). *Sierra Leone,* world reports, human rights developments. Retrieved from the Human Rights Watch website http://www.hrw.org/wr2k1/africa/sierraleone.html

Kreitzer, L. (2002). Liberian refugee women: A qualitative study of their participation in planning camp programmes. *International Social Work 45*(1), 45-58.

Leigh, J. (1998, June 11). Sierra Leone Ambassador to the United States, *Reconstructing Sierra Leone.* Testimony before the Subcommittee on Africa, Committee on International Relations, Rep. Edward R. Royce, California, Chairman, United States House of Representatives. Retrieved from http://www.sierra-leone.org

Leslie, H., & Millard, A. (2000, January). Rethinking trauma healing: Local practices in post-conflict reconstruction. *World confrontation now.* Retrieved from: http://www.worldconfrontationnow.com/archive/11/1trauma.htm

McCallin, M. (1999). Understanding the psychosocial needs of refugee children and adolescents. In A. Ager & M. Loughry (Eds.), *The refugee experience: Psychosocial training module.* Retrieved from the Refugee Studies Centre, University of Oxford website http://earlybird.qeh.ox.ac.uk/rfgexp/rsptre/student/natconf/toc.htm

Mollica, R., Wyshak, G., Marneffe, D., de Khuon, F., & Lavelle, J. (1987). Indochinese versions of the Hopkins Symptom Checklist-25: A screening instrument for the psychiatric care of refugees. *American Journal of Psychiatry, 144*, 497-500.

Office of the United Nations Commissioner on Human Rights (OHCHR) (2001, February 1). Fifty-eighth Session, *Situation of human rights in Sierra Leone* (pp. 4-8). UN Document: E/CN.4/2001/35.

Office of the United Nations Commissioner on Human Rights (OHCHR) (2002, February 18). Fifty-eighth Session, *Situation of human rights and fundamental freedoms in any part of the world, Situation of human rights in Sierra Leone* (para. 19-21). UN Document: E/CN.4/2002/37.

Parson, E. R. (1985). Post-traumatic accelerated cohesion: Its recognition and management in group treatment of Vietnam veterans. *Group, 9,* 10-23.

Reis, C., Amowitz, L., Lyons, K. H., & Iacopino, V. (2002). *War-related sexual violence in Sierra Leone: A population-based assessment, Physicians for human rights.* Retrieved from the Physician for Human Rights—USA website http://www.phrusa.org/research/sierra_leone/report.html#1

Ressler, E. M. (1993). *Children in war: A guide to the provision of services.* A study for UNICEF (pp. 113-140 & 165-208).

Revolutionary United Front's Apology to the Nation (1997, June 18). Delivered on SLBS. Retrieved on March 20, 2002 from http://www.sierra-leone.org/rufapology.html

Rice, S. (1999, March 23). Assistant Secretary for African Affairs, Testimony, (para. 1). House International Relations Committee, Subcommittee on Africa, Washington, DC. Retrieved from Sierra Leone Web on March 20, 2002 http://www.sierra-leone.org/usds032399.html

Smith, H. (1998, November). *Despair, resilience, and the meaning of family: Group therapy with exiled survivors of torture from Africa.* Symposium presentation at the 14th Annual Meeting of the International Society for Traumatic Stress Studies, Washington, DC.

Summerfield, D. (1998). The social experiences of war and some issues for the humanitarian field. In P. Bracken & C. Petty (Eds.), *Rethinking the trauma of war* (pp. 9-37). London: Free Association Books/Save the Children Fund.

Swiss, S., & Giller, J. (1993). Rape as a crime of war: A medical perspective. *Journal of the American Medical Association, 270*(5), 612-615. Retrieved from Physicians for Human Rights—USA, http://www.phrusa.org/research/health_effects/humrape.html

United Nations General Assembly (1999, March). Fifty-fourth session, *Report of the United Nations High Commission for Refugees,* Supplement No. 12 (A/54/12).

United Nations General Assembly (1999, October 1). *Promotion and protection of the rights of children,* Fifty-fourth session, Agenda item 112 (para. 131), United Nations Document: A/54/430.

United Nations General Assembly (1999). *Fifty-fourth session, Report of the UN High Commission for Human Rights,* Supplement No. 36 (para. 13) (A/54/36).

United Nations High Commissioner for Refugees Global Report 2000 (2001, July 1).

United Nations OCHA Integrated Regional Information Network (IRIN) (2002, May 8). *Sierra Leone: Refugee students get help*. Abidjan.

Van Damme, W. (1999). How Liberian and Sierra Leonean refugees settled in the forest region of Guinea. *Journal of Refugee Studies 12*(1), 36-53.

van der Veer, G. (2000). Empowerment of traumatized refugees: A developmental approach to prevention and treatment, *Torture, 10*(1), 8-11.

Victorian Foundation for Survivors of Torture (1996). *A guide to working with young people who are refugees: Strategies for providing individual counseling and group work*. Victoria, Australia: Victorian Foundation for Survivors of Torture.

World Bank Group (2002, March 27). *World Bank approves transitional support strategy and HIV/AIDS project for Sierra Leone*. New Release No. 2002/260/AFR, 27.

Wessells, M. (1999, August). *Child soldiers in Angola: Entry, reintegration, and traditional healing*. Symposium presentation at the 107th Annual Convention of the American Psychological Association, Boston, MA.

Yassen, J., & Glass, L. (1984). Sexual assault survivor groups. *Social Work, 37*, 252-257.

4

Internally Displaced Cambodians: Healing Trauma in Communities

Willem A. C. M. van de Put and Maurice Eisenbruch

Civil war and ruthless experiments in social engineering created terror for decades in Cambodia. During the most intense years of the conflict, a large portion of the population was uprooted and displaced, one in four Cambodians died, and when the worst of the conflict was over, 20 more years of low-intensity warfare followed. Amidst all of this, the international community expects Cambodians to rebuild their country. However, the psychological scars left by organized violence and abuse prevent many from participating in social processes, and the culture of Cambodia has to be reinvented for a globalizing world. Nevertheless, traditional ideas and healing methods still exist and remain relevant at the core of Cambodian communities. It is from these kernels of traditional culture that it is possible to design meaningful and effective interventions that can help people help themselves.

BACKGROUND

Sociopolitical Context

The history of Cambodia unfolds as a complex mixture of conflict and violence, picturesque peasant life and colorful ceremony, religious rhythm and international interference. Toward the end of the 1960s, external events such as the Vietnam war and internal power abuse drove the country into civil war. The subsequent rule of the infamous Khmer Rouge is described as being different in quality to anything before or after. It brought with it the "Cambodian holocaust," a total disruption of everything that had constituted normal life in Cambodia.

The Khmer Rouge attempted to completely remold Cambodian society and its institutions with a radical experiment in social engineering. Every aspect of daily life was disrupted. Monks were defrocked and forced to marry, cities emptied, and villages replaced. Ritual life was halted, Buddhism denied, and family life disrupted. Practically all families were forced to resettle. The first victims were the urban elite, the *new* people, who were seen as needing re-education to fit them into the pastoral ideal. Driven into the countryside, they were forced to share every aspect of life with the rural peasants, known as the *old* people, and were threatened with execution if they proved to have the wrong political affiliations. The rural population, for whom life seemed to change but little in the first months, was eventually forced to participate in work collectives, lost control of their homes and food production, and even had to give up sharing meals as a family when everyone was forced to eat collectively. There was very limited access to education and health care and no justice system, and any attempt to help one's neighbor was seen as betrayal to the system. People died of illness, malnourishment, and direct violence from leaders who felt helpless to change a situation in which heavily armed Khmer Rouge cadres threatened them. No escape from the grip of the *Angkar* (i.e., the Organization or the Khmer Rouge system) was possible.

In 1979, after 3 years, 8 months and 20 days of Khmer Rouge rule—all Cambodians can quote these figures by heart—Vietnamese troops overthrew the Khmer regime and the three-quarters of the population that survived found themselves scattered over the countryside—often far from their original homes or in refugee camps on the Thai side of the border. Vietnamese rule brought its own instability to Cambodia—with low intensity warfare continuing between Vietnamese troops and Khmer Rouge guerrillas even after a peace was brokered in 1991. In 1993, the United Nations intervened with a massive peacekeeping force to oversee elections, but armed factions continued to roam the countryside, and the coalition between former enemies arising from the election fell apart in July 1997. The UN mission did succeed, however, in repatriating some 1.5 million Cambodians who had spent up to 14 years in the Thai border camps. Pol Pot, leader of the Khmer Rouge, did not die until April 1998. His followers were finally militarily defeated and new elections were held that concentrated power in the hands of one party. A period of relative political calm has ensued and reforms in the public sector—covering macroeconomic and public finance management, civil service restructuring, and military demobilization—have gained momentum. State reforms laid the foundation for the first ever local commune elections in February 2002, confirming the power of the ruling Cambodian People's Party.

The Cambodian population of 11.5 million is currently growing at about 2.5% per year, and one third continues to live below the basic needs poverty line. Income inequalities continue to be much higher than in most other Asian countries. Women represent 53% of the active labor force and head 25% of Cambodian households. The high incidence of HIV/AIDS (169,000 cases reported in 2000; UNDP Global Human Development Report, 2001) poses a major threat to development.

Although the mental health problems of the hundreds of thousands of Cambodians who fled to other countries have been documented (Boehnlein, Kinsie, Ben, & Fleck, 1985; Eisenbruch, 1990a, 1990b; Eisenbruch & Handelman, 1989; Kinzie, Boehnlein, Leung, & Moore, 1990; Mollica, 1994; Mollica et al., 1990), less is known about how those who remained in Cambodia coped with psychosocial and mental health problems. A program to implement the community mental health approach of the Transcultural Psychosocial Organization (TPO; de Jong, 1997) in Cambodia began in 1995, with the aim of identification, prevention, and management of psychosocial problems. The program developed interventions to enable Cambodian people and communities to overcome the effects of traumatic events.

In this chapter we describe the community-oriented aspects of the TPO intervention—how psychosocial problems and coping strategies were identified and interventions designed to bring relief to the stress experienced at the community level. We begin by outlining the need for psychosocial intervention in Cambodia, and then discuss the concept of community in Cambodia and why we chose to take a community-based approach to intervention.

Mental Health and Psychosocial Implications

Assessing the Level of Dysfunction

Small communities in Cambodia have the kind of problems common to all developing countries. A fragile economic system, lack of job opportunities, and chronic poverty are the most obvious, and beneath these lie a score of related issues such as domestic violence, alcohol abuse, and poor health. Many of these difficulties are viewed simply as part of everyday life, and villagers know that only a dramatic and unlikely income increase would alleviate them. In a similar way, after the terrors of genocide and a long war, psychosocial dysfunction has been so much part of Cambodian life it has ceased to be thought of as a changeable condition. When the TPO project team—initially a small group of nurses, doctors, teachers and social workers—went into the villages to assess the level of psychosocial dysfunction, symptoms like sleep disruption with recurrent nightmares were so common they were not considered worth reporting. Families with more severe problems had, in many cases, lost all their possessions in their search for help. Approximately 20% of families in the villages assessed by the project team were considered to be dysfunctional by their fellow villagers, and this included anything from alcoholism to extreme poverty, from not being able to take care of children in the household to recurrent violence, abuse, or chronic disease.

Using the Cambodian Taxonomy

The team decided to use an indigenous taxonomy in order to obtain a better grasp of the problems as perceived by the Cambodian people themselves. Violations of moral codes proved to be an important category of problems for them. Examples of these included "madness of the dhamma" (*ckuət thoa*) stemming from wrong thinking about the Buddhist dhamma and "wrong healer" (*cku Bt khoh kruu*) where the culprit was a *kruu* who had violated his code (Eisenbruch, 1992). In a world so devastated by conflict, illnesses which Western health workers might call psychosomatic disorders or paranoid psychosis were seen by the Cambodians as caused by the interference of supernatural agents and known as "magical human intervention madness". In "sorcery madness" for example, it was the intention of the sorcerer to make the victim die a horrible death, and the patient's symptoms often suggested catastrophic physical injury, such as shattered bones or dangerous foreign bodies that hit the victim with the force of a missile.

Workers familiar with Cambodian refugees in the 1980s were accustomed to the complaint "thinking too much," sometimes called simply the Cambodian sickness, although it does in fact share similarities with a mental disorder described throughout Southeast Asia. Of all the types of mental disorders, this illness known in Khmer as "madness of the *sa?te? ?aaram*", seemed to be most closely linked to the stress, loss, and bereavement, as well as the social and economic deprivation and family disruption villagers had endured in relation to the war. All these factors were named as contributing causes to the slow destruction of the mind that "thinking too much" progressively entailed. There were terms for each stage of this illness. It began with demoralization, literally "small heart", *tooc cət,* and progressed to worries causing broken thoughts known as *khooc cət,* literally "broken down heart-mind". This then progressed to *lap,* a term implying mental distraction, and later to its more serious version *lap lap.* Further deterioration led to utter muddling and "lost and confused intellect or cognition." So common was this condition that anyone might have this mental state and not yet be counted as mentally ill (Eisenbruch, 1999).

Using the Western Taxonomy

Assessments using the indigenous taxonomy were backed up by appraisals using Western classifications of emotional disorders. In a sample of 610 randomly selected and interviewed Cambodians aged 15 to 65 years, lifetime prevalence of post-traumatic stress disorder (PTSD) was 28%, and 11.5% were found to suffer major depression. In 9% of the sample, PTSD and major depression were present together. Disorders were more common in people who were exposed to war events in the past or current family and community violence. Trauma-related stress, grief, and cognitive impairment were found to be important risk factors for psychological disorders. The prevalence of emotional disorders was higher in geographic areas that had witnessed more social upheaval due to war events, or that were undergoing social structural change at the time of the assessment. Forty percent of the sample met criteria for anxiety disorder (14.4% for men, 49.1% for women), and more than half of all people interviewed (53.4%) met criteria for anxiety disorder, PTSD, mood disorder, or somatoform disorder.

These rates of dysfunction meant that every household bore the scars of warfare, violence, and repression. It was striking to hear so many people say that the only hope they had left was not to be born a Cambodian in the next life. More worrying still was the fact that 14% of all respondents had actually attempted suicide in a country where it is generally believed that suicide engenders negative consequences for the following 500 lives.

Local Beliefs and Practices

Many mental health and psychosocial interventions focus on the individual. However, in designing the TPO program in Cambodia, earlier investigations, as well as our ethnographic experiences in Cambodia, led us to believe that a community-based approach would be most effective. Some of the assumptions for this approach had been verified in 1993 before the TPO program was launched. The first assumption was that traumatic events were experienced widely in the Cambodian population; the second assumption was that there was a need to understand something of the Cambodians' larger cosmology and taxonomy of suffering to truly understand the expression and effects of these experiences. For example, rather than assessing the psychosocial and mental health status of individuals by applying a Western nosology and assessment tools, we felt that an approach that encouraged Cambodian people to express themselves in terms that were meaningful to them, rather than us, would be more useful. We needed to know more about the way Cambodians expressed distress, and how they coped with their problems. As we interpreted the data from initial assessments, group discussions, and focus group interviews, we discovered that in addition to scarce resources (Cambodia had almost virtually no trained health staff or functioning health system) there were basic epistemological considerations urging us to go beyond an individual clinical approach. To truly comprehend what was keeping community members from coming to terms with their trauma-related experiences, we had to understand not only how they defined themselves as individuals, but how they functioned in their communities, and what exactly constituted a community. The latter point is now discussed.

Definitions of Community

Pre-Revolutionary Cambodia was 80% peasant, 80% Khmer, and 80% Buddhist. First, it was an overwhelmingly rural economy. Its village society was decentralized, its economy unintegrated, dominated by subsistence rice cultivation. Compared to Vietnam, its villagers participated much less in village-organized activities. They were often described as individualistic; the nuclear family was the social core. (Kiernan, 1996, p. 5)

In a nutshell, such was traditional Cambodian life. As such, for planning and development purposes, officials had always experienced difficulties finding a "unit of analysis" for community-based work in Cambodia.

On the administrative level, a Cambodian district is divided into *khum*, which in turn are subdivided into anything between 4 and 20 *phum*, most readily translated as *villages*. May Ebihara, an anthropologist who wrote about Cambodian rural life in the 1960s, described a *phum* as a social unit, or:

[an] . . . aggregate of known and trusted kinsmen, friends, and neighbors. Within the realm of social relationships, family and kinship were of great importance. There were several types of families to be found (nuclear families, stem families, and extended families). Apart from the family/household, there were no organized groups, whether formal associations, clubs, political parties, or the like. Neither were there major class strata within the community. (Ebihara, 1987, p. 19)

This lack of community integration had been noted also by Chandler (1993), writing about 19th-century Cambodia: "In . . . Cambodian villages . . . there were no durable functionally important groups or voluntary associations aside from the family and the Buddhist monastic order or Sangha" (Chandler, 1993, p. 104).

Due to forced relocation and other social changes brought about by the Khmer Rouge, the majority of families that lived in *phum* by the early 1990s would have been much more scattered only a few decades previously into small clusters or hamlets (*krom*) of 8 to 12 houses, inhabited by matrilineal relatives. Government decrees, warfare, and insecurity had occasionally forced people together, but many still carry a nostalgic and perhaps idealized notion of their original homeland as tiny hamlets separated from other such clusters of homes by patches of forest. They will point to a small mound in what is now a rice field and say that is where their family lived. When people were forced to combine for defense or festivals into larger groups, these units rarely endured beyond the specific need for which they came into being. *Krom* dwellers' relations with outsiders and with government authorities were sporadic and unfriendly. Quarrels were settled by conciliation rather than by law, and they often smoldered for years (Chandler, 1993). Given this history, it is not surprising that avoidance proved to be a common coping mechanism when trauma occurred and rural social organization traditionally has not encouraged community-based initiatives.

On top of these historic patterns of social fragmentation, the Pol Pot regime relocated the whole Cambodian population on a large scale. *Phum* were rebuilt on the orders of the Khmer Rouge cadres, only to be moved again when new cadres were appointed. People were forcibly relocated or fled from their homes and often had no means to return after the war was over. As a result, different types of *phum* have come into existence. In some, a number of kin have managed to stay together over time. They have experienced the hardships as a group and have some sense of belonging. Such *phum* typically consist of three or four clans, headed by the older men and may be called "old" *phum*. When reference is made to "new" people in such *phum*, these turn out to be the husbands who have moved in from other *phum* and other families, no matter how long ago. "Mixed" *phum* consist of a number of related families who can be seen as the core of the community and who have been joined over time by influxes of refugees from border camps unable to trace their original *phum* and others dislocated at various stages of the lengthy conflict. A third type of *phum* is the "new" *phum*. These were created either in the 1990s specifically for returnees, or earlier for families in need of new land, or as a result of government efforts at control. In these villages people may or may not be related and their capacity to create a sense of community and stabilize sufficient income for basic needs has varied considerably.

Against this recent historical backdrop of often extreme social disruption, it was obvious that even the political and economic security and emergence from isolation brought about in Cambodia in the 1990s would not repair the shattered cosmology that had defined traditional Cambodian peasant social relationships in terms of close family bound to small, well-defined geographical sites. When the TPO commenced its community health program, traditional views on life, moral conduct, relationships, and health had been threatened by events that shook the foundations of Cambodian society to its very core. Yet, at the same time, the memories of what had constituted traditional order and outlook were often all that was left, all that had kept Khmer identity alive amidst terror and social destruction. In order to understand the problems of Cambodian communities, it was necessary to know how things once had been, and whether traditional avenues of healing could be called upon to help rebuild Cambodian society. Therefore, the TPO team set about identifying potential community resources to help with healing.

Identifying Available Resources

Local Committees, Associations, and Helping Customs

The most respected villagers in any *phum* were members of the "pagoda committee," and together with the *achaa*, the ritual assistant of the monks, plus the head of one of the important families in the village, these men were important in the village associations that provided the blueprints for organizing mutual support. Examples of village associations and ways of working together included the "pots and pans group" (*samakum chaan chhnang*); the funeral association; the construction association; the rice bank groups, and the parent associations. The presence and functioning of these associations was closely related to the type of *phum*: The closer the relationships between the people who made up a community (as in the old *phum*), the greater the number and higher the level of functioning of these associations.

Another avenue for social support was provided by the Cambodian custom of reciprocal work, usually called *provas dai* (giving a helping hand). In addition, there were formal authority figures, such as the village chief (*mee-phum*), and members of various village committees, as well as informal leaders and respected community members who acted as patrons for others. All these local people had well-defined roles in traditional Cambodian society, and even though the social situation had been severely disrupted, they still enjoyed some authority, which gave them a capacity to help alleviate some of the villagers' psychosocial distress.

The Pagoda

Pagodas, the place where milestones in life are marked by appropriate ceremonies, have always been the center of religious life in Cambodia. They are found all over the countryside, usually located between villages. Several villages use the same pagoda and, in some sense, such a group of villages can be viewed as making up a community. The pagoda is a place of worship, education, meetings, and rituals. In the pagoda, one finds monks, novices, and sometimes nuns.

The importance of a pagoda for the community depends largely on the activities of the monks present, and these are not the same everywhere. There are many pagodas where the activities of monks may be strictly religious and there is hardly any activity outside the fortnightly prayers and the large annual ceremonies. A monk may restrict himself to explain to people the *toah*, the code of conduct according to the Buddhist principles. This may help people understand and accept their suffering. However, there are also pagodas where monks help people with social and health problems. Some of these are famous for their capacity to deal with specific problems, such as mental health problems (e.g., *Wat Andouk* in Battambang). And some monks have earned a reputation for initiating community development work (e.g., in Battambang, Svay Rieng, and Siem Reap). A prior ethnographic investigation (Eisenbruch, 1992) of traditional healers revealed their potential to contribute to the community healing approach that guided the TPO intervention, and this is now discussed.

Traditional Healers

During the early 1990s, Eisenbruch (1992) carried out an ethnographic study of several hundred traditional healers in Cambodia and identified three main groups:

1. *Mediums* had no formal training but acted as vehicles for healing forces. This group included those possessed with healing powers through healing spirits—which could be ancestral spirits or guardian spirits from the forest. These mediums were known as *kruu chool ruub*. Such "informal" healers, mainly women, had become healers after perhaps a single episode of possession, and from then on acted as mediums. Not only did they act as general psychosocial supports, they also helped to ameliorate the problems of patients afflicted by serious and acute psychiatric derangement such as "magical human intervention" and spirit possession. Mediums were often women who had gone through a particularly difficult period, such as an illness, and found that a spirit had come to help them as long as they, in turn, would help the spirit help others. The spirit that was the ac-

tual healing power and used the *kruu cool ruup* as a medium, thus
chose its own time in staying with the person it had chosen.

2. *Kruu Khmer*: These were the trained traditional healers. Whereas the
   spirit mediums had no training or defined codes of behavior, the
   traditional healers undertook years of formal study and followed a
   strict code. The *kruu Khmer* had been apprenticed and acquired formal knowledge of healing theory and ritual. There was at least one
   kruu in every village. The *kruu*, like the monks, were an integral part
   of the community and highly respected among most villagers. If
   monks and *kruu* carried out similar healing rituals, the monks were
   seen as spiritual healers, the *kruu* the medical ones. The *kruu* treated
   people who suffered from physical illness and mental disturbances;
   the latter included *çhkuet*, the vernacular term for serious behavioral
   disorders and insanity. The *kruu* also dealt with psychosocial problems. They carried out a range of work that included magical healing. *Kruu* worked in their homes, where they grew medicinal plants,
   saw their patients, and taught their disciples.

3. *Buddhist monks*, known as *preah sang*, and their ritual assistants, the
   achaa, worked largely from the pagoda. Most villages had their own
   Buddhist pagoda, the *wat*, a community place with moral, educational, and social functions. Although the pagoda was where the
   Buddhist monks did most of their work, in the 1990s some noteworthy monks broke out of the pagoda-based tradition to set up training
   and support elsewhere in the community. Behavior toward the
   monks was even more closely tied to rules of conduct than with the
   kruu. Monks could treat more patients at the same time, and a personal relationship between the monk and his patient depended entirely on the personality of the monk. The ritual assistants described
   and analyzed the technical details of healing rituals that the monks
   performed. Not constrained to the same extent as the monks, the assistants were sometimes a freer source of information about the
   magical aspects of Buddhist healing practiced in the pagoda.

In some villages there were exceptionally effective traditional healers.
Some based in Buddhist pagodas enjoyed nationwide fame. Some managed up to 10 or 15 inpatients at a time, and their outpatient clinics could
handle more than 100 patients per day. The healers did not claim they

could cure all serious psychiatric illnesses, but they believed they could ameliorate symptoms in a majority of cases. For the most part, patients did not pay more than they would have paid to visit the local hospital.

The Public Health System

When the 1995 TPO intervention in Cambodia began, public systems of care were weak in all respects. Ministries of women's affairs, social welfare and veterans affairs, culture and religion, and rural development had existed since the United Nations Transitional Authorities in Cambodia were installed in 1992. It would be beyond the focus of this chapter to give a detailed overview of the efforts in all these ministries to set up systems of care for the most vulnerable groups in society. What they all had in common, however, was a fundamental lack of means to effectively cater to the large size of the target groups.

When the Khmer Rouge seized power in 1975, the only existing mental hospital, *Takmou*, which had provided mainly custodial care, was closed, as were most other medical services. Few traditional healers and monks who had provided care for the mentally ill were allowed to continue (Eisenbruch, 1994). After the fall of the Khmer Rouge regime in 1979, public health care was modeled on that of Vietnam. This effort to introduce a nationwide system resulted in a situation in which too many staff had had too little training and were scattered too thinly throughout the country with neither the means nor the supervision needed to deliver effective care. Once again, the traditional healing sector, although affected by years of war and terror, was able to regain a central place in the options for health care after 1979. In 1995, at the time the project started, psychiatric care and mental hospitals were simply nonexistent.

Low salaries not only make it difficult for health workers to devote themselves fully to their public duties but also severely limit the impact of training efforts to bring about behavioral change. The efforts of the TPO project to help install basic mental health skills in integrated primary and secondary health care settings are described by Somasundaram, van de Put, Eisenbruch, and de Jong (1999) and the TPO project's attempts to develop community-based mental health interventions to complement traditional forms of healing are described in this chapter. There was simply no viable public health system in place to address the massive traumatization that had occurred and a community-based approach that incorporated, as well as complemented, the work of local healers and helpers was utilized by the TPO team.

INTERVENTION

Theory and Rationale

The TPO team drew on traditional Cambodian understandings of health and illness to design the intervention. Although traditional worldviews were severely shaken, Cambodians still had some framework of meaning that incorporated ancient explanations for illness and evil and attributed specific significance to birth and death. Behavior, and therefore health, was embedded in beliefs about natural and supernatural forces in the environment of the village itself and the surrounding fields and forests. The worldview of Cambodians stresses the continuous cycle of lives, the importance of b'aap bon (good karma) in reincarnation, and the reality of the impact of spirits and ancestors on the environment. The importance of conducting the right rituals for the dead and the need to restore disturbed relations with the spiritual world were always essential elements of coping with disrupting events in Cambodia, and there was evidence that these mechanisms were still playing a role in controlling distress. These practices could be tapped into and used as points of departure for a sustainable intervention designed address trauma at the community level. The respect and familiarity given to traditional healers in Khmer society, the continuing relevance of ancient explanatory belief systems and cosmology, the wide coverage offered by traditional healing options—even the most remote villager could access some type of healer—were obvious inducements to the team to take advantage of traditional sector resources in setting up their community program to ameliorate trauma or PTSD.

Another reason for focusing on a nonclinical approach to healing trauma-related distress, such as symptoms of PTSD, was that this type of suffering often does not produce the severe, incapacitating dysfunction of psychotic illness, and a mental health clinic was unlikely to be seen by the sufferers as an appropriate venue to seek help. It could be expected that many with PTSD manifesting through somatic complaints (Kirmayer, 1996) would seek help in the traditional sector. The team also knew that a PTSD diagnosis in the usual public health services was likely to be overlooked because of inadequate training and experience, as well as the possible role of transference as an obstruction in asking about trauma.

The challenge then became how to devise interventions at the community level that would *complement* and not corrupt existing avenues of coping with trauma. Traditional ways to deal with the effects of trauma at the community level are revealed in the following analyses of sorcery and infractions against ancestral spirits.

At the level of the village and community, individuals and groups inevitably come into conflict, and such conflicts are often given the label of "magical human intervention". This is the same phenomenon as what is commonly described as sorcery and is not unusual in Southeast Asia (Eisenbruch, 1999). Sorcery as an explanation for distress has not waned in Cambodia even with modernization, which brings in its wake complications in work, marriage, and sexual relations and induces its own forms of social strain. Referrals to traditional healers because of sorcery are as numerous as ever, and sorcery is understood as a key marker of social and domestic disharmony whose ritual treatment is geared specifically to restoring social harmony. In Cambodia, sorcery is understood to lead to the acute onset of bizarre and socially disruptive behavior in the victim, which traditional healers appear to be able to ameliorate. Cambodians may blame sorcery that they believe was instigated by human hands, as opposed to spirit intervention, for the breakdown of community relationships. Various types are distinguished on the basis of agent (nonhuman or human), mechanism (invading spirits, a spell, or projected foreign bodies) and physical effect (swelling, caused by disrupted body elements, or pain, caused by the effects of foreign objects).

One can see that traditional understandings of sorcery are used to explain fairly violent forms of community strain in Cambodia, such as the indiscriminate violence facing the society in the wake of war—two friends playing cards, or a married couple, suddenly in disagreement, and one shoots the other at point blank range with a B-40 rocket launcher. The other feature affecting the victims of sorcery—peculiar somatic symptoms—could be (mis)interpreted by psychiatrists as psychosomatic or somatoform disorders, but experienced by the patient and family as a sign of a community disorder. We had to train our core TPO staff to understand and work with these two points of view.

"Ancestral spirit disorder" is another example of a traditional affliction that reflects community disruption and is treated by community intervention. In Cambodia, ancestral spirits function as *regulators* of social conduct and, in their capacity as moral policemen, when they are not properly treated they withdraw protection and leave the descendant open to sorcery attack, initiated by the aggrieved family. In this way, the person's ancestors act in concert with the community (Eisenbruch, 1997). The spectrum of ancestral spirit disorders can be treated by a ritual sequence: The calendrical ritual offerings to the ancestral spirits— performed on behalf of the whole community in a ritual known as "erecting the pavilion"—can be seen as a "general vaccination" of the whole community. This ceremony, rather than curing an individual patient, helps everyone: The emphasis is on the periodic "vaccination" of the whole community. The local *kruu* and medium may collaborate to treat an individual patient and, at the same time, they inoculate the community against harm. Impoverished people, preoccupied with eking out an existence and avoiding landmines, can forget these ceremonies and the affliction might reflect their sense of moral negligence. Again, the TPO group needed to know how to link these types of local idioms of distress with their intervention to alleviate traumatic suffering.

Implementation

Developing Complimentary Interventions

The TPO intervention drew upon local explanatory models of distress and healing, as well as existing ethnographic data on the healing rituals of traditional healers, mediums, and monks. The explanatory models pointed the way to the right resources for help. Identifying these resources, and knowing what they did and how they could be approached, helped bridge the gap between a family in distress and community resources for healing. Knowledge about people's roles and social hierarchy informed us about how best to access various resources for helping. Also, knowledge about the various types of *phum* (i.e., old, new, or mixed) helped us plan what type of intervention approach would be most effective (e.g., in mixed and new *phum* age-old Cambodian community relations needed restoring).

The benefits of working with traditional healers were numerous. They were successful as counselors (e.g., the mediums), and in providing a productive link between the cosmological framework of meaning and the daily suffering of families (e.g., the *kruu* and the monks). But social change triggers a mismatch between the problems people face and the capacity of traditional healers to ameliorate them. A lesson learned in Cambodia was to experiment with the composition of the teams of *phum* volunteers used for psychosocial work. Outreach activities—from identifying families at risk to organizing group sessions and psychoeducation campaigns—needed to be carried out by individuals who had easy entry into homes—including those of the most marginalized. *Phum* volunteers were modest people, often widows who had been diagnosed as in need of help and who had been convinced of the profound difference that could be made by connecting distressed people to existing resources. The stumbling block was that such people lacked authority—and therefore, in Cambodia, lacked security. The solution lay in teaming them with monks or ritual assistants who provided the necessary authority, and this pairing of *phum* volunteers proved ideal for instigating community-based psychosocial work.

Nevertheless, with the passage of time, health beliefs were changing in Cambodia, as were patterns of help-seeking behavior. Traditional healers began to face competition from other sectors that offered help. Both their explanatory models and their livelihoods came under threat. They had families to maintain and, like other small-time entrepreneurs in a rapidly globalizing society, they faced economic annihilation and were forced to try and adapt. Those that were able changed along with their clients. Their taxonomy of disorders proved to be neither frozen nor fossilized. Their treatments could be extended to cover the new range of personal problems that modernization triggered. As the TPO project developed, we heard both from healers who felt at a loss trying to ease the contemporary emotional problems of their clients and from those adept at expressing their classifications and explanations in more contemporary idioms.

Despite the adaptive powers of some healers, it became clear that new interventions—complementary to the traditional healing system—also were needed to address psychosocial distress. The TPO team sought to find culturally appropriate solutions aimed at strengthening local resources to identify and manage psychosocial problems by:

1. Forming teams of villagers (chosen from those who had been trained and proved most effective in the pilot phase of the project) to provide psychoeducation and refer families for further help if necessary;
2. Offering training to local health workers and NGO staff by providing psychoeducational materials to build awareness of psychosocial and mental health problems;
3. Forming self-help groups, where women and men could find a "niche" in village life and a safe place talk about their emotions.

The following section describes various components of the intervention and discusses its effectiveness.

Training for Group Work

The TPO intervention aimed at enabling Cambodians themselves to identify and manage psychosocial problems through supportive, psychoeducational group work. On first entering a *phum*, the TPO team sought contact with the local authorities, respecting the existing local hierarchical order. The team explained the idea of psychosocial work as trying to address the problems of the "heart–mind" (*khooc cat*). In each village, people who were already in position to assist families in distress were then identified. These included teachers, village chiefs, monks, *achaas*, traditional healers, staff of government agencies, NGOs, the public health sector, and ordinary villagers. These core groups of individuals were offered psychoeducational training by the TPO team, and curricula were developed especially for the Cambodian situation and laid an emphasis on achieving realistic possibilities. A training manual was developed that guided this work, and it included sections on (and attempted to integrate ideas from) basic psychiatry and psychology, Cambodian idioms and taxonomies of distress, and the role of various traditional healers. Attempting to work across two vastly different cosmological systems of healing (Western versus Buddhist/Brahmanic/animistic)—not to mention the technical problems confronted in translating between English and Khmer—presented challenges that ultimately led to a greater understanding of potential points contention and overlap of between the two systems of healing.

Depending on the type of village entered, the initial intervention approach consisted of either psychoeducational training for anyone interested, individual case work aimed at strengthening local resources for help, or individual casework to build a basis for a group approach. Specifically, if a traditional, "old" *phum* with a majority of related people was encountered, it was easy to contact healers and other resources for help and to organize group sessions where the problems of the heart–mind could be discussed. Psychoeducational materials—posters, videotapes, and presentations on particular psychosocial themes—developed by the project staff were used to encourage people to shift the angle of interpretation of their daily problems. Building on the existing relations in the village, the team organized training for interested helpers in the community, and group work came almost automatically.

In mixed villages, however, the TPO team had to take a more careful approach. The unrelated villagers were best approached separately, and the team took pains to discover through interviews of key informants (teachers, village leaders, monks) the social history of the group. In these *phum*, building individual relationships between healers, helpers, and people in need meant building up a sense of mutual trust that was the essential basis for group sessions. In "new" *phum*, the most effective approach was for the team to start individual casework and identify individuals who had common interests. Once brought together, the various groups were provided psychoeducation and supportive relationships between community members began to seem and be possible.

In all villages, *phum* volunteers agreed with the suggestion of the project team to visit families that were known to be in distress. At the house of an identified family, for example, a discussion about their problems and causes would be pursued along the following lines: The family was asked what was typically done to find solutions to their problems, then the project team member asked to come along to the house, market, or hospital where help was found. There the healer, health worker, or any other local resource was asked to comment upon the problem and give her/his views about the causes and potential chances of healing. Because the majority of people had visited several health sectors, it was often possible to reconstruct the help-seeking path and see the reported problem from several angles.

Self-Help Groups

"Group therapy is defined as a professionally led therapeutic activity occurring in a group setting employing techniques varying from educational to those in which specific interactional and dynamic issues are examined" (Kinzie, 1997). Group sessions were the first step in developing self-help initiatives at the community level. The group approach was primarily a response to the sheer quantity of people needing help. It was also a chance to reinforce an important message, namely that people can actually help themselves and do not need an extra layer of "psychosocial workers" to do it for them. Group work also provides an opportunity to search for meaning, or an acceptable explanation, for the events of the past and the present. Exchanging opinions on this fosters cohesion and becomes a force for mutual empowerment and community building.

In preparatory discussions of group sessions with Cambodians, it had been remarked that differences in cultural values—such as respect for authority, the need for smooth relationships, traditional interdependent family relationships, and harmonious living with nature—are important in the psychotherapeutic relationship and could pose difficulties for a positive outcome (Kinzie, 1997). There is certainly no cultural analogue in any of the Asian healing ceremonies to the type of self-disclosure encouraged in psychotherapy group sessions.

The TPO team attempted to steer around these potential obstacles with the following measure: Groups were composed of individuals from the same social strata. For example, women in comparable social positions discussed their problems together, often for the first time in their lives, because they found themselves in a safe setting that was not automatically available in communities marked by displacement and isolation. Participants experienced these groups as a welcome opportunity to discuss problems they thought other women in the same situation would not have been willing to listen to. The introduction of these female self-help groups revealed some surprises. It was sometimes difficult for outsiders to believe that despite daily contact female kin from the same *phum* and with a shared history of traumatic events had never broached the subject of their sufferings with each other. Discussion of trauma was avoided partly because of the strict hierarchical organization of society which impedes free talk with those who are in a superior or a lesser position, and partly because the culture had never explored the therapeutic effect of talking to people who shared similar dilemmas and pain. Cambodian villagers did not traditionally seek or expect help or advice from people at the same level in the social hierarchy and, even more significantly, did not generally indulge in in-depth discussion of emotional problems. In addition, this was not a society where some had suffered and others had not, and many felt it was difficult enough to avoid "thinking too much" about their own problems for fear of going down the path to losing one's mind. The prevailing attitude was that one should try not to think, but enjoy life as it is and "be happy you are still alive."

In one of the group sessions we organized for Cambodian war widows, we asked them what they thought they would need to have a better life. They answered that first of all, there should be no more war; second, they should have enough to support their families; and third, what they needed was more friendly relations with other people. It turned out that they felt they were being looked down upon and their poverty excluded them from friendly contacts with other people.

The behavioral changes among group participants noticed by TPO staff indicated that something important was happening to them. In many cases women insisted on continuing their weekly sessions, and even rejected suggestions to start planning other activities such as income-generating initiatives. Rejection of income-generating activities was admittedly partly a result of memories of the pernicious experiments in communal work of the Khmer Rouge era, but it also seemed related to the women's sheer relief to be talking for the first time about their daily emotional problems and they seemed reluctant to put this at risk by embarking on potentially disruptive communal economic enterprises. The women were at a stage that could not be rushed, where repetition of their life stories served the purpose of giving meaning to what had happened and rebuilding mutual trust. As the project developed, women increasingly revealed the profound relief they experienced in sharing similar problems and their consequences with others. As a result, other self-help groups began to emerge—for example, for male alcoholics.

From today's perspective it is evident that short-term mutual interest between individual villagers and families is acting as an organizing principle for community life in many Cambodian villages and this has replaced older systems as a practical survival mechanism. For instance, widows in the same position—with small children, lack of income, and living outside their original *phum*—were often isolated from the community. But, as some self-help groups have shown, these women have been able to create networks of friends in similar circumstances that stretch much farther than the *phum*. These networks eventually link up and crisscross communities, so that the whole network of women comes to function as a mutual support group.

Counseling

In addition to the group work at the heart of the TPO intervention, training the team members in individual counseling skills was an important intervention component aimed at ameliorating suffering among villagers. The basic elements of communication between healer and sufferer that were detected in traditional healing relations indicated to the TPO team that there was common ground on which to build. Counseling training could even be used as a way of improving communication within the team itself, and counseling could be a start for developing a common language for describing helping activities. It offered the core group a set of basic therapeutic skills, such as listening skills, for helping in general. Furthermore, the very basics of counseling were expected to be of particular use for people working with the most vulnerable clients.

However, the therapeutic value of talking with, or even just listening to people talk about the problems they faced was not readily accepted among Cambodians. Healing was traditionally seen as a process requiring specific activity from the healer. The role of the Cambodian team members was at stake when they were asked to visit people and families in distress, in order to just listen to them or talk with them. As educated people and NGO workers they felt they had to live up to the expectations people would have, and either give material support or sound and clear advice. This was at least partly because in the interactions between patients and healers in the traditional Cambodian sector advice is at the center of the transaction. People ask for advice from healers and expect clear answers. The answers partly point at the cause of the problem, and always provide clear guidelines on what to do.

Training the core group of the project in counseling turned out to be a time-consuming affair. However, after 2 years the core group members had developed self-confidence in this new role, and came to understand that there are many shades between the extremes of "telling people what to do" and taking a completely passive role. In addition, to the surprise of the core group members, many local people actually liked being offered a chance to talk about their problems. The notion that a counselor does not solve the problems of a client *for* him/her appears to have been more difficult for the counselors to accept than for the clients.

In describing common factors in the many brief psychotherapeutic approaches, Bergin and Garfield (1994) listed the following basic general therapeutic factors: the therapeutic relationship, helping the client to understand and confront his/her problems, emotional release, reinforcement of client responses, giving information and reassurance to the client, promoting successful coping, and emotional involvement of the client. The TPO team's experience with the Cambodian caseload indicates that these same factors apply in Cambodia, and the team members could make use of them all.

This does not mean that counseling has proved itself a wholly effective tool for addressing the psychosocial problems of the large numbers of people in Cambodia. Training the team to spread the counseling skills was difficult—especially because of the difficulty of the concept of talk-therapy, the need for a new role to be created for the counselors-to-be, and the actual time counselors were required to invest in their individual clients. The individualized therapeutic work done by local healers, such as mediums, may be more efficacious and sustainable, is definitely more cost-effective, and is already in existence and readily accessible throughout the country.

CONCLUSIONS

Psychosocial problems in Cambodia have had a paralyzing effect on so-cial rehabilitation. Although mental health clinics are helpful for some individuals and families that need psychiatric treatment, this type of health coverage is limited and the treatment offered often does not relate to Cambodian people's understanding of their problems. The challenge, as shown by this chapter, is how knowledge about the traditional func-tioning of Cambodian society might be harnessed to develop interven-tions aimed at community healing, reconciliation, and rehabilitation.

The work of the 1995 TPO intervention is still going on in Cambodia. A team of Cambodians formed an organization to take over the original project tasks, and they currently are extending the work all over the country. At the community level, however, there is still evidence of dys-function. The ongoing lack of cohesion between groups is readily detect-able. Returnees are often among the most vulnerable. Refugee literature finds that the phenomenon of resettlement does not necessarily bring relief (Muecke & Sassi, 1992). Neither is the process of rebuilding Cam-bodia a short-term project. It is more likely that it will take decades for the Cambodian people to recover from the civil war and the genocidal Khmer Rouge regime. Public mental health programs will need to give careful consideration to the consequences of the conflict for years to come.

The first generation of Cambodians that has not been through a se-ries of traumatic events is now coming of age, but what is striking is their continuing sense of cultural and personal loss (Lipson et al., 1995; Schindler, 1993). From the perspective of our experience, we would urge those who try to help them to stress the importance of retaining a grip on their cultural identity, as there is evidence that those who do so fare best in post-conflict situations (Berry, 1991; Cheung & Spears, 1995; Eisen-bruch, 1986; Moon & Pearl, 1991).

In addressing the problems in Cambodia at the community level, we tried to make use of the hidden reserves at that level. An individualized, psychiatric approach would not have adequately addressed the numbers of those experiencing traumatic suffering or the need to restore the bonds of trust between people. Beneath the nationwide destruction of social infrastructure, some tenuous and fragile threads of trust and respect had been preserved. The traditional healers had safeguarded them, and when the cataclysm lifted, these healers could bear witness that the core of traditional Khmer society had not been completely broken.

We learned that interventions that complement the traditional systems of healing were not easy to develop. The assumption in successful complementarity is that the other party needs additions. The Cambodian villagers did not automatically see this need. We had to demonstrate that self-help groups could ease distress and build trust, and that counseling could help individuals regain more optimal psychosocial functioning. Only then were we able to add to the work already done by traditional healers whose value as trauma therapists could not be denied and, indeed, had to be supported and built upon (Bracken, Giller, & Summerfield, 1995; Gibbs, 1994; Wilson, 1989). Traditional healers provided and continue to provide a therapeutic mode that for some is simply more agreeable than those of the classical public health system and Western psychiatry.

In contrast to the villagers, the traditional healers early on did see the value in adding new techniques and ideas to their repertoire. The community turned out to be not only a useful "unit of analysis" to discover how a complex history of warfare and terror affected the personal and social functioning of the individuals that formed it, but also proved to be the reservoir of potential solutions—solutions that were valid and in harmony with a context in which people are rebuilding not only their own lives, but also the world that they live in.

REFERENCES

Bergin, A. E., & Garfield, S. L. (1994). *Handbook of psychotherapy and behavior change* (4th ed.). New York: Wiley.

Berry, J. W. (1991). Refugee adaptation in settlement countries: An overview with an emphasis on primary prevention. In L. A. Frederick & L. A. Jean (Eds.), *Refugee children: Theory, research, and services* (pp. 20-38). Baltimore, MD: Johns Hopkins University Press.

Boehnlein, J. K., Kinzie, J. D., Ben, R., & Fleck, J. (1985). One-year follow-up study of posttraumatic stress disorder among survivors of Cambodian concentration camps. *American Journal of Psychiatry, 142*(8), 956-959.

Bracken, P. J., Giller, J. E., & Summerfield, D. (1995). Psychological responses to war and atrocity: The limitations of current concepts. *Social Science and Medicine, 40*(8), 1073-1082.

Chandler, D. P. (1993). *A history of Cambodia.* Boulder, CO: Westview Press.

Cheung, P., & Spears, G. (1995). Psychiatric morbidity among New Zealand Cambodians: The role of psychosocial factors. *Social Psychiatry and Psychiatric Epidemiology, 30*(2), 92-97.

de Jong, J. T. V. M. (1997). *TPO Program for the identification, management, and prevention of psychosocial and mental health problems of refugees and victims of organized violence within primary health care of adults and children.* Amesterdam: Transcultural Psychosocial Organization. Internal document.

Ebihara, M. M. (1987). Revolution and reformulation in Kampuchean village culture. In D. A. Ablin & M. Hood (Eds.), *The Cambodian agony* (pp. 16-61). Armonk, NY: M. E. Sharpe.

Eisenbruch, M. (1986). Action research with Vietnamese refugees: Refugee, befriender and researcher relationships. *Journal of Refugee Studies, 7*(2), 30-51.

Eisenbruch, M. (1990a). Cultural bereavement and homesickness. In S. Fisher & C. L. Cooper (Eds.), *On the move: The psychology of change and transition* (pp. 191-205). New York: Wiley.

Eisenbruch, M. (1990b). The cultural bereavement interview: A new clinical research approach for refugees. *Psychiatric Clinics of North America, 13*(4), 715-735.

Eisenbruch, M. (1992). The ritual space of patients and traditional healers in Cambodia. *Bulletin de l'Ecole Française d'Extrême-Orient, 79*(2), 283-316.

Eisenbruch, M. (1994). Mental health and the Cambodian traditional healer for refugees who resettled, were repatriated or internally displaced, and for those who stayed at home, *Collegium Antropologicum, 18*(2), 219-230.

Eisenbruch, M. (1997). The cry for the lost placenta: Cultural bereavement and cultural survival among Cambodians who resettled, were repatriated, or who stayed at home. In M. van Tilburg & A. Vingerhoets (Eds.), *Home is where the heart is: The psychological aspects of permanent and temporary geographical moves* (pp. 119-142). Tilburg: Tilburg University Press.

Eisenbruch, M. (1999). Culture and illness—Clinical presentation and management of somatoform disorders in Cambodia. In Y. Ono, A. Janca, & N. Stratorius (Eds.), *Somatoform disorders: A worldwide perspective* (pp. 153-162) Tokyo: Springer-Verlag.

Eisenbruch, M., & Handelman, L. (1989). Development of an Explanatory Model of Illness Schedule for Cambodian refugee patients. *Journal of Refugee Studies, 2*(2), 243-256.

Gibbs, S. (1994). Post-war social reconstruction in Mozambique: Re-framing children's experience of trauma and healing. *Disasters, 18*(3), 268-276.

Kiernan, B. (1996). *The Pol Pot regime: Race, power, and genocide in Cambodia under the Khmer Rouge, 1975-79.* New Haven, CT: Yale University Press.

Kinzie, J. D., Boehnlein, J. K., Leung, P. K., & Moore, L. J. (1990). The prevalence of posttraumatic stress disorder and its clinical significance among Southeast Asian refugees. *American Journal of Psychiatry, 147*(7), 913-917.

Kirmayer, L. J. (1996). Confusion of the senses: Implications of ethnocultural variations in somatoform and dissociative disorders for PTSD. In J. M. Anthony et al. (Eds.), *Ethnocultural aspects of posttraumatic stress disorder: Issues, research, and clinical applications* (pp. 131-163). Washington, DC: American Psychological Association.

Lipson, J. G., Hosseini, T., Kabir, S., Omidian, P. A., & Edmonston, F. (1995). Health issues among Afghan women in California. *Health Care Women International, 16*(4), 279-286.

Mollica, R. (1994). Southeast Asian refugees: Migration history and mental health issues. In J. M. Anthony et al. (Eds.), *Amidst peril and pain: The mental health and well-being of the world's refugees* (pp. 83-100). Washington, DC: American Psychological Association.

Mollica, R. F., Wyshak, G., Lavelle, J., Truong, T., Tor, S., & Yang, T. (1990). Assessing symptom change in Southeast Asian refugee survivors of mass violence and torture. *The American Journal of Psychiatry, 147*(1), 83-88.

Moon, J., & Pearl, J. H. (1991). Alienation of elderly Korean American immigrants as related to place of residence, gender, age, years of education, time in the U.S., living with or without children, and living with or without a spouse. *International Journal of Aging and Human Development, 32*(2), 115-124.

Muecke, M. A., & Sassi, L. (1992). Anxiety among Cambodian refugee adolescents in transit and in resettlement. *Western Journal of Nursing Research, 14*(3), 267-285.

Schindler, R. (1993). Emigration and the Black Jews of Ethiopia: Dealing with bereavement and loss. *International Social Work, 36*(1), 7-19.

Somasundaram, D. J., van de Put, W. A., Eisenbruch, M., & de Jong, J. T. (1999). Starting mental health services in Cambodia. *Social Science and Medicine, 48*(8), 1029-1046.

Wilson, D. (1989). African contributions on AIDS/HIV, AIDS care. *Psychological and Socio-Medical Aspects of AIDS/HIV, 1*(2), 195-198.

5

Internally Displaced Sri Lankan War Widows: The Women's Empowerment Programme

Rachel Tribe and the
Family Rehabilitation Centre Staff

This chapter describes a community-based intervention for internally displaced widows living in refugee camps in Sri Lanka as a result of the 19-year-long civil war. The Women's Empowerment Programme was one of a series of interconnected programs run by the Family Rehabilitation Centre (FRC), a Sri Lankan nongovernmental organization committed to promoting ethnic harmony and community development, and to assisting victims of war by providing medical and psychological care and increasing socioeconomic knowledge. The FRC advocates a holistic, psychosocial model and philosophy and views mental health as embedded in a broad matrix of well-being and functioning. This matrix of interrelated factors encompasses psychological, social, and community functioning, cultural or spiritual belief and support systems, as well as economic and sociopolitical factors.

The Women's Empowerment Programme offered brief, small group, supportive interventions designed to empower Sri Lankan war widows by providing them with access to information, facilitating individual and community-level coping strategies, and drawing on the considerable inner resources of the women themselves. Although the program is no longer active due to a shift in FRC funding priorities, the WEP held more than 40 interventions in most of those areas within Sri Lanka containing refugee camps.

BACKGROUND

Sociopolitical Context

Sri Lanka is located to the south of India, close to the equator, and is an independent nation state. It gained independence in 1948 after approximately four centuries of colonial rule (1505–1948), first by the Portuguese, then the Dutch, and finally the British. It has a population of nearly 19.5 million, comprised of the Sinhalese majority (approximately 74% of the population), who are mainly Buddhist and live mostly in the south and west of the country, and the Tamils (approximately 18% of the population), who are mainly Hindu and live predominately in the north and east of the country. There are also smaller populations of Moors, Malay, Vedda, and Burghers (descendants of the European colonialists) in Sri Lanka. Approximately 8% of the population is Christian, represented by members of all ethnic groups, and 7% are Muslim (*CIA World Factbook*, July 2001).

Sri Lanka has been involved in an on-going, armed civil conflict since 1983 (*Sri Lanka Monitor*, 2000). The Liberation Tigers of Tamil Eelam (LTTE or Tamil Tigers) are fighting the Sri Lankan government for control of the north and east of the country, which they want to become an independent Tamil state.[1] The conflict has been brutal, and a large number of reports have detailed human rights violations by both sides (Amnesty International Annual Report, 1999; *Sri Lanka Monitor*, 2001). These violations include the failure to adhere to the legal conventions on the conduct of war, imprisonment without trial, rapes, disappearances,

---

[1]For a further discussion of the conflict, readers are referred to Dissanayaka (1995) or Somasundaram (1998).

and torture (Amnesty International, 2001; *Sri Lanka Monitor*, 2002). As a result of military action and violence, approximately 64,000 men, women, and children from all the ethnic groups have lost their lives (Refugee Council, 2001). Hundreds of individuals are missing and many others have suffered injuries (Amnesty International, 2000). More than 170,000 Sri Lankans applied for asylum in Europe and North America between 1990 and 1998 (UNHCR, 1999).

In February 2002, an initial agreement was signed by the Prime Minister of Sri Lanka and the LTTE to work toward a negotiated peace between the two sides. The negotiated cease-fire, which began in February 2002, has held fairly well since then. Peace talks between the LTTE and the Sri Lankan government, facilitated by Norwegian mediators, took place in Thailand on September 16th and November 2nd of 2002. The outcome of these meetings has been the establishment of a political committee to discuss Tamil claims for self-determination, as well as two joint committees concerned with security issues and the management of development aid (Reuters, 2002). The situation is looking very positive and some refugees and internally displaced people are beginning to return to their homes (UNHCR, 2002), although uncleared land mines continue to be a major worry (Harrison, 2002).

According to UNHCR (2000), the number of internally displaced people of all ethnic groups within Sri Lanka, at the end of December 2000, was approximately 706,000. Most of these people have been living in Sri Lankan refugee camps where conditions are frequently poor, with acute overcrowding, little privacy, and no proper sanitation (Sivayogen & Doney, 1991). In addition, during the years of civil conflict, parts of the north and east of the country were under regular bombardment and many essential supplies were unavailable due to the politics of war (*Sri Lanka Monitor*, 2000); while a number of serious bomb attacks in the south of the country resulted in death, injury, property damage and considerable emotional distress to the people living there.

The Family Rehabilitation Centre (FRC)

Within this context of ongoing, often unpredictable violence, the Family Rehabilitation Centre (FRC), a Sri Lankan nongovernmental organization, was established to provide a broad range of psychosocial and medical support services to victims of the war. In addition to the Women's Empowerment Programme for war widows, the FRC has run children's play activity groups, programs for military personnel, torture survivors and their families, families of the disappeared, detainees and ex-detainees, and direct victims of war (e.g., bomb blast survivors).

In working with these various groups, the FRC views mental health and well-being as dependent on a number of interrelated factors. These factors include psychological, social, and community functioning, cultural or spiritual belief and support systems, and economic and sociopolitical factors. The FRC model of well-being loosely reflects Maslow's (1971) model of a "hierarchy of needs," in which primary needs (e.g., health, safety, and security) serve as preconditions for higher order needs (e.g., occupational satisfaction, skill mastery, and self-actualization). Therefore, the FRC assists various war-affected groups by providing services that address basic health care (e.g., running mobile and project-based medical clinics and physiotherapy) and material assistance (e.g., providing sewing machines or poultry to enable individuals to start self-employment businesses), as well as more advanced job skill training, personal empowerment, and psychological education and support groups.

The FRC is a diverse organization with staff drawn from all of the different ethnic groups in Sri Lanka. Most staff members have had many years of experience working within the community and a number of them are internally displaced people themselves. This has made it much easier for the FRC and its various programs to gain access to, and acceptance by, the different ethnic communities caught up in the civil conflict.

Mental Health and Psychosocial Implications

Research has demonstrated a connection between exposure to violent conflict and psychological problems in combat veterans and civilians (Boman, 1986; Figley, 1986; Green, 1993; Solomon, 1993). Additionally, various studies have noted the adverse effects of becoming a refugee on mental health (Fuller, 1993; Kinzie & Sack, 1991). However, research on refugees concentrates almost exclusively on the 17% of the world's refugees who have resettled in industrialized countries, while the majority of refugees either remain displaced within their own country or cross national borders into neighbouring developing countries. Although internally displaced people (IDPs) are often difficult to access, it is crucial that more attention be paid to the compromised psychological well-being of the millions of IDPs worldwide.

During 19 years of civil conflict in Sri Lanka, many civilians have become internally displaced and have been emotionally affected or traumatized, either by direct involvement in the conflict, or by fear of its potential effect on their lives. A comprehensive overview of the main presenting problems of civilians in war-affected parts of Sri Lanka can be found in Somasundaram and Sivayokan (2000), Somasundaram (1998), and Arulananthan, Ratneswaren, and Sreeharan (1994).[2] To summarize, these authors have documented a range of trauma-related reactions in the Tamil community living in the war zone, including an increase in alcohol and drug consumption, depression, somatic complaints, evidence of developmental problems, and sleep disturbances. Many family members have been separated from one another, and normal community and social supports have been compromised.

The situation for women in Sri Lanka is especially difficult. According to Sivachandran (1994), Sri Lankan women have faced many psychological and physical burdens during the war, and Somasundaram (1994) noted that statistical data collected in Jaffna (in Northern Sri Lanka) on clinical attendance, in-patient treatment, and community surgeries suggests that women are at increased risk of developing psychological disorders. Somasundaram surmised that the reasons for this are "due to migration, death, detention, disappearance, or direct involvement in the conflict by young males, as well as the increased burden and responsibilities placed on the females to run the homes and look after children single-handedly" (p. 27).

As for mental health service provision, there are very few psychiatrists or psychologists in Sri Lanka: approximately 33 for a population of

---

[2]All of these authors were working with the Tamil community. The Sinhalese and Muslim communities have also suffered from the war, but it is difficult to find comprehensive studies based on these communities. In view of this, the findings may not generalize to the wider war-affected Sri Lankan community.

almost 20 million, with few practicing in the conflict zones (P. de Silva, personal communication, July, 2002). Although this highlights the inadequacy of existing professional mental health services in Sri Lanka, it fails to capture the range of local individuals available to provide important support for individuals suffering psychological distress. In rural areas, those identified as healers and helpers may be community or religious leaders, indigenous Ayurvedic doctors, or other members of the community. These local healers provide vital psychological support and may even serve communities in ways that Western-trained psychologists and psychiatrists cannot. For instance, they are usually easily accessible to community members and are not associated with notions of mental illness or psychological difficulties, which may carry a negative connotation within the community. Because of this, indigenous healers are encouraged to participate actively in FRC programs such as the Women's Empowerment Programme, and they make an extremely valuable contribution in helping to re-establish traditional networks of helping and healing in displaced communities.

Population of Focus

The war has forced many thousands of Sri Lankan civilians into refugee camps for internally displaced people. Direct attacks on homes and villages have left many homeless, while others, fearing army or LTTE attacks or reprisals, have left their homes for the uncertain safety of the refugee camps. There are thousands of widows living in refugee camps in Sri Lanka, many of whom are still in their 20s or 30s. In addition to coping with the grief of losing loved ones who were frequently the breadwinners, Sri Lankan women widowed by the war are faced with numerous socioeconomic, health, and legal problems. The Director of the Centre for Women and Development in Jaffna, Sri Lanka, wrote:

> [T]he tension and trauma created by this war have badly scarred many of our children and women. Women . . . live with high levels of tension. They fear that their children will join the liberation movement and die in combat. (Sivachandran, 1994, p. 48)

Women from the different ethnic groups face common difficulties. Numerous women have reported incidents of sexual harassment; some have been sexually assaulted or threatened, while others have been robbed. In addition, many women are pressured to take political positions or engage in political activities. Many women who have lost their husbands are left destitute with no way of earning a living to support their families. In addition, the widows may face considerable gender discrimination and a general lack of social and economic opportunities. In our work with the FRC, we found that war widows were frequently so distressed by the ongoing conflict that they often were unavailable to their children for emotional and basic support. We also found that many parents found it extremely difficult, if not impossible, to tell their children that a relative was missing or dead. This appeared to be because they themselves had difficulty accepting this information. The uncertainty around and difficulty coping with loss was quite understandable, given that individuals in Sri Lanka often go missing and information about what has happened to them is frequently inaccurate, scarce, or unavailable. In Sri Lanka, as in other situations of civil conflict, accurate information is often withheld as part of the politics of war, and incorrect information is used as psychological propaganda.

In attempting to cope with the uncertainty regarding the whereabouts of missing loved ones, many widows creatively filled the information gap themselves or for their children. For example, some shared narratives with us that a relative had gone to work abroad, and others related hopes of relatives returning home after many years. One frequently told narrative, which may or may not be apocryphal, related to a "widow" re-marrying after her husband had been missing for many years, only to have her first husband suddenly return, leading to the ruin of her life and that of the families. This type of shared narrative and "unknowing" kept many women fearful of moving on with their lives after losing a husband.

Given the extreme stressors faced by Sri Lankan women, particularly widows, the target group for the Women's Empowerment Programme was women whose husbands had died or were missing as a result of the ethnic conflict. Program participants were resident in refugee camps and represented all of the major ethnic groups in Sri Lanka. All Women's Empowerment Programme participants volunteered to take part after learning about the program through local community leaders and other organizations working in their geographical areas.

INTERVENTION

Theory and Rationale

Community mental and public health practitioners, as well as those taking an ecological or eco-systemic perspective, advocate harnessing existing community and cultural resources to promote well-being, rather than merely targeting individual level difficulties (MacLachlan, 1997; Sarason, 1974). Vinck (1994) asserted that public health workers forming coalitions and collaborating with communities are better able to enhance and promote well-being than those who fail to do so, and research from various regions of the world indicates that community-based health promotion campaigns focusing on both psychological and physical health have been effective (e.g., Ager & MacLachlan, 1998; Nakshani, Tatara, & Fujiwara, 1996).

The Women's Empowerment Programme (WEP) was designed as a short-term, therapeutic, community-based intervention for Sri Lankan war widows with the goals of maximizing resources and building capacity among participants. After participating in the program, it was hoped that the widows would then set up their own self-help groups with the support of the FRC's area office. Minuchin and Minuchin (1974) have stressed the importance of short-term therapeutic group work in mobilizing strengths, as have community mental health practitioners around the world; we drew on these ideas in our program. The community-based approach allowed us to reach far more individuals than would a traditional, individual therapy model. Working in and with the communities of war widows also increased the cultural appropriateness, acceptance, and sustainability of the intervention, and the WEP provided a context for participants to develop a normative understanding of the difficulties faced by widows and sensitized others in the community to their dilemmas, as well as their remarkable strengths. The WEP targeted communities of women, rather than individuals, because offering individual women help might have been viewed as pathologizing their difficulties and might have had less impact on precipitating positive change.

Organizing Principles and Goals of the WEP

The promotion of psychological health and well-being among Sri Lankan war widows was the main overarching aim of the WEP. The FRC was made increasingly aware of the need for such a program through research and collaboration with community groups, as well as through a needs analysis and feedback from other FRC projects. In accordance with the philosophy of the FRC—that mental health is influenced by individual, community, sociopolitical, and economic factors—the fundamental organizing principles of the WEP represent a blend of ideas designed to promote the well-being of program participants at multiple (i.e., individual, family, *and* community) levels. The organizing principles and goals of the WEP are based on traditional models of both individual and group psychological theory, as well as theories of individual and community empowerment. In its design of the WEP, the FRC gathered input about the needs and concerns of displaced Sri Lankan war widows from the widows themselves, from local community leaders, and from staff who had considerable experience working with Sri Lankans affected by the civil conflict.

The three major goals of the WEP were to increase ethnic harmony among women of different ethnic groups; to provide psychoeducation about trauma and build adaptive coping skills; and to help develop long-lasting support systems and community resources among program participants.

Toward the promotion of ethnic harmony, women from the four main ethnic groups (Sinhalese, Tamil, Muslim, and Burgher) were invited to attend WEP groups together. The rationale was that helping develop supportive relationships among women from the different sides of the conflict would create opportunities for them to reframe perceptions, negative attitudes, and stereotyped beliefs about one another. In his contact hypothesis, Amir (1969; and more recently Cairns, 2001) proposed that relationships between groups who are in conflict may be enhanced if they are given opportunities to spend time together in a safe and contained environment. The WEP hoped to help shift negative and divisive attitudes, build supportive bridges between the diverse program participants in the safety of small, participatory groups, and reduce the social isolation felt by many of the widows.

The WEP also was designed to promote psychoeducation and the use of adaptive coping skills among participants. For example, it has been argued that assisting people who have been traumatized to develop a belief in the predictability of their lives, their safety, and their ability to deal successfully with crises, affords them the confidence to cope more adaptively with traumatic events (Mitchell & Everly, 1993). One component of this is to normalize the experience of traumatic distress through education around how traumatic reactions may be normal reactions to abnormal events. Developing this awareness helps increase tolerance and acceptance of these reactions, and enhances feelings of affinity among those experiencing a disaster together.

In addition, the WEP was designed to maximize social support among participants. The WEP provided numerous opportunities for participants to develop a sense of a supportive community of women and to strengthen their collective potential. Light (1992), writing about Guatemalan refugee women who had lived in refugee camps in Southern Mexico for 10 years, noted that women organized themselves into productive co-operative groups over time and were subsequently able to use this collectivism to their advantage. Influenced by this work, we believed that the Sri Lankan women also might experience similar benefits after the empowerment program.

Social support has been shown to be important during times of stress, by providing opportunities to develop helping networks, friendships, and collaboration. The role of social support as a protective factor in psychological well-being has been noted by Yule (1998), Gorst-Unsworth and Goldenberg (1998), McCallin (1992), Brown and Harris (1978), Ressler, Boothby, and Steinbock (1988), and Davidson (1980), among others. Indeed, Bisson and Deahl (1994) go so far as to suggest that social support may be more important in preventing traumatic reactions after a trauma than the provision of psychological interventions soon after the event. Additionally, Hobfoll et al. (1991) claimed that social support benefits not only the recipient but also the giver.

The WEP attempted to mobilize participants as resources for one another by organizing self-help groups and encouraging collaborative endeavors, such as starting businesses. Participants also were encouraged to reflect on strategies they had used in the past to overcome difficulties and to share these with other widows in the program. The WEP included supportive activities and social events to provide a context for participants to develop networks for sharing difficulties, ideas, and strategies throughout and after the program.

Another program component involved the empowerment of widows through the acquisition of contextually relevant knowledge and skills. The WEP encouraged women to take control of their futures by providing them with information about how to access and manage resources relevant to their specific concerns and priorities. The widows identified a range of topics as important, including a need for more information about employment and resettlement opportunities outside the refugee camp, their children's and their own health and development, self-employment procedures, and the legal statutes relevant for widows (such as the issue of death certificates). Relevant local experts and knowledgeable FRC staff provided program participants with information about these topics and skills training to help them access relevant resources and maximize employment opportunities.

To encourage the continued development of long-lasting, empowering, and supportive community networks, an integral part of the WEP design was the cascade or waterfall learning method of training individuals who then teach or pass on their knowledge and skills to other women in their communities. In accordance with this model, after participating in the WEP, some women volunteered to be "be-frienders" and received intensive training in the capital of Sri Lanka with emphasis on leadership, cascade learning methods, and community work. These women were then employed by the FRC at local extension offices to disseminate information and assist other women affected by the war. As well as providing social support, the be-frienders tried to maintain contact with relevant authorities to ensure that any bureaucratic problems that the women were experiencing were addressed. The be-frienders also were expected to facilitate any follow-up from the program, such as giving advice and providing support around self-employment opportunities and endeavors.

Implementation

As stated previously, the shortage of highly trained professional personnel is often seen as a major problem in providing mental health services in situations of civil conflict, such as that seen in Sri Lanka. In our view, the model used in the WEP offers an approach that enables the implementation of such services with limited expert staff.

Preliminary Groundwork

Prior to the implementation of the WEP in any given area, the FRC networked with local organizations and discussed the program to see if it would be useful and/or accepted in different regions of Sri Lanka. This initial assessment process was termed a "fact–finding mission" and took place some weeks or months before individual programs were implemented. We found that it was vital, at the outset, to work with local organizations rather than around or across them. If local community organizations wished the WEP to take place and believed it would be beneficial, then it went ahead. If they did not believe it would be helpful, then it did not. To encourage community acceptance and participation, local community leaders frequently organized the logistics, provided resources, and/or participated in the program as facilitators.

Process

Each WEP was held over a period of 3 to 5 days as a residential program close to the refugee camps. WEP seminars had no more than 35 women drawn from all of the ethnic groups resident in any one geographical area and were run with simultaneous translation into the two national languages, Sinhalese and Tamil. Although each program followed a similar general formula, the specifics were tailored to the particular needs of the women living in that area. Each WEP combined (1) practical information and skills training, which had immediate relevance to the widows, with (2) helping the women increase their awareness and understanding of the common psychological issues and problems facing them, with the overarching goal of creating a safe and supportive environment for the women to develop and strengthen social networks and learn from one another.

The empowerment programs were run using a range of teaching and learning methods including didactic talks, experiential exercises and role-plays, mini intensive workshops, small group discussions, and whatever format appeared relevant to the particular group of women involved. Each new program utilized feedback from the last and so was constantly evolving. A range of community members and local experts (such as lawyers and Ayurvedic doctors) were used as resources and invited to speak at the empowerment programs whenever possible— partly because they often played key roles in assisting widows in their communities, and partly to sensitize the larger community to the issues facing the widows.

The well-known adage commonly used by the FRC staff to encompass the empowerment vision of the program was, *"We do not give them fish, but teach them how to fish."* Indeed, the WEP was designed to empower participants to use and develop their knowledge, skills, and resources, to build adaptive coping strategies, and to create a network of support among the women and their communities. Toward these goals, the WEP seminars covered a range of topics identified during the fact-finding missions as important to war widows. These topics included financial and employment matters, primary health care, and mental health. Local lawyers talked with the women about their rights, entitlements, and how to get legal assistance, while staff from local Government Agents offices spoke to the women about compensation issues related to the loss of their husbands. Staff from the FRC or other relevant local NGOs spoke to participants about financial concerns, and worked with them on job-finding skills and self-employment opportunities. Local medical officers or matrons and indigenous Ayurvedic doctors helped address the women's concerns regarding primary health care and first aid. Psychoeducation around mental health issues (e.g., adaptive coping and normalization of traumatic reactions) was provided by FRC staff and, if available, local resource people.

During the day, women participated in the various seminars and groups, and in the evenings, there were opportunities for informal discussions, recreation, and individual counselling and consultation with the FRC team or relevant resource persons. Participants often spent their evenings together playing games or organizing entertainment, such as variety shows. During this time, many friendships appeared to grow as the women continued to get to know each other in a relaxed, unstructured atmosphere.

On the final day of the program, women who had been through the WEP before were invited to return to the groups to share their experiences, both positive and negative, regarding what had happened to them since they had participated in the program. Many former participants took this opportunity to reflect on their experiences of the WEP, and to offer advice and encouragement to the group. Several former participants offered to act as mentors and advisers to members of the new group of women. These relationships appeared to offer practical and psychological benefits to both parties. The mentors were able to share their experiences and knowledge with their mentees, provide important support and encouragement, and act as role models. Conversely, the mentees gained personal and social support and knowledge from their more experienced mentors.

In addition, the WEP model was designed to ensure that the learning among and support for war widows did not end with the 3 to 5 day intensive programs. As previously discussed, the WEP relied on cascade learning methods to ensure that as many widows as possible could access the program if they so wished. The cascade model involved setting up a system for those WEP participants who undertook more intensive training in advocacy and support to work at local FRC extension offices and to serve as "be-frienders" to other women, who, in turn, could pass on what they learned to even more women in their communities.

CHALLENGES AND LESSONS LEARNED

A number of organizational, ethical, political, and cultural concerns and challenges arose while planning and implementing the WEP. At the organizational level, we found that staff changes can affect a program significantly. Two of the women who were instrumental in establishing the

WEP left the organization, and this changed the organizational culture[3] and priorities.

When setting up any program, we would stress the importance of thorough groundwork, ensuring that all the necessary parties are met and the ideas discussed. It is very important to be aware and respectful of organizations, community, religious, and support groups already in existence, and to try and work with them rather than across them. We found it was essential that initial partnerships were formed and trust was established between WEP staff and local community leaders, health and education workers, and other service providers before the implementation of any programs. This was especially critical in the Sri Lankan context, where civil conflict had broken trusting and cooperative working relationships between many community members.

We also found that before the implementation of a program, any reservations that are raised by community members need to be listened to, and program organizers must be prepared to change their ideas in response to feedback. The FRC team had gained a comprehensive understanding of Sri Lankan spiritual, cultural, and sociopolitical issues and mores over many years of working in the community, and fortunately, the positive reputation of the FRC and its staff went before us. This helped us considerably in setting up the WEP.

The process of networking with community leaders and service providers when setting up a community-based intervention can reveal surprising "clashes" between local community members and organizations (such as the FRC) about how best to assist a target population. For example, an unexpected dilemma we encountered in setting up the WEP in one location was a helpful male community leader who assured us that the most useful thing we could do to empower war widows was to find them husbands. In his sincere desire to help, he had even selected a number of potential "husbands" from his community. This situation lead to a number of discussions among the FRC team, and we eventually decided to explain respectfully to the community leader that finding the

---

[3]Organizational culture is understood by major theorists in this area to be the rules, beliefs, and ways of doing things that become established over time and may be decided initially by the task of the organization and the personalities of the key players in the organization.

women husbands was not our task, but an individual choice for each woman if she wished to find or be found a husband. It is not easy to prepare for the various conflicts of interest that can arise when setting up a community-based intervention, and not always clear how they should best be handled.

Within a refugee camp there is frequently an undercurrent of fear and suspicion, with uncertainty about whom to trust. Anyone working in a refugee camp in a context of civil war must be cognizant of the fact that people from opposing sides of the conflict are likely to be resident there, and that they may hold a range of views, ranging from sympathy to outright hostility and hatred, about those from the "other" side (Tribe, 1998). This needs to be appreciated when introducing a psychological intervention into such a situation. Such potential challenges should be assessed and addressed as close to the planning stages and outset of an intervention as possible.

Along these lines, FRC staff had to be self-consciously aware of both their own political opinions and the wider social and political context of their work. The FRC is a nonpartisan, nongovernmental organization with a humanitarian mission to improve ethnic harmony as one of its aims. Therefore, although staff members held personal political opinions, these had to remain personal and not influence their work in any significant way. This was sometimes a challenge for staff, but necessary in remaining true to the goals of the nonpartisan FRC and for avoiding the perception among community members that FRC staff were aligned with one political position or another.

Unexpected obstacles and challenges always arise during the implementation of an intervention, and it is necessary to be flexible and think laterally about how to address such problems. For example, in one of our programs, entry into the refugee camp was restricted after 4 o'clock in the afternoon, and when women gave birth after this time, there was no medical attention available. We therefore arranged for one of the medical practitioners to run a session during which the women learned how to deliver a baby should the need arise. This training had not been in our original program, but it was important that we responded flexibly to the immediate needs that arose.

We also found it essential to respect cultural differences in all their forms and to take time to consider their implications. Almost all the members of the FRC are Sri Lankan nationals; however, diverse ethnic groups with different cultural and religious practices are represented among the staff. In addition, at various times, individuals from outside of Sri Lanka were involved in the program and they needed to consider clearly their cultural positioning. This was sometimes as simple as considering different dress codes. As an example, a few years ago, an American psychologist working with the FRC attended a meeting wearing a baseball cap the wrong way around, as was common among young people in the West. A senior Sri Lankan colleague interpreted this, however, as an indication that the man had severe problems, as he was unable to even dress himself correctly or appropriately. Such cultural misunderstandings abound in this field, and we have found it necessary to encourage cultural competence and open communication among and between program staff and community members around such issues.

EVALUATION

Due to the ethnic conflict, we have undergone many hardships. [During the WEP] *I have been able to share my problems with others. We learned so much we did not know. Now we realize that the most important thing is to be united and work hard to achieve something.*

— A WEP participant

Throughout the program, participants were asked to offer verbal feedback and suggestions to the FRC team through the use of semistructured interviews and open group discussion at the end of each day of the program. In addition, at the end of each program, a sample of participants was interviewed and their comments were recorded and later reviewed by each program's facilitators.[4] With hindsight we believe we could have devised an evaluation questionnaire before implementing the first program, and used this consistently throughout each program to enhance the thoroughness of the evaluation process. However, the nature of our evaluation can be attributed to the ongoing civil war and the concomi-

---

[4]The information was collected in whichever language the participants wished to speak, and was then orally translated and discussed by the FRC team.

tant difficulties associated with this; for example, issues of trust and confidentiality may be compromised in a civil war. Other factors included a variety of literacy levels among the widows, as well as pressures of time, the fact that two or three staff members would have been needed to help us deal with the different languages and back-translations, and the fact that the project was seen primarily as a community-based intervention rather than a research-led project.

The WEP was able to monitor the effects of the program by maintaining contact with many former participants. For example, during each program, women from previous programs were invited to report on their progress and on any difficulties they had encountered since undertaking the program. This became an opportunity for program staff to hear how former participants were using the knowledge, skills, and support they gained from the program—and to hear about ways the program might be improved. FRC also maintained follow-up contact with many of the participants by letter, telephone, or by team visits, through the extension offices and through other NGOs.

Through feedback from participants and follow-up contact, we learned that there have been a number of positive outcomes from the WEP. These include the establishment of a women's group and several participant-run credit unions. In addition, many of the widows were able to obtain financial compensation for the loss of their husbands. Also, a number of small-scale co-operative ventures have taken off. These include projects for the making and mending of clothes, mat weaving, catering projects, growing vegetables and herbs, and making paper bags to sell to local stall holders and shops. One participant noted that the WEP assisted her and other participants in using their skills and encouraged them to "be brave and courageous" so that others would respect what they had to say. In so doing, she added, "We can be role models." Other comments from the participants in the WEP are offered as a primary data source:

> I came with the hope that I will be able to solve my problems. Now I understand that there are others like myself from other ethnic groups who have undergone the same problems and hardships.

After my husband was killed, I had no love for life. I was beside myself. . . . After attending the FRC seminar, I began to realize that there were many others affected like me. The kindness, compassion, and training given by FRC helped me to stand on my own two feet. I have learned a lot from these programs and now have the courage to face the future and look after my child.

We had problems trying to obtain death certificates for our husbands. I am happy to learn from the lawyer who spoke to us how to obtain the death certificates.

I have decided to form a co-operative society, when I return to the camp, we will start with a small amount. . . . This will enable us to give loans to members for self-employment such as mat weaving or poultry keeping.

After the WEP had been running for approximately 1 year, a formal qualitative evaluation was conducted on behalf of an international NGO that had funded the WEP. The evaluation was a condition of future funding, and employed independent researchers who spoke to women currently participating in the program, those who had completed it, and those who had been appointed to work in the extension offices. The evaluators travelled to a variety of sites in the country where the program had been implemented and spoke to a sample of staff and community members involved in running the program.

The evaluators wrote in their report that they hoped "that the findings . . . will be of use to FRC in making more effective the important and opportune task they have dedicated themselves to." With regard to the war widows, the evaluators noted that, "FRC is filling a very important gap by recognizing and targeting this marginalized group. This phenomenon in our country's recent history has yet to reach the public consciousness. As such, FRC's work is certainly both pioneering and opportune."

The full written evaluation report was submitted to FRC and was available to all relevant staff. Overall, the evaluation was positive. However, the report touched on a number of important dilemmas related to the role of women in Sri Lanka, and to the sustainability of the project. In particular, the report raised concerns about an overemphasis by the WEP on the women in their roles as mothers. The evaluators noted, ". . . if the program is to 'empower' the women psychologically, then it is vital that the women are imbued with the notion of the self (as a woman) first as well as a mother." This concern was addressed by a change in the focus of the intervention toward a more central focus on the women's needs and futures. Indeed, it was appreciated that if too much focus remained on women in their roles as mothers, this would put too much pressure on both them and their children. The evaluators also suggested that FRC might consider lobbying more actively for the women locally and nationally, thus working at the macro, as well as the micro level.

The evaluators also suggested that the balance between relief and rehabilitation be further considered:

> As an evaluation team, one problem we faced in particular was the disparity in the value placed by us and by the participants on the psychological aspect of the program. While we feel that this focus of the program reflects a crying need that is addressed by FRC, it is only natural that the participants and to see their most immediate needs as being solely economical. Combined with their general experience of NGOs being entirely relief oriented, the participants did not place equal value on this kind of [psychological] support. Nevertheless, it is our opinion that these women need more intensive and regular counselling and the program is able to satisfy this to a certain extent.

This evaluation gave FRC much to consider, and detailed discussions around the WEP intervention priorities followed. The staff team eventually decided that there were many organizations offering economic relief, and the WEP had been set up primarily to address the issue of rehabilitation and assisting survivors of the conflict. Indeed, this was the major objective of our funding agencies. It was decided, therefore, that we should network more with relief oriented agencies, so that we could refer easily and appropriately to them (and vice versa) to ensure that the basic economic needs of the women were addressed, while we focused more centrally on the psychological well-being of the women.

In the end, the important question of whether we were prioritizing what was really important to the war widows, or inadvertently imposing what we (or our funding agencies) thought should be important continued as a dynamic and lively tension within the program, as it does for many humanitarian agencies around the world. We hoped to address the dilemma through coordinated service provision with other organizations, but continued to struggle with the tensions.

Overall, the feedback from the independent evaluation was extremely useful to us. The evaluation report gave us an opportunity to discuss important criticisms raised about the WEP, and made us aware that our desire to assist the widows and provide the program had, perhaps, led us to "roll it out" rather too quickly, without sufficient forethought around some issues. It also provided us with an opportunity to make some improvements in the WEP to address these concerns.

The WEP was designed with sustainability in mind. It was hoped that the cascade model, which involved setting up extension offices staffed by participants who had undergone further training, would promote the long-term effects of the program. This was the case for a period of time, but a change of staff and direction by the FRC management to working almost exclusively with torture survivors meant that the WEP did not fit the remit for which FRC was funded. In consequence, it was discontinued. However, other NGOs in Sri Lanka have adapted many of the ideas developed by the WEP and are running similar programs independently. In addition, a staff member who had been one of the key players in establishing the WEP moved to another organization, and has continued to implement numerous components of the WEP there.

SUMMARY

The Women's Empowerment Programme (WEP) was one of a series of interconnected programs run by the Family Rehabilitation Centre (FRC), a Sri Lankan nongovernmental organization committed to promoting ethnic harmony, community development, and to assisting victims of war by providing medical and psychological care and socioeconomic knowledge. The overarching goal of the WEP was to improve the mental health and well-being of displaced Sri Lankan war widows, and our preliminary needs analysis led us to realize that we needed to be innovative and responsive to the expressed needs of our target population, rather than rely on a traditional health clinic model to offer mental health services to individual women. Drawing on a multilevel blend of ideas pertaining to psychological knowledge, group dynamics, community resources and support, plus an empowerment model, the WEP was designed as a brief, supportive intervention focused on building strengths among widows at the small group level. The primary goals of the intervention were to improve ethnic harmony, support and build adaptive coping strategies, and increase socioeconomic knowledge and skills among the women participants. In addition, to help participants develop their community networks and resources, and to reach as many women as possible, the WEP used a cascade model in which a number of program participants received further training and were employed by local extension offices to provide ongoing support, advice, and advocacy for women in their communities.

Feedback from former program participants and outside evaluators has been generally positive, and many women have made positive changes in their lives after participating in the WEP. Unfortunately, the program is no longer running due to a change in FRC administration and a subsequent change in funding priorities. However, the program ran on more than 40 occasions throughout most of the areas of Sri Lanka containing refugee camps, and aspects of the WEP have been adopted by other programs and will hopefully continue to impact the lives of Sri Lankan women in positive ways. The widows of the war have played an extremely heavy price for the continuing civil conflict in Sri Lanka. Many women and children have little or no experience of life in peacetime or outside a refugee camp. Our hope is that the WEP has contributed to minimizing the adverse effects of living in conditions of ongoing violence and deprivation, by facilitating healing and promoting resilience and positive adaptation among the many women who participated in the program.

REFERENCES

Ager, A., & MacLachlan, M. (1998). Psychometric properties of the Coping Strategy Indicator (CSI) in a study of coping behaviour amongst Malawian students. *Psychology and Health, 13,* 399-409.

Amir, Y. (1969). Contact hypothesis in ethnic relations. *Psychological Bulletin, 71,* 319-342.

Amnesty International Annual Report (1999, 2000). London: Amnesty International.

Arulanantham, K., Ratneswaren, S., & Sreeharan, N. (1994, September). Victims of war in Sri Lanka: A quest for health consensus. *Proceedings of the International Conference on Health.* Manning Hall, University of London Union, London.

Bisson, J., & Deahl, M. P. (1994). Psychological debriefing and prevention of post-traumatic stress—More research is needed. *British Journal of Psychiatry, 165,* 717-720.

Boman, B. (1986). Combat stress, post-traumatic stress disorder, and associated psychiatric disorder. *Psychosomatics, 27,* 567-573.

Brown, G., & Harris, T. (1978). *The social origins of depression.* London: Tavistock.

Cairns, E. (2001). War and peace. *The Psychologist, 14,* 292-293.

CIA World Factbook. (2001). Retrieved July, 2001, from http://www.cia.gov/cia/publications/factbook/geos/ce.html

Davidson, S. (1980). The clinical effects of massive psychic trauma in families of Holocaust survivors. *Journal of Marital and Family Therapy, 6,* 11-24.

Dissanayaka, T. D. A. (1995). *War or peace in Sri Lanka.* Colombo: Government Press.

Family Rehabilitation Centre (1993). *Empowerment programme for women affected by organised violence.* Colombo: Family Rehabilitation Centre.

Figley, C. R. (1986). *Trauma and its wake* (Vol. 2). New York: Brunner/Mazel.

Fuller, K. L. (1993). Refugee mental health in Aalborg, Denmark: Traumatic stress and cross-cultural treatment issues. *Nordic Journal of Psychiatry, 47,* 251-256.

Gorst-Unsworth, C., & Goldenberg, E. (1998). Psychological sequelae of torture and organized violence suffered by refugees from Iraq. *British Journal of Psychiatry, 166,* 360-367.

Green, B. (1993). Identifying survivors at risk: Trauma and stressors across events. In J. P. Wilson & B. Raphael (Eds.), *International handbook of traumatic stress syndromes.* New York: Plenum Press.

Harrison, F. (2002). Trauma haunts Sri Lanka. *BBC News* [On-line]. Retrieved from http://news.bbc.co.uk/1/hi/world/south_asia/2018602.stm

Hobfoll, S. E., Speilberger, C. D., Folkman, S., Lepper-green, B., Saranson, I., & Van der Kolk, B. (1991). War-related stress: Addressing the stress of war and other traumatic events. *American Psychologist, 46,* 848-855.

Kinzie, J. D., & Sack, W. (1991). Severely traumatised Cambodian children: Research findings and clinical implications. In F. L. Ahearn & J. L. Athey (Eds.), *Refugee children: Theory, research, and services*. Baltimore, MD: John Hopkins University Press.

Light, D. (1992). Healing their wounds: Guatemalan refugee women as political activists. *Women and Therapy, 13*, 281-296.

MacLachlan, M. (1997). *Culture and health*. Chichester, England: Wiley.

Maslow, A. (1971). *The farther reaches of human nature*. New York: Viking.

McCallin, M. (1992). The psychological well-being of refugee children: Research, practice, and policy issues. Geneva: International Catholic Child Bureau.

Minuchin, S., & Minuchin, P. (1974). *Families and family therapy*. London: Tavistock.

Mitchell, J. Y., & Everly, G. S. (1993). *Critical incident stress debriefing*. Ellicott City, MD: Chevron.

Nakshani, N., Tatara, K., & Fujiwara, H. (1996). Do preventative health services reduce eventual demand for medical care? *Social Science and Medicine, 43*, 999-1005.

Refugee Council (2001). Information obtained from The Press and Information Office, London.

Ressler, E., Boothby, N., & Steinbock, C. J. (1988). *Unaccompanied children: Care and protection in wars, natural disasters, and refugee movements*. New York: Oxford University Press.

Sarason, S. B. (1974). *The psychological sense of community: Prospects for a community psychology*. San Francisco: Jossey-Bass.

Sivachandran, S. (1994, September). *Health of women and the elderly: Victims of war in Sri Lanka, a quest for health consensus*. Conference proceedings of the International Conference on Health, Manning Hall, University of London Union, London.

Sivayogen, S., & Doney, A. (1991). *Assessment of health status of refugees in Colombo, Sri Lanka*. Presented at the Third International Conference on Health, Political Repression, and Human Rights, Santiago, Chile.

Solomon, Z. (1993). *Combat stress reaction*. New York: Plenum Press.

Somasundaram, D. (1994, September). Mental health in northern Sri Lanka – An overview. In K. Arulanantham, S. Ratneswaren, & N. Sreeharan. *Victims of war in Sri Lanka: A quest for health consensus*. Conference Proceedings of the International Conference on Health, Manning Hall, University of London Union, London.

Somasundaram, S. (1998). *Scarred minds: The psychological impact of war on Sri Lankan Tamils*. Colombo: Vijitha Yapa.

Somasundaram, D., & Sivayokan, S. (2000). *Mental health in the Tamil Community*. Jaffna: Transcultural Psychosocial Organisation.

Sri Lanka Monitor (2001). Sri Lanka Project, The Refugee Council, 3, Bondway, London

Terr, L. (1994). *Unchained memories: True stories of traumatic memories, lost and found.* New York: Basic Books.

Tribe, R. (1998). What can psychological theory and the counselling psychologist offer in situations of civil conflict and war overseas? *Counselling Psychology Quarterly, 11,* 109-115.

UNHCR (United Nations High Commission on Refugees; 1999, 2000, 2002). Retrieved from http://www.unhcr.ch/cgi-bin/texis/vtx/statistics

Vinck, J. (1994, July 17-22). *The role of health psychology in the promotion of public health.* Paper presented at the International Congress of Applied Psychology, Madrid, Spain.

Yule, W. (1998). Psychological adaptation of refugee children. In J. Rutter & C. Jones (Eds.), *Mapping the field: Initiatives in refugee education.* Stoke on Trent, U.K.: Trentham Books.

6

Internally Displaced East Timorese: Challenges and Lessons of Large-Scale Emergency Assistance

Kathleen Kostelny and Michael Wessells

The attacks by the Indonesian paramilitaries on the people of East Timor in September of 1999 created mass displacement, destroyed most homes and property, and amplified poverty and hunger nationwide. The brutality of the attacks, which followed decades of oppression of the East Timorese and the betrayal of the UN referendum process for safe elections, created emotional and social wounds that needed to be addressed as part of the peace building agenda. Children and youth[1] were at significant risk for a number of negative outcomes. Children were largely unsupervised, as schools had been destroyed and parents were consumed with procuring basic necessities, and were at risk for physical injury from mines and broken glass while playing and scavenging in dangerous buildings and streets. Youth, who had played a key role in

---

[1] For this project, children are defined as people under 13 years of age, while youth include people between the ages of 13 and 24 years. Targeting this group allowed the inclusion of people who were at important decision points in their lives and who had the potential to contribute much in the peaceful reconstruction of their country.

the liberation struggle but had few prospects for jobs or positive life options, were frustrated, alienated, and at risk for engaging in delinquent and violent behavior. Both children and youth were at risk for disease and bad health from lack of shelter, as well as the emotional distress that accompanies homelessness.

To address this situation, a consortium of three NGOs (nongovernmental organizations)—Christian Children's Fund (CCF), International Rescue Committee (IRC), and Save the Children Federation (SCF), conducted an 18-month, national program of community-based psychosocial support for the care and protection of East Timorese children and youth. This chapter, which focuses primarily on the work of CCF, describes how psychosocial support was provided through the mobilization of communities to support children, the organization of structured recreational activities that strengthened children's resilience and reduced risk factors, and youth's participation in meaningful and economically productive activities.[2] Recognizing the interaction of physical and psychosocial needs in a complex emergency, the chapter also describes the integration of psychosocial support with shelter assistance to help meet basic needs, reduce stresses associated with homelessness, and enable sustainable return.

A key task of the chapter is to analyze the enormous challenges associated with working in East Timor following September of 1999. These challenges and obstacles are explored not to detract from the project, but to highlight the struggles and problem solving that characterized the project implementation. This discussion is offered in the spirit of increasing understanding of the complexities associated with humanitarian assistance in complex emergencies.

BACKGROUND

Sociopolitical Context

East Timor, a small country of approximately 800,000 people consists of half the island of Timor (West Timor is part of Indonesia), which lies 200

---

[2] The views expressed in this chapter are solely those of the authors and do not necessarily reflect those of CCF.

miles northwest of Australia. More than half its population is under 15 years of age. The East Timorese are primarily agrarian with a strong sense of identity and a strong sense of kinship. Tetum is the primary language, although 22 indigenous languages are spoken throughout the country. People live in small communities (aldeias) which are typically clustered together in groups of 3 to 6 to form a larger suco (with populations typically between 300–1000 people) with leadership from the suco chief (chiefe de suco). In addition to the suco chief, strong leadership at the clan level also exists. A council of elders, typically male, arbitrates local disputes and conflicts through a process of extended dialogue, negotiation, and mediation.

Cultural practices are grounded in a belief system in which spirituality is prominent. The East Timorese belief system, which is dynamic and reflects ideas from a variety of cultural systems, is part of a wider system of traditions and practices that confer identity and provide meaning regarding the world. Adults pass on this system of traditions to young people around the age of puberty through gender-specific rituals and instruction in traditions. Especially in rural areas, people believe that events in the visible world are caused by the unseen spirits of the ancestors who must be honored through traditions and rituals. Most extended families have a sacred family house that preserves the family history, houses sacred family objects, and serves as a bridge that connects the living members of the family with the family ancestors. Families perform rituals in the houses to thank the ancestors for a successful harvest and build the harmony with the ancestors on which good fortune depends. These local practices are interwoven with Catholicism, which the Portuguese established through four centuries of colonization. Today, more than 90% of East Timorese are Catholic. The Catholic Church has provided health services, education, orphanages and assistance to the poor, and has introduced beliefs and activities related to Catholicism that are a strong source of emotional and social support for many East Timorese.

The East Timor Crisis

The East Timor crisis is rooted in domination and mistreatment by outsiders, a pattern that has, over the years, created both strong internal cohesion among East Timorese people and deep fear and suspicion of outsiders. The Portuguese colonized and dominated East Timor from the 16th century until 1974. When the Portuguese withdrew in 1974, East Timor enjoyed a brief independence that was shattered by the Indonesian invasion in 1975. The Indonesian military occupation employed political repression, intimidation, torture, disappearances, political killings, and human rights abuses on a massive scale (Taylor, 1999). The East Timorese people launched an independence movement, the strength of which was based in part on the maintenance of traditional patterns of leadership and activity (Pinto & Jardine, 1997).

The Indonesian military fought young East Timorese independence supporters repeatedly and used arrests, detentions, and torture in hopes of weakening the movement. In November of 1991, the military massacred 273 East Timorese who had gathered at a memorial Mass to honor a young student who had been killed in the liberation struggle. Frustrated over its inability to eradicate or control the independence movement and the resistance of groups such as Fretilin, the Indonesian government turned control of East Timor over to Kopassus, the Indonesian army's Special Forces unit. In 1991, the occupation became increasingly brutal. The Indonesian army increasingly used "irregular" troops and allowed the activity of so-called paramilitaries, including infamous "ninja" gangs, who intimidated communities through torture, killings, and abductions. An estimated 200,000 people—approximately one fourth of the population—were massacred or allowed to die of starvation from 1975 until 1999. In 1998 and 1999, the Indonesian paramilitaries brutally attacked and assaulted villagers with machetes, knives, and guns, villages suspected of harboring liberation supporters (Taylor, 1999).

As international pressures for peace increased, the UN organized a referendum allowing the East Timorese to vote for either independence or an "autonomous" arrangement under Indonesian control. On August 29, 1999, 98% of the population voted, with 78% voting for independence. This outcome triggered a volcanic eruption of violence by pro-Indonesian paramilitaries supported by the Indonesian government. During this period of horrific violence in September of 1999, civilians were attacked on a wide scale by paramilitaries who brutalized and killed men, women, and children, and raped young girls and women. Rampaging through cities and the countryside, they attacked unarmed groups, killed opposition leaders, and burned nearly every building. In the capital, Dili, they destroyed more than 70% of the homes and businesses. Country-wide, there was an enormous loss of agricultural production, making food extremely scarce.

The paramilitary attacks displaced nearly half of the 800,000 people of East Timor. By mid-September of 1999, hundreds of thousands of people had fled their homes and were hiding in the mountains in East Timor, while approximately 150,000 others had been forced across the border into Indonesia-controlled West Timor, where they lived with great insecurity in refugee camps. During flight, many family members became separated from one another, leaving people to wonder about the safety of their children and other loved ones. While in flight or hiding, most people experienced fear of death and profound hunger, which is often what people in war zones report as their most difficult circumstance (Wessells & Monteiro, 2000).

With the arrival of international peacekeepers in late September of 1999, the militia fled back to West Timor and other parts of Indonesia, and the UN established the United Nations Transitional Authority in East Timor (UNTAET). Although disarmament and security were achieved relatively quickly, tensions remained high in many areas, particularly border areas. In addition, powerful needs existed for humanitarian assistance, including psychosocial support, throughout East Timor.

Mental Health and Psychosocial Implications

In complex humanitarian emergencies, many psychologists view their role within a mental health and illness idiom that focuses on traumatic symptoms and Western concepts of healing. In fact, ample evidence exists that armed conflict and displacement can lead to significant increases in traumatic symptoms as manifest in nightmares, flashbacks, avoidance of people and situations associated with life-threatening events, and hypervigilance (Marsella, Borneman, Ekblad, & Orley, 1994; Marsella, Friedman, Gerrity, & Scurfield, 1996; van der Kolk, McFarlane, & Weisaeth, 1996). In addition, the violence and displacement of armed conflict can lead to depression, anxiety, and other problems that are comorbid with traumatic symptoms (Apfel & Simon, 1996; Mollica et al., 1999).

Although no empirical reports existed when the authors first visited the capital of Dili in mid-October of 1999, it is likely that traumatic distress and depression were not uncommon among the East Timorese. The paramilitary assault had exposed large numbers of people to traumatic experiences such as attack, exposure to violence and death, uprooting, and sexual violence. In addition, many East Timorese had experienced repeated traumas during the occupation, making it more appropriate to speak of continuous (rather than post) traumatic stress (Straker, 1987). Indeed, CCF staff who had been working in East Timor reported sleep difficulties, exhibited sadness and lethargy, and expressed a strong sense of hopelessness about their situation.

For numerous reasons, however, trauma and the mental illness idiom provided a weak starting point for psychosocial assistance in East Timor. Trauma approaches cast people into victims' roles and emphasize deficits, whereas the East Timorese are survivors who have significant resilience. To label, as some psychologists have done, the East Timorese as a traumatized people is to pathologize and stigmatize individuals who have survived in the face of enormously difficult circumstances. In addition, the trauma idiom tends to medicalize problems having deep political, social, and historical roots (Bracken & Petty, 1998; Punamäki, 1989; Summerfield, 1999).

Through discussions with local people, it became clear that the current situation in East Timor—with its challenges of rebuilding community and struggling to meet the needs of families—provided stresses as great as those associated with armed conflict and direct experience of violence. Group discussions conducted by the authors with elders, women, and youth immediately after the September violence, revealed that their biggest stress was the lack of adequate shelter, which forced people to live in very crowded conditions, increased economic stresses, and exposed them to disease. People also identified poverty and hunger as priority issues, reminding us that armed conflict and its emotional sequelae were not necessarily the most impactful aspects of people's experiences.

Furthermore, it was learned by the authors (after building trusting relationships with community members) that another significant source of stress was the inability to conduct their traditional rituals and ceremonies. After the Indonesian militias attacked, they looted and destroyed many family houses (sacred structures which were not residences, but where traditional rituals were performed and special family objects were kept), damaging priceless family treasures and the spirits believed to reside within them. This spiritual calamity was amplified by the theft of gold items, which poor families could ill afford to replace. The failure to conduct regular rituals was a major source of stress and was believed to have caused sickness and other problems in the communities. This suggested to us that the traditions of the East Timorese were vital sources of psychosocial support and that the disruption of traditions was an important source of distress. Local people also reported that significant suffering and violence arose from disputes at the family and community levels. Difficult economic circumstances, together with population movements, suspicions about who had collaborated with the Indonesians, chronic poverty, and rising expectations and frustrations, created a climate ripe for the outbreak of local disputes among family and community members and associated stresses.

A trauma approach did not provide the holistic framework needed to encompass these various dimensions related to people's suffering and resilience. Furthermore, it focused mostly on past wounds rather than the current situation. A high priority in psychosocial programming is to help meet people's basic needs, the lack of which is a significant sources of stress. In addition, the trauma idiom provided a weak point of departure for psychosocial assistance to children, who are important resources in the post-conflict reconstruction of countries. Although anecdotal reports by some parents suggested that some East Timorese children exhibited problems such as nightmares and lack of concentration, many children and parents alike reported that lack of food and shelter were their most pressing needs. As in many post-war contexts, significant problems arose from the separation of children from their parents and families and also from the lack of parental supervision. Initial, direct observation by the authors and reports from Church personnel who worked with children indicated that parents were so preoccupied with gathering food and trying to meet basic needs that many children spent large amounts of time unsupervised on the streets, which posed risks of physical injury from playing in dangerous debris as well as risks for involvement in delinquency and crime. A trauma focus afforded little attention to these issues and did not point toward the need to mobilize communities around meeting children's needs.

A trauma approach also did not seem a fitting strategy for working with youth, who play a key role in the reconstruction of East Timor for peace. Youth had played a lead role in the liberation struggle, but felt alienated following liberation, as they were seldom consulted or centrally involved in high-level decisions about the reconstruction of East Timor. Moreover, since they lacked the technical skills and education required for employment by the influx of humanitarian organizations and the UN, their prospects for jobs and earning an income were bleak. Experience in many post-conflict environments indicates that youth have enormous potential to do good or to cause harm (Wessells & Kostelny, in press; Women's Commission, 2000). Not uncommonly, former youth combatants turn to violence as a means of meeting their basic needs and expressing their frustration following the signing of a peace accord (Boothby & Knudsen, 2000; Wessells & Jonah, in press). To focus on trauma as their central issue is to stigmatize youth who exhibit considerable agency and to orient psychosocial assistance toward counseling or other means of reducing trauma. What young people often need most, however, are skills and values for meaningful participation in society, means of meeting their basic needs, and a positive social role in their communities. Trauma and mental illnesses comprise a small part of a much wider mosaic of psychosocial issues facing such youth.

Issues of culture, power, and fear of outsiders also made a trauma approach a questionable starting point for psychosocial assistance in East Timor. East Timorese people, although very friendly, are wary of outsiders and attach great value to their own spiritual cosmologies and cultural modes of coping with difficulties. Many people reported that the practice of traditional ceremonies, such as harvest and burial rites, had provided significant psychosocial support during the Indonesian occupation, which often tried to suppress cultural practices that gave people strength (Kostelny & Wessells, 2002). In this context, to bring in outside concepts such as a trauma approach would risk doing damage to local practices. In a situation of desperation, local people often silence their own cultural practices, cling to Western approaches that have the imprimatur of science, or "play along" by giving the appearance of accepting outside approaches in hopes of getting food or money from powerful outsiders.

Too often, this begins a postcolonial process of undermining local under-standings and practices and of strengthening the influence of outsider ideas at the expense of local strengths and resources (Dawes, 1997; Wessells, 1999). Tacitly, a damaging message sent is that local views and practices are inferior. In the authors' field experience, this message can strengthen a colonially implanted sense of inferiority and weaken local people's belief that they have the capacity to build their own positive future. A high priority, then, is to start with local people's own under-standings of their situation and modes of coping.

Unfortunately, numerous problems can thwart this approach of starting with local understandings and modes of coping. First, emergencies pose enormous pressures for immediate action, making it difficult to learn about local modes of coping and resilience. Second, well-intentioned outsiders may adopt romanticized views of local culture, some of which may be harmful. Third, donor priorities often call for trauma approaches, which hold appeal in part because they yield measurable results, whereas the impacts of holistic approaches are more difficult to measure. Fourth, psychologists trained in clinical psychology are understandably reluctant to reach beyond their areas of training and expertise. Starting with people's own experience and coping mechanisms can often lead into territory more traditionally associated with anthropology. Constructed with awareness of these problems, this project assumed that each cultural system has discernible strengths and weaknesses and that outsider concepts and tools may have a role to play in assisting people.

Population of Focus

The project, called the Child and Youth Development Project (CYDP), focused on the children and youth of East Timor. The definition of highly specific vulnerable groups was avoided since nearly all children and youth had been affected by displacement, poverty, and hunger. Further, in the Timorese context, it was vital to avoid privileging some groups over others. Thus, all children and youth in a community were eligible to participate in the program. Recognizing that in many emergencies, outside agencies often help in cities more than in rural areas, this project supported not only urban but also rural areas that exhibited enormous needs.

INTERVENTION

Theory and Rationale

The CYDP was grounded in a risk-resilience framework that conceptualized risks as multiple, interacting, and demanding a holistic approach. During armed conflict children experience numerous risks, including attacks, the destruction of home, repeated and prolonged violence, injury, and the death of family members (Apfel & Simon, 1996; Cairns, 1996; Garbarino & Kostelny, 1993; Kostelny & Garbarino, 1994). While symptoms such as sleep disturbances, flashbacks, withdrawal, aggression, difficulty concentrating, and anxiety may result, it is the long-term developmental consequences that are the most devastating to children's social and emotional well being (Garbarino, Kostelny, & Dubrow, 1991a, 1991b; Garbarino & Kostelny, 1994). Armed conflict destroys the families and communities that provide security and structure in children's lives, and it violates the interpersonal trust needed for healthy social development (Wessells, 1998b; Wessells & Kostelny, 1996). Young children also suffer from their mothers' exhaustion, high levels of stress, and inability to provide emotional nurturance. Youth suffer loss of social trust, hopelessness, and are at risk for becoming perpetrators of violence (Wessells & Kostelny, in press).

These risks can only be understood, however, when they are situated in the context of powerful, chronic stressors such as poverty, malnutrition, and hunger. Among the worst chronic stressors throughout a child's development is poverty. Poverty adds significantly to the suffering of families already struggling to acquire basic necessities such as food, shelter, and health care. The risk-resilience framework accommodates these chronic and acute risks and recognizes their interaction with various protective factors. In these respects, it offers a useful, holistic model with which to view the situation of children in conflict and post-conflict situations (Garbarino et al., 1992; Wessells & Kostelny, 1996).

A risk accumulation model posits that the likelihood of developmental damage increases exponentially as the number of risk factors accumulate, particularly when the number of risk factors is already high (Garbarino et al., 1992a; Garbarino, Dubrow, Kostelny, & Pardo, 1992; Wessells & Kostelny, 1996). Research by Rutter (1979) found that the accumulation of three or more risk factors can produce ten times the negative outcomes than result from the presence of a single risk factor. In addition to the number of risk factors, their frequency and severity also influence the likelihood of developmental damage.

At the same time, protective factors and sources of resilience can buffer children from negative developmental outcomes. In conflict and post-conflict situations, children's well-being and level of resilience depends on the balance of risks and protective factors (Rutter, 1985, 1987). Children who experience a similar event, such as displacement, may react very differently depending on protective factors at the individual, family, and community levels, as well as cultural and spiritual supports available (Garbarino, Kostelny, & Dubrow, 1991a). For example, children exhibit significant variation in their temperament and their ability to cope with adversity. Furthermore, a child's age affects their response to stress, as young children have less cognitive competence than older children in making sense of stressors in their environment (Garbarino, Kostelny, & Dubrow, 1991b; Garbarino & Kostelny, 1996). At the family level, a stable emotional relationship with a nurturing caregiver is an important protective factor, while at the community level, social and emotional support from informal networks of women, groups of youth, and religious organizations function as protective factors (Lösel & Bleisner, 1990; Wessells & Kostelny, 1996).

In addition, cultural and spiritual supports often serve a protective function and enable resilience—as traditions, familiar rhythms, and normal daily practices confer a sense of meaning and continuity in life. Because stress as well as protective factors are culturally constructed, specific events such as loss or killing may have different meanings and risk values in different cultures (Wessells & Monteiro, 2001). Thus, when considering appropriate steps for intervention in a crisis, knowledge of cultural specific risk and resiliency factors is crucial.

The CYDP aimed to reduce risks and strengthen resilience through facilitating culturally grounded activities conducted by and for East

Timorese people at the community level. The well-being of children and youth is intertwined with the health of their communities. Thus, constructing healthy, low-risk communities is one of the highest priorities in and following armed conflict—as it is in such a context that children develop a sense of continuity and security, and youth develop the capacity for hope and social integration (Boothby, 1996; Wessells & Monteiro, 2000). Situation analyses by the consortium partners (CCF, IRC, and SCF) conducted in October and November of 1999 in urban and rural East Timor found that nearly all children and youth had been affected powerfully by displacement from their homes and by the destruction of their schools. Young children suffered from the disruption of stable caregiving routines, because their parents were focused on obtaining food and shelter, while youth—many of whom had been leaders in the liberation struggle—were now without constructive roles and responsibilities. These youth spent time idling and they expressed frustration over their marginalization in the new political process and their inability to receive skills training or obtain jobs.

The goal of the CYDP project was to enable East Timorese children and youth to resume healthy development through protection, psychosocial, and reconciliation activities that encouraged participation across gender, ethnic, socioeconomic, and geographic lines. The project strategy consisted of six elements:

1. Provision of a holistic response by linking psychosocial assistance with material support

Shelter was a high priority because 70% of East Timorese homes had been destroyed and children and families who lacked shelter were at risk for poor health and contracting diseases. In addition, parents who were preoccupied with obtaining shelter did not have the emotional resources to provide the necessary care and nurturance for their children. Accordingly, the project sought to address the physical, social, and emotional needs of children, youth, and communities by linking psychosocial supports with material assistance in the form of shelter. Although shelter construction was not part of the design of the CYDP, this complementary element was linked with a UNHCR-funded program of participatory shelter construction in communities served by the CYDP. Providing housing was an important element in reducing physical risks and emotional distress for children, in strengthening children's resilience by promoting a sense of security and stability, and in promoting greater supervision and emotional availability of parents and adults in children's lives.

2. *Community mobilization on behalf of children and youth through structured activities for children and development activities for youth*

Mobilizing communities on behalf of children is an important catalyst for healing, empowerment, and peace building. Armed conflict displaces people, destroys social trust, and disrupts normal patterns of community life. During and after the fighting, there is often a mixture of hopelessness, passivity, collective distress, and lack of community participation that are antithetical to the promotion of healthy child development. To reengage communities in effective development and peace building, it is vital to take an empowerment approach that enables communities to reassert control over their circumstances, to build hope, and to heal their emotional and social wounds (Wessells & Monteiro, 2000). Community-based programs can do this by mobilizing communities around the needs of children and youth, enabling adults and parents who may have been minimally functioning to become more fully engaged as parents and stewards of future generations.

A particularly useful way of mobilizing communities around children is via programs that help to restore a sense of safety, predictability, play, and emotional expression. This can be achieved by engaging children in structured activities appropriate to their age and culture—such as traditional songs, games, and traditions—while re-engaging parents, family, and community members around facilitating these activities and meeting children's needs (Gibbs, 1997; Reichenberg & Friedman, 1996; Wessells & Kostelny, 1996). For children, engaging in structured, supervised activities reduces their exposure to risks in the environment and increases their exposure to protective factors. This is especially important in post-conflict or emergency situations, as children often lack a sense of normalcy and structure, have little protection from dangerous activities or events, and lack strong emotional and social support from parents and other caretakers who themselves may have been strongly affected by the conflict (Boothby, 1988; Cairns, 1996).

Youth also need normalizing activities to restore healthy development and increase competencies and positive behavior through peer interactions. Some East Timorese communities had reported that youth were engaged in vandalism, interpersonal violence, verbal harassment, and drunkenness. Activities such as intervillage soccer matches supported the development of cooperative behavior, nonviolent conflict resolution skills, and positive social interaction, while reducing idling behavior and risks of engaging in delinquent and criminal activities.

3. Support for youth through positive roles and responsibilities

The project sought to engage youth in meaningful activities that helped them acquire a positive role in the community. Few, if any, opportunities existed for them to express their thoughts and feelings. Youth were strongly affected by the loss of important educational opportunities and by experiencing their communities ripped apart by suspicion, hatred, and violence. To enable positive youth development promoting tolerance, teamwork, and peace, the CYDP aimed to teach life and vocational skills, to promote youth leadership, and to provide positive roles and responsibilities. The project strove to enable youth to avoid negative developmental outcomes and to pursue positive developmental pathways leading to education, jobs, social integration, and poverty reduction.

4. Increasing geographic coverage via interagency collaboration that extended assistance into rural areas where needs were great

In most emergencies, NGOs compete for funding, and often cluster in the capital cities rather than in rural areas where needs are usually greatest. To enable coordination and wide geographic coverage, the Christian Children's Fund (CCF), the International Rescue Committee (IRC) and Save the Children Federation (SCF), worked as partners in a consortium. To provide assistance on a national scale, the three consortium partners worked together within a common theoretical framework using a geographic spread approach wherein each agency assumed responsibility for particular districts. The CYDP covered 9 of the 13 districts in East Timor.

5.   *Building capacities of East Timorese to provide community based psychosocial assistance*

Local communities provide a wealth of resources for supporting children. However, during conflict and post-conflict situations, these resources are often strained. Strengthening existing community resources helps to build local capacity on behalf of children. Moreover, community capacity building is vital for program sustainability beyond the funding period and for avoiding dependency on humanitarian organizations.

6.   *Rapid assessment and response*

This project sought to build local capacities by conducting rapid assessments, providing assistance, mobilizing communities. The foundation for the project was developed through initial situation assessments in October and November of 1999 by psychosocial consultants from the three consortium partners. Information was gathered on the current situation of children and youth, and needs and resources were identified at the community level and guided the CYDP. During project implementation, upon entering each community, a further rapid assessment was conducted to assess the immediate physical, social, emotional and cognitive needs of children and adolescents. The project then rapidly mobilized local adults to provide structured, normalizing activities that addressed these needs.

Implementation

Staffing

The overall staff structure included a *psychosocial coordinator* who had overall responsibility for the project and took on the project manager role. Technical assistance from *psychosocial consultants* was provided throughout the program from CCF headquarters with periodic in-country visits. The psychosocial coordinator supervised *program developers*, local staff who were trained in community-based development approaches and were responsible for community mobilization and training. The program developers, in turn, supervised *community and youth animators*, individuals from local communities who facilitated structured activities for children and youth, as well as the promotion of youth groups and activities. Other CCF staff provided logistical and financial support.

The Four Steps of the CYDP Program

The CYDP was implemented in four main steps, as outlined below.

Step One

The project hired as program developers 27 local East Timorese staff, including women and men who were mostly in their 20s and 30s and came from districts throughout East Timor. At the beginning of the project, external psychosocial consultants provided for the program developers a 2 week, intensive training on topics of child development, sensitizing adults to the effects of violence on children, implementing structured activities with children, conducting assessments, and keeping records.

The training was conceptualized as an opportunity for exchanging East Timorese and Western ideas about how to support children, assuming that each cultural system (East Timorese and Western) had particular strengths and weaknesses. Through asking elicitive questions about how local people view healthy children or what local activities families like to provide for children, expatriate consultants encouraged program developers to share local concepts of children's development, as well as songs, stories, and games that local people viewed as useful resources for children. The expatriate staff shared Western methods, such as expressive drawing and drama, as well as ideas and strategies about gender equity. The project strove to use a combination of Western and local tools to support children and adolescents in difficult circumstances while maintaining a stance of critical awareness. Through dialogue, the group decided which tools and approaches were most appropriate in the local context. Associated with the training were field activities and follow-up support that enabled the program developers to implement the activities in communities without constant field oversight.

Step Two

Having obtained the support of the village chief, the program developers facilitated group discussions with community leaders, parents, women, and youth to identify both their priorities and their existing community-based resources, such as women's groups and youth groups, for addressing the protection and psychosocial needs of children and youth. The goal was to understand and build on existing local resources, strengthening communities' and families' coping mechanisms and natural resilience.

Because East Timorese identified mothers as an important resource for supporting children and youth, mothers support groups were established and topics identified by local women were addressed in group discussions with the program developers and a community liaison (who was also a nurse and community worker). Discussion topics included health, child rearing, discipline, and nutrition issues.

In communities that already had an institution or group, such as the school or Church, that organized activities for children, the project supported these institutions as the center of activities. This proved to be valuable since in some communities, the September attacks had interrupted child-focused activities previously provided through the Church. The project provided materials such as recreation kits containing balls and other items, gained the support of influential adults, and introduced additional psychosocial concepts and resources to these local institutions.

Step Three

A key element of the CYDP was mobilizing communities to provide structured activities that would support children's healthy development. Community animators were identified who would provide regularly scheduled activities for both children and youth. Through dialogue at the community level, program developers recruited adults and youth who were respected in their communities and demonstrated ability and enthusiasm to work with children and youth. The selected people, called animators, then organized activities such as drawing, group discussions, theater and music, sports, and informal educational activities. In many cases, the community animators were already youth leaders whom the community had called on previously to engage youth in activities such as soccer. The program developers conducted 1- to 3-day trainings for the community animators based on the psychosocial training they had received during the project. The training focused on how to conduct activities that address children's psychosocial needs, support healing, promote healthy child development, and help develop positive social interactions with peers and adults.

Working outdoors in spaces that could accommodate many children, the animators organized activities such as singing and cooperative games. Children and youth participated in the identification of culturally appropriate activities, and the program developers provided technical assistance and training on the rationale behind the activities, which also included a Western perspective. For example, community animators thought it was useful to engage in music and dance because it made children happy and kept them out of trouble. Having learned this, the program developers organized discussions and showed examples of how music is an important cultural resource, provides emotional expression, and enables cooperation and a sense of solidarity.

In their community work, the animators adopted a human rights approach and encouraged age and gender inclusiveness. As this was not always congruent with local norms, the animators tried to avoid imposing outside ideas and created, instead, a dialogue with influential community members in which both sides brought ideas for discussion and mutual learning. This process enabled community members to think through how they might want to apply and adapt Western ideas in their local context, and allowed CCF staff a deeper understanding of local customs and practices.

The activities facilitated by the animators incorporated a holistic, ecological, culturally grounded approach that was structured to reduce risks and enhance protective factors. The goal was to create predictable routines and supervision by caring adults who provided safety, security, and structure for children in an environment that had been chaotic and dangerous. In addition, cooperative games and recreational activities fostered physical development through improved perceptual and motor skills, and social development and integration through developing friendships, communicating with adults, and strengthening conflict resolution skills. Group storytelling and free drawing allowed children to express feelings and emotions in a safe, non-threatening manner and supported emotional healing.

Step Four

To promote youth development, program development teams engaged youth in a dialogue about their aspirations, concerns, and reactions to the conflict. These discussions encouraged youth to reflect on their role in the community and share their own vocational, social, and emotional needs. These discussions generated ideas that subsequently were implemented with the help of the program developers. Youth activities included organization of activities for younger children, construction of youth centers, development and implementation of community service activities, establishment of interest-based groups, and provision of life skills and vocational training. Depending on the nature of the activities and using small grants provided by the CYDP, these groups addressed various interpersonal and developmental needs of youth and participated in income generating activities. In sum, the youth groups provided an expressive outlet through sports, drama, and music; helped youth plan for a more productive future through skills training and apprenticeship opportunities; and fostered the sense of capacity for community service through socially conscious activities.

CHALLENGES AND LESSONS LEARNED

Although the implementation of the CYDP went reasonably well in several areas, it was problematic in others. In a spirit of sharing, learning through experience, and wanting to improve humanitarian response in emergency situations, this section outlines in some detail a number of the challenges encountered and the lessons we learned along the way.

Laying the Groundwork:
Helping the Helpers

Before implementing a new program, such as the CYDP, CCF needed to attend to the needs and experiences of the existing local CCF staff. These staff, who had experienced the violence and destruction of September of 1999, would provide key logistics, security, and related support for projects such as the CYDP. A first line of defense in post-conflict situations should be to support and help the local staff, who often work under stressful conditions and are in need of training, support, and help in managing their experiences. However, such help is rarely available (Danieli, 1996; Garbarino, Dubrow, Kostelny, & Pardo, 1992; Wessells, 1998a).

A situation analysis conducted by the authors immediately following the violence in September of 1999 revealed that the local CCF staff were in need of help and support. Many staff members had been forced to flee from their communities, had their homes destroyed, and were missing family members. Some had suffered from hunger, subsisting on leaves and grass while hiding in the mountains from the Indonesian militia. The staff spoke of how they felt isolated, unsure of their roles and responsibilities, and anxious that they may be "mentally ill" or "traumatized."[3]

An immediate question was which priority was higher: responding to the staff's needs or conducting a situation analysis that would guide a psychosocial intervention for East Timorese children and youth. Although providing an intervention for the staff had not been part of the original plan, given the desperation of the staff, we requested from headquarters that the mission be changed to provide a brief, psychosocial intervention to the project's local staff, delaying the situation analysis. Having received permission to do so, we struggled with the question

---

[3]Based on remarks made by foreign staff and consultants with no psychosocial or mental health expertise.

of which type of intervention would be most beneficial to the staff. We had not come prepared to conduct a staff-focused intervention, and not knowing the culture, we were also unsure which support strategies might be effective in this particular context. However, in discussions with the staff, they quickly identified two sources of resilience—activities and rituals connected with the Catholic Church and their solidarity as East Timorese working together for the future of their country. However, as priests had fled and been dispersed, staff had not been able to participate in any Church related activities since before the September attacks. Our personal views of the Catholic Church as a patriarchal institution that did not afford the women equal rights led us to question whether to utilize the Church in supporting the staff. Eventually, however, we decided to suspend our personal doubts and to respect local views. This led to a twofold strategy of first organizing a solidarity Mass and then engaging the local staff in cooperative, normalizing activities that would strengthen their sense of solidarity. The normalizing activities aimed to mobilize staff members on behalf of children through a program of training and implementing recreational activities for children. We decided to offer the Mass and training as strictly voluntary activities, and all staff who had returned to the capital of Dili participated.

We also struggled with how to deal with previous comments made by expatriate CCF team members that had been interpreted by the local staff to mean that they were traumatized, needed therapy, and could not work for at least 6 months. Unfortunately, the previous team, whose mission was to locate CCF staff who had been dispersed, had not included anyone with psychosocial expertise and were not in a position to make diagnoses. However, we did not want to confuse the local staff or diminish the confidence and trust that they had developed with both teams—so we ended up explaining that in our experience in other extreme situations, some people show traumatic symptoms and benefit from therapy, but often many people benefit from sources of support in their family, community, and culture. We also explained that we were not qualified to provide therapy, but could assist with organizing a Mass and providing training for them to help local children return to normal life.

The intervention sought to promote the healing and recovery of staff through empowerment, solidarity, and finding meaning in their roles and responsibilities. The solidarity Mass built on aspects of resilience and reconnected local staff with an important practice that had previously been a key source of meaning and rhythm in their lives. The Mass enabled them to mark the end of their flight and horror, and it demarcated the transition to a time of freedom. Social support was promoted through a 2-week training and organization of children's activities that promoted teamwork, socializing, and highly participatory activities. Having completed the training, the staff set up a Child Friendly Space that provided structure and culturally appropriate activities such as singing, drawing, and playing local games. This combination of training and organization of normalizing activities enabled the staff to support each other and to recover their own capacity for laughter and play. Moreover, they were able to recover their role as effective staff, fostering feelings of empowerment and providing meaning for past, present, and future activities. Within CCF, this provided a platform for the development of the consortium's community-based program.

Working as a Consortium

Numerous challenges arose in connection with the consortium partners (CCF, IRC, and SCF) at the field level. Despite agreement at headquarters level on vision, strategy, and implementation of the project, the partner agencies and their field directors developed the project in radically different directions on the ground. The local directors differed in their interpretation of the current situation in East Timor and their vision of how to best implement the project. For example, in Dili, one agency director viewed East Timor as no longer representing an emergency situation but one that required a long-term development response. The agency therefore changed the original strategy from implementing normalizing activities and small youth projects toward development activities such as building a large youth center in each of the districts it served. A second agency initially wanted to conduct an extended assessment of communities rather than implement a rapid assessment and rapid response model. These decisions affected the rapidity with which each of the agency's psychosocial coordinators were hired and brought in, and thus what the coordinators did. Moreover, despite agreement at headquarters level between two of the partners to share an office during the first months of the consortium, this proved to be unworkable in the field.

With regard to staffing, the original intent of the project at headquarters level was to retain each agency's distinct characteristics with its own personnel and office space, while sharing training, finance, and logistical support. However, a decision was made in the field, urged by the psychosocial consultants at the time, to integrate the staff into a unified program, the CYDP. Although the East Timorese staff had wanted this decision, which enabled staff to see themselves as CYDP employees and as part of the same solidarity system, this decision reduced the distinctiveness of the three consortium partners' contributions. Although the three agencies shared office space for the CYDP project, problems related to command structure, personnel policies, and personality differences resulted in closure of the CYDP office after the first 4 months of operation. Two of the agencies retained a number of the program developers, but some were let go due to the change of strategy wherein one agency decided to build youth centers and to employ fewer program developers. Despite multiple explanations to the staff about the changes in policy and strategy, the closing of the office and the letting go of staff nevertheless caused confusion and a loss of morale when, in fact, their solidarity and unity within CYDP had been a source of pride and resilience.

Staff Issues

Local Staff Recruitment and Training

Although we wanted to open the recruitment to all qualified individuals, the hiring of local staff proved challenging in a number of ways. First, the consortium consultants struggled with how to recruit in a fair manner. Initially, the plan had been to post a notice for the positions of 27 program developers, describing their main responsibilities and necessary qualifications. However, this was discouraged on advice from CCF's country director (an expatriate East Timorese) because of the risk of violence. In one case where an NGO (nongovernmental organization) had posted a job, more than 4,000 people showed up and demanded to be interviewed, despite not having the required qualifications. A riot ensued when interviews were not given to everyone. Therefore, although "word of mouth" recruiting seemed biased, it was nevertheless used since people were desperate for jobs and the risk of violence was high. In the end, hundreds of people showed up and demanded to be interviewed, despite the fact that most lacked the qualifications of experience working with children, youth, or communities. To reduce the workload and mollify the crowd by interviewing most people, the consortium consultants interviewed people in groups, but in-depth interviews were not possible.

A further selection issue was that the massive destruction of infrastructure and chaos within the country made it impossible to check on references and qualifications. Many East Timorese had worked for the Indonesians, who had now fled the country and, even if found, could not be expected to provide accurate information. Another challenge was the low skill level of the local population. Despite the number of people who showed up to be interviewed, the overwhelming majority, due to their experience of marginalization and deprivation under the Indonesian occupation, lacked the skill level needed to implement the project. In the end, 27 program developers with a range of experiences and skills were hired. Whereas some program developers proved to be skilled at working with children and youth and mobilizing communities, others were not, and this was reflected in the inconsistency of project quality across communities.

Another underlying challenge was the resentment by local East Timorese toward the expatriate East Timorese who had left more than 20 years ago during the Indonesian occupation, but who had now returned to help rebuild the country. Because the expatriate East Timorese had technical skills and spoke English, they easily obtained highly coveted jobs with much higher salaries than local people could obtain. They were viewed by some as not only having abandoned the liberation struggle, but as now reaping the benefits denied to those who had stayed and suffered.

Furthermore, the UN and other non-NGOs had offered significantly higher salaries than what NGOs offered and had already hired the most skilled and qualified East Timorese by the time the project had begun. Thus, finding competent translators was an ongoing problem throughout the project period. In addition to not being able to compete with the salaries offered by the UN, it was not possible to find translators who not only could translate between Tetum (the official local language) and English, but who also knew the distinct dialects spoken in the rural project areas. Finally, finding a qualified East Timorese project manager had been viewed as a key part of capacity building. However, this proved impossible given the intense competition by the UN and other agencies, who could pay several times what NGOs were allowed to pay (NGOs had reached a common understanding regarding pay scales for jobs for the East Timorese). A project manager was hired initially, but left after a few weeks to take a better paying job.

Difficulties also arose in training the program developers. For one thing, psychosocial assistance was a new concept. Although the training aimed to be participatory and promote social support, 27 program developers was too large a group for the in-depth training that needed to occur. While there were three consultants at the time to do training, they did not speak the local language, and because only one translator could be found at the time, training in smaller groups was not possible. Thus, when it became apparent that much of the training had not "taken," a second "training of trainers" approach was implemented a few weeks later. In the latter, five of the program developers who had demonstrated leadership abilities were further trained by two of the consortium consultants in specific steps of participatory assessment, conducting focus groups, and community mapping. These staff, using a team approach, in turn trained the remaining 22 program developers.

Training continued throughout the program to reinforce key psychosocial concepts and skills. Frequently reinforced topics included the effects of violence on children, social and emotional requirements for healthy child development, engaging in emotionally expressive activities (e.g., free drawing without being graded or corrected), promoting gender equity, alternatives to physical punishment, and structuring activities in a way that promotes teamwork, cooperation, and nonviolence. These subsequent reinforcement trainings were most effectively carried out in the context of field visits to support learning and decision making about how to handle difficult situations. In one case that occurred early in the project, a debriefing following a community visit revealed that the local teacher had used a big stick to keep order and punish the children. In discussion, the staff agreed unanimously that threat and physical punishment were the only ways for adults to achieve "respect" from children. Exploration of their own experiences of physical punishment as children, however, revealed that they had felt anger and humiliation in response to such punishment. This opened the door for an exploration of alternative methods of discipline and the use of different strategies for managing behavior.

Although we wanted to "blend" local and Western concepts and approaches, the agenda of the authors and other consultants often conflicted with local norms. One of the biggest challenges was in training the program developers in child development—conveying the idea that young children had special needs and that engaging in developmentally appropriate activities was important for young children. Local program developers and communities saw youth as needing activities and jobs, but thought young children would be fine if left on their own. Consequently, on field visits, it was not uncommon to find young children on the sidelines watching older ones play. Local staff felt young children were "learning by watching," whereas Western trained child development specialists saw a strong need for engaging the children in physically stimulating, participatory activities with peers and adults.

Furthermore, the program developers' skill level was not always sufficient to allow effective training, monitoring, and evaluation of the community animators. Field visits by the technical consultants found that the training by program developers had not always "taken," and that corrections and adjustments to benefit the program had not always been made. For example, in one visit to a community, the authors observed the community animator grading free drawings (intended to be at children's discretion) using criteria such as accuracy and neatness and comparing equally the drawings of 5-year-olds with those of 12-year-olds. Not surprisingly, the younger children received "bad" marks.

A breakdown in training for both program developers and animators also occurred when all but one program developer quit 4 months before the completion of the project due to perceived differences in the consortium partners' policies requiring staff to pay taxes on their salaries. The hiring of new program developers coincided with the hiring of a new psychosocial coordinator who had skill in delivering psychosocial kits and implementing small start up grants but who lacked experience in psychosocial assistance. This led to a gap in training the new group of program developers in psychosocial concepts. In turn, the program developers did not adequately train the community animators in conducting activities with children. For example, during a field visit by one of the consultants, the community animator proudly showed the visitor all the new, untouched drawing supplies given by the project that he was keeping in a locked cabinet until the local school reopened; however, the intent had been to organize activities outside of school.

Expatriate Staff and Consultants

The original strategy was for each agency to have its own short-term technical consultants as well as a psychosocial coordinator who was responsible for providing long-term psychosocial assistance in the form of training, support, and supervision. However, a number of issues, including the level of urgency felt by the agency staff at field level, interfered with getting psychosocial coordinators in a timely and coordinated manner. It also proved difficult to find, on short notice, qualified, experienced individuals who could relocate to East Timor for at least a year. Until each agency found a long-term psychosocial coordinator, it sent in consultants and short-term coordinators who varied in their vision and skills. Some had decades of experience in humanitarian crises, while others were graduate students who had experience in developing countries but not in post- conflict or emergency situations. The consultants and short-term coordinators also varied in the amount of time they spent in the field (ranging from 2 to 6 weeks), thereby producing gaps in the project and making it difficult to give an effective hand-off to the next person.

It was 6 months before all three agencies had a permanent psychosocial coordinator. Moreover, because an East Timorese project manager was never found for two of the agencies, including CCF, the management role fell on the psychosocial coordinators. Furthermore, the departure after 5 months of the long-term psychosocial coordinator for CCF was followed by the hiring and departure (after another 3 months due to a family emergency) of a second psychosocial coordinator. A third coordinator, hired for the last 3 months of the project, was experienced in emergency situations and efficient in the distribution of materials, but did not have a psychosocial background. The departure of coordinators and the gaps in program resulting from a lack of good hand-off, resulted in frustration by the program developers and disruptive discontinuities in the project.

Implementation in Communities

Although the project was successful in providing normalizing activities for children and development activities for youth, numerous challenges arose during the implementation of project activities. First, many of these communities suffered "assessment fatigue" from repeated visits by international groups, who wanted to know their "needs," but whom communities perceived as not delivering. A major expectation upon entering communities is that help will be given, even if explicit promises are not made. Similarly, delays in implementation are viewed as a sign of a lack of commitment. Unfortunately, delays in the delivery of materials by UNHCR in the shelter assistance program were perceived by communities as "broken promises" by CCF, which hindered progress in providing the psychosocial component of the project. In addition, delays in the implementation of the psychosocial project occurred due to a lack of transportation during the first months of the project until purchased vehicles arrived from overseas. These transportation problems prevented staff from consistently reaching project communities and forced them to rely on vehicles borrowed from other agencies, which had their own emergencies and changes of plans. Failure to return to communities when expected because of lack of vehicles (telephones in rural communities were non-existent and thus calls to inform communities could not be made) were interpreted by community members as a lack of commitment by the project.

Delays experienced in the distribution of psychosocial kits—comprised of basic education supplies and recreational and sports equipment—also produced frustration in the communities, the program developers, and the psychosocial coordinators. Procurement of supplies went through the consortium partner that was managing finances and logistics, and their rules and restrictions prevented rapid acquisition of materials. Getting the requisite number of price quotes for supplies from overseas took valuable time, even though, in some cases, materials were available locally. When materials finally arrived, communities were sometimes disappointed even further. For example, the procurement officer ordered children's soccer balls instead of regulation size balls, insulting youth and frustrating the children who wanted "real" equipment. In another instance, boxes of thread for a women's weaving project to make the tais (traditional cloth), consisted of only white thread instead of the multitude of colors they had requested. These problems raised questions about the sensitivity of the project to the views of children, youth, and women. Fortunately, many of these issues were reduced when each agency took on their own finance and procurement responsibilities later in the project. For example, women in the weaving project were given a fixed amount of money and allowed to purchase supplies locally, thereby giving them control by enabling them to compare prices locally and select their own materials.

Urban–rural issues also affected the project implementation. Although the CYDP was headquartered in the urban capital, Dili, where large numbers of unskilled youth had streamed into the city looking for scarce jobs, it was implemented mainly in distant rural districts. While CCF hired drivers and security guards from the urban community for the Dili office, the number of youth having needs in the city was great. At one point, a group of angry youth had threatened staff at the CCF headquarters. The country director was able to address the needs of the angry group in a small way by providing them with soccer balls and organizing soccer competitions between groups of youth. CCF also supported urban youth associations, such as IMPETTU, a group of university students that provided a wide array of recreational, educational, and skills training opportunities for more than 200 children and youth. CCF supplied IMPETTU with tables, chairs, and books, and also provided materials to fix the windows and doors of a building that had been destroyed. These tangible improvements, implemented in an area outside that of the CYDP, were important in building good relations with area youth and enabling a large number of youth to receive support.

Unintended Consequences

Although the Western staff strove to be culturally sensitive and to support local cultural resources, the time urgency associated with the rapid response made it difficult to conduct a careful cultural assessment. Many issues were circumvented by the guidance of the CCF country director, an East Timorese expatriate. Still, lack of a thorough understanding of East Timorese culture contributed to tensions and misunderstandings throughout the project. For example, during the initial intervention with CCF staff, a modest lunch was provided to the staff. Because food was scarce, the authors, as psychosocial consultants, left during lunch so that there would be more food for the staff. However, we learned later that the staff viewed our behavior as a lack of solidarity with the staff and that they would have preferred us to be "all together" with little food rather than "separate" with sufficient food. It took time to establish the trust and relationship needed for the East Timorese expatriate country director to feel comfortable "correcting" us in such matters, as East Timorese consider such directness towards foreigners as rude.

Given the East Timorese's history of oppression and domination by the Portuguese and Indonesians, communities were also distrustful of the "mali" (outsiders) and, in the beginning, did not share many cultural rituals or traditions with us. Learning in significant depth about culture and rituals was also something we did not do well in the rapid response situation we faced, since building trust takes time. In some cases, we did not know that we did not know something. For example, psychosocial consultants initially expressed a desire to work with local healers and persistently raised this option with communities. Local people often listened politely and even agreed, but the doors did not open. Subsequently, we learned that local people held beliefs that healers would be contaminated by associating with outsiders. Learning about the local culture required building stronger relationships, which took time to develop. As another example, it was only midway through the project that the authors learned of the importance of the family houses. It was still later that the authors learned of the psychosocial support provided by the rituals performed in the houses and the significance of the stresses associated with not performing the rituals. Having this information earlier would have impacted the design of the psychosocial intervention, but local people felt comfortable disclosing their beliefs and practices only after they had had longer relationships with the authors.

In some situations, we thought we were following the correct cultural script, only to discover later that the situation involved more complexities than had been envisioned. For example, we followed the advise of East Timorese expatriates to seek permission from the *suco* chiefs (the political heads of villages) as a means of gaining entry into communities to implement the project. Subsequently, we learned of another community and cultural structure, the clan chief, who wielded different power and respect in the community and was capable of thwarting the initiatives of 'the *suco* chief. In retrospect, the initial process of gaining permission and showing respect also should have involved the clan chiefs.

Another tension concerned our privileged status as foreigners. Although international workers faced difficult conditions, they were very well off compared to the East Timorese. A huge discrepancy existed between expatriates' salaries and those of local people. For example, international workers could easily afford multiple daily meals at the restaurants that had sprung up and catered to the international humanitarian and development agencies. Eating even once in such a restaurant was beyond the means of nearly all the East Timorese.

In addition, agency policy sometimes contradicted cultural norms. For example, it was customary for the East Timorese, if they had a vehicle, to give a ride to those who needed one. However, the policies of most agencies, CCF included, prohibited staff from giving rides to nonstaff or to local staff during nonwork hours. Although this policy was designed to insure staff protection, it created the appearance that every foreigner had their own new, air conditioned vehicle at their disposal and were unwilling to help local people, who lacked basic transportation. As the white vehicles passed by, East Timorese people experienced incredulity, frustration, and feelings of being treated as second-class citizens in their own country. The East Timorese people's sense of relief over the initial arrival of peacekeepers and humanitarians slowly gave way to attitudes of bitterness and resentment. Within 1 year, some East Timorese even referred to the influx of humanitarian groups as the "third occupation" (after the Portuguese and Indonesians).

The presence of humanitarian groups also had a profound effect on local norms and social interactions. Although the project had assumed initially that community members would willingly volunteer their services for the good of children and youth, this proved to be extremely problematic in some communities. First, in some communities, the concept of volunteerism applied at the family level, but not the community.

Second, the influx of the UN and international groups operating with enormous sums of money created expectations of pay that undermined volunteerism. For example, in delivering sewing machines to communities in one district, problems arose when community members wanted to be paid a relatively large amount of money for unpacking the sewing machines, while the CYDP assumed that the community would naturally volunteer their labor. Of course, children and youth also needed money. Some children skipped school in order to watch the cars of UN workers while they ate lunch in hopes of getting an occasional dollar. Other East Timorese people told us that begging was unknown before the arrival of foreigners. Thus the arrival of foreigners with large sums of money had unforeseen negative consequences.

Challenges also arose in connection with divergent understandings of "youth." For example, youth were defined in East Timor as young men who were not yet married, while girls, who typically married young in the rural areas, were no longer considered youth. Thus we found groups of 30-year-old men taking over recreational equipment meant for children and adolescents, while young girls did not participate in activities because of their status and responsibilities as wives and mothers. Incorporating additional activities for girls required creativity and initiative that varied from community to community and depended on the skill and motivation of each team of program developers.

Lessons Learned

Six key lessons emerged from our experience in East Timor:

1. A holistic response is necessary in providing psychosocial assistance in emergency situations. Without the provision of shelter and material assistance, the CYDP would have achieved far less impact. In addition, local people related their stresses to lack of material goods and inability to meet basic needs.

2. To prevent assessment fatigue and frustration, agencies need to provide immediate assistance from the time they enter a com-

munity. The provision of structured activities that enable safety, play, predictability, and positive interactions and that can mobilize adults on behalf of children is a very useful starting point in community empowerment and assistance. This strategy would have been even more helpful if additional time had been taken for the hiring of local staff.

3. Helping the helpers is a high priority. CCF could not have undertaken their community-based work if it had not taken care of its existing staff who provided a platform for the CYDP. Too often, helping the helpers, if done at all, is an afterthought. However, in situations of conflict and post conflict, caring for the needs of local staff should be an integral part of humanitarian organizations' response.

4. When working as a consortium, it is best to allow each agency operational autonomy. Giving each agency leeway to follow their own procedures and policies minimizes difficulties and tensions while maintaining the unique characteristics of each agency.

5. Working with local cultural resources requires significant trust and understanding of local beliefs and practices. Both of these are difficult to construct quickly in the heat of an emergency. A key priority for teams, in advance of their departure, is to access the anthropological literature on the area of interest or to dialogue with cultural experts in advance.

6. Work with youth is crucial in post-conflict reconstruction for peace. The CYDP was the only international response to the needs of youth, and a much wider, integrated response was required. The needs of youth in Dili had proven to be a serious gap in the response of humanitarian organizations. This gap subsequently led to an escalation of frustration and violence.

This last lesson provides an important note of caution in future emergencies. Following political violence, waves of criminal violence often occur, and much of it is committed by youth who lack education, job skills, and positive life options. Images of youth as troublemakers and as people who exercise little responsibility have undermined donors' faith in youth. As this project illustrates, however, youth have significant capacity to help in emergency situations and to contribute to their communities. International agencies would do well to recognize that it is youth who will either continue cycles of violence or become agents of peacebuilding.

EVALUATION

An evaluation of the CCF project was conducted by two members of the CCF Technical Assistance Group. The methodology included direct observation, key informant interviews (with program and field staff, teachers, youth leaders, and community leaders), focus group discussions (with youth, women, and community leaders), and general community discussions. In addition, for all 181 communities in which CCF worked, the evaluation team reviewed available documents—including monthly field reports, quarterly project reports, proposals from communities, and reports and memos written by psychosocial coordinators, program developers, program managers, consultants, the community liaison officer, and the country director. In-depth interviews and group discussions also were conducted with the program developers, the psychosocial coordinator, the program manager, community animators, the community liaison officer, and the country director for the program.

The evaluation was designed to achieve wide geographic coverage, stimulate self-reflection, and enable intensive learning about the project in a small number of communities. The evaluation team selected and visited a representative sample (n = 20) of the 181 *aldeias* in which CCF had worked. The sample was constructed with the intention of including a mixture of rural and more urban communities, representing very different situations. Also, the team used reports from staff to identify and include in the sample a mixture of communities in which program success had been relatively strong and communities in which numerous difficulties had been encountered. This mix of successes and difficulties was intended to reveal important lessons that might have implications for emergency work in other contexts.

In different communities, different evaluation methods were used, depending on the amount of time available and the ease of access to community members. In all 20 communities, data were collected through community and youth group discussions. A subsample of four communities was examined in greater depth and a more intensive, multimodal data collection procedure was applied—which included additional discussions with community groups, women's groups, and gender specific groups for young men and young women. Key informant interviews with teachers, youth group leaders, project volunteers, religious leaders, leaders of women's cooperatives, and *suco* and *aldeia* chiefs were also conducted.

Although the evaluation revealed mixed results, major accomplishments in three areas were found. First, the structured activities provided a sense of normalcy, continuity, and hope that helped young children cope in an environment saturated with uncertainty and discontinuity. They also provided a catalyst for organizing communities and groups that, under great stress, had lapsed into relative inactivity and disorganization by helping to structure daily life. More than 20,000 children and 17,000 youth participated in the activities, and many reported that before the project, few if any activities had been available. Interviews revealed that prior to the structured activities children and youth spent their time idling or engaged in delinquent behavior, such as throwing rocks at cars. Parents and community members reported that the activities provided structure to the children's days, and that the children were happier and more content as a result of being able to participate.

Second, leadership activities and vocational and employment opportunities for more than 500 youth were provided. The inclusion of more than 200 youth in the design and implementation of the psychosocial program for younger children was an important element in promoting youth's self-esteem and leadership. As youth were mobilized and given key roles in their communities, their perception of themselves as active members in the rehabilitation of their communities increased greatly. Discussions with youth and key informants indicated that the skills and vocational training for more than 300 youth had reduced their risks of marginalization, feelings of helplessness and boredom, and contributed to feelings of renewed hopefulness about their future and self-efficacy. The small grants for income generation projects were remarkably successful in providing opportunities where few had existed before. The following is one example, which illustrates a successful youth income generation activity.

In one community in Lautem district, 60 youth maintained a chicken cooperative. The chicken cooperative existed before the referendum in August 1999 but had been destroyed by the Indonesian militia. CCF supplied 91 chickens to the cooperative, while the youth constructed the chicken houses from local trees, gathered food, and fed them. The youth generated income through the sale of eggs and young chickens. Subsequently, they expanded the project community-wide, and the youth mentored other young people in starting their own chicken farms at home to assist with the family income. The youth also modeled tolerance, peacebuilding skills, and reconciliation at the community level. The president of the cooperative had been active in the resistance movement, while the vice-president of the cooperative had been employed by the Indonesian army. Now, however, they worked together "to be one community again" and "to develop our new country."

A third accomplishment was that the project created a reasonably holistic response to a complex emergency. Although shelter construction was technically part of a parallel project, it had intentionally been implemented as a complement to the psychosocial project. The shelter construction process was participatory in that the communities selected which shelters to rebuild, and local people donated much labor. Local people said these activities, which helped to build trust in CCF, had made them more hopeful toward the future.

As could be expected on the basis of the challenges outlined above, however, weaknesses and inconsistencies occurred. Because of the low skill level of the program developers and the gaps in service of the psychosocial coordinators, monitoring and evaluation of the project was weak, and this reduced the ability to adjust the project when necessary. For example, although gender equity for participation in structured activities and for engaging community and youth animators was achieved in some activities, equity was not achieved in the most popular activities, such as guitar playing and soccer. In addition, males dominated the vocational skills training and employment opportunities. Too often, older children benefited most from the structured activities. In the majority of communities, group games and activities catered to older children (aged approximately 8 and above) while younger children sat on the sidelines and watched. In future interventions, much more training and attention needs to be given to younger children and how to creatively address gender inequities.

REFERENCES

Apfel, R. J., & Simon, B. (Eds.). (1996). *Minefields in their hearts: The mental health of children in war and communal violence.* New Haven, CT: Yale University Press.

Boothby, N. (1996). Mobilizing communities to meet the psychosocial needs of children in war and refugee crises. In R. J. Apfel & B. Simon (Eds.), *Minefields in their hearts: The mental health of children in war and communal violence* (pp. 149-164). New Haven, CT: Yale University Press.

Boothby, N., & Knudsen, C. (2000). Children of the gun. *Scientific American, 282*(6), 60-65.

Bracken, P. J., & Petty, C. (Eds.). (1998). *Rethinking the trauma of war.* London: Free Association Books.

Cairns, E. (1996). *Children and political violence.* Oxford: Blackwell.

Danieli, Y. (1996). Who takes care of the caretakers? In R. J. Apfel & B. Simon (Eds.), *Minefields in their hearts: The mental health of children in war and communal violence* (pp. 189-205). New Haven, CT: Yale University Press.

Dawes, A. (1997, July). *Cultural imperialism in the treatment of children following political violence and war: A Southern African perspective.* Paper presented at the Fifth International Symposium on the Contributions of Psychology to Peace, Melbourne, Australia.

Garbarino, J., Dubrow, N., Kostelny, K., & Pardo, C. (1992). *Children in danger: Coping with the consequences of community violence.* San Francisco, Jossey-Bass.

Garbarino, J., & Kostelny, K. (1993). Children's response to war: What do we know? In L. Leavitt & N. Fox (Eds.), *The psychological effects of war and violence on children* (pp. 23-40). Hillsdale, NJ: Lawrence Erlbaum Associates.

Garbarino, J., & Kostelny, K. (1996). The effects of political violence on Palestinian children's behavioral problems: A risk accumulation model. *Child Development, 67*, 33-45.

Garbarino, J., Kostelny, K., & Dubrow, N. (1991a). *No place to be a child: Growing up in a war zone.* San Francisco: Jossey Bass.

Garbarino, J., Kostelny, K., & Dubrow, N. (1991b). What children can tell us about living in danger. *American Psychologist, 46*, 376-383.

Kostelny, K., & Garbarino, J. (1994). Coping with the consequences of living in danger: The case of Palestinian children and youth. *International Journal of Behavioral Development, 17*(4), 595-611.

Kostelny, K., & Garbarino, J. (2001). The war close to home: Children and violence in the United States. In D. Christie, R. Wagner, & D. Winter (Eds.), *Peace, conflict and violence: Peace psychology for the 21st century* (pp. 110-119). Upper Saddle River, NJ: Prentice Hall.

Kostelny, K., & Wessells, M. (2002). *Mapping local cultural resources for psychosocial support in East Timor: A pilot study.* Richmond: CCF International.

Lösel, F., & Bliesener, T. (1990). Resilience in adolescence: A study on the generalizability of protective factors. In K. Hurrelmann & F. Losel (Eds.), *Health hazards in adolescence.* New York: Walter de Gruyter.

Marsella, A., Bornemann, T., Ekblad, S., & Orley, J. (Eds.). (1994). *Amidst peril and pain: The mental health and well-being of the world's refugees.* Washington, DC: American Psychological Association.

Marsella, A., Friedman, M., Gerrity, E., & Scurfield, R. (Eds.). (1996). *Ethnocultural aspects of posttraumatic stress disorder.* Washington, DC: American Psychological Association.

Mollica, R. F., McInnes, K., Sarajlic, N., Lavelle, J., Sarajlic, I., & Massagli, M. P. (1999). Disability associated with psychiatric comorbidity and health status in Bosnian refugees living in Croatia. *Journal of the American Medical Association, 282,* 433-439.

Pinto, C., & Jardine, M. (1997). *East Timor's unfinished struggle: Inside the Timorese resistance.* Boston: South End.

Punamäki, R. (1989). Political violence and mental health. *International Journal of Mental Health, 17,* 3-15.

Rutter, M. (1979). Protective factors in children's responses to stress and disadvantage. In M. W. Kent & J. E. Rolf (Eds.), *Primary prevention of psychopathology* (Vol. 3, pp. 49-74). Hanover, NH: University Press of New England.

Rutter, M. (1985). Resilience in the face of adversity: Protective factors and resistance to psychiatric disorder. *British Journal of Psychiatry, 147,* 598-611.

Rutter, M. (1987). Psychosocial resilience and protective mechanisms. *American Journal of Orthopsychiatry, 57,* 316-331.

Summerfield, D. (1999). A critique of seven assumptions behind psychological trauma programmes in war-affected areas. *Social Science and Medicine, 48,* 1449-1462.

Taylor, J. (1999). *East Timor: The price of freedom.* London: Zed Books.

van der Kolk, B. A., McFarlane, A. C., & Weisaeth, L. (Eds.). (1996). *Traumatic stress: The effects of overwhelming experience on mind, body, and society.* New York: Guilford.

Wessells, M. G. (1998a). Humanitarian intervention, psychosocial assistance, and peacekeeping. In H. Langholtz (Ed.), *The psychology of peacekeeping* (pp. 131-152). Westport, CT: Praeger.

Wessells, M. G. (1998b). The changing nature of armed conflict and its implications for children: The Graça Machel/U. N. Study. *Peace & Conflict: Journal of Peace Psychology, 4*(4), 321-334.

Wessells, M. G. (1999). Culture, power, and community: Intercultural approaches to psychosocial assistance and healing. In K. Nader, N. Dubrow, & B. Stamm (Eds.), *Honoring differences: Cultural issues in the treatment of trauma and loss* (pp. 276-282). New York: Taylor & Francis.

Wessells, M. G., & Jonah, D. (in press). Reintegration of former youth soldiers in Sierra Leone: Challenges of reconciliation and post-accord peacebuilding. In S. McEvoy (Ed.), *Youth and post-accord peacebuilding.* South Bend, IN: University of Notre Dame Press.

Wessells, M. G., & Kostelny, K. (1996). *The Graca Machel/U.N. study on the impact of armed conflict on children: Implications for early intervention.* Working paper prepared for UNICEF.

Wessells, M. G., & Kostelny, K. (in press). The plight of children in conflict and post-conflict societies. In A. Schnabel & A. Tabyshalieva (Eds.), *Women and children in post-conflict peacebuilding.* Tokyo: U. N. University for Peace.

Wessells, M. G., & Monteiro, C. (2001). Healing wounds of war in Angola: A community-based approach. In D. Donald, A. Dawes, & J. Louw (Eds.), *Addressing childhood adversity* (pp. 176-201). Cape Town: David Philip.

Women's Commission for Refugee Women and Children (2000). *Untapped potential: Adolescents affected by armed conflict.* New York: Women's Commission.

PART II

PROGRAMS IN SOUTH AND NORTH AMERICA

7

Internally Displaced Colombians: The Recovery of Victims of Violence Within a Psychosocial Framework

Jorge Enrique Buitrago Cuéllar [1, 2, 3]

In this following chapter we describe the psychosocial focus and recent experience of a pioneering organization in Colombia, that has developed its work as a nongovernmental organization (NGO) since its foundation in 1992, under the name Corporación AVRE (Apoyo a Víctimas de Violencia Sociopolitical pro Recuperación Emocional—Support and Emotional Recuperation for Victims of Sociopolitical Violence). We describe the focus of the intervention, which is characterized by the interaction and coordination of organizations that provide support to individuals and communities affected by political violence. In addition, the intervention provides services directly to organizations of people who have

[1]The author wishes to express his appreciation to the following members of Corporación AVRE for the invaluable assistance they provided in the preparation of this chapter: Elena Martín Cardinal, Gloria Amparo Camilo, Óscar Gómez, and Dora Lucía Lancheros.

[2]The editors wish to thank Jaime Iniguez for his work on the translation of this chapter from Spanish into English.

[3]Corporación AVRE has published a variety of training materials in Spanish and English based on the work described in this chapter. Interested readers can contact Corporación AVRE at the address listed on the Author Affiliations page.

themselves been affected by acts of violence. A central theme in our work is an understanding of emotional support as dynamically linked to community processes, sociopolitical and cultural contexts, and the resources of those affected and their families and social networks. The three modalities that comprise the Corporation's model of psychosocial intervention include the following: procedures and actions for strengthening community-based organizations; the provision of direct clinical services; and the training of Popular (i.e., paraprofessional) Therapists (PTs) and Multipliers of Psychosocial Action, Mental Health, and Human Rights (MPAs). Each of these modalities is described next.

In this chapter, we focus particularly on the important and most recently developed modality, the training of the PTs and MPAs. By training community members to work as PTs and MPAs, we are able to significantly expand the reach of our mental health, psychosocial, and human rights activities. Both the PTs and the MPAs are capable of recognizing the impact that sociopolitical violence has on people's mental health as well as on the fabric of society, and both are capable of providing assistance in the form of therapy (psychological "first aid") or complementary psychosocial activities provided within a framework of institutional coordination, designed to counteract the effects of the violence.

The training of PTs and MPAs is a project that is currently in development. A pilot implementation of the training has been conducted and evaluated, and the training has been adjusted based on that pilot experience and is now being implemented again. In addition, a publication with the complete description of the training process and the materials needed to carry it out it is currently being prepared, so that it may be reproduced by other organizations and individuals, with the adaptations that are considered appropriate for each context.

BACKGROUND

Sociopolitical Context

Colombia has a population of 42 million inhabitants living in an area of 1,200,000 square kilometers. The country has very favorable conditions for its socioeconomic and political development due to its location, in the northwest region of South America, with coasts along the Atlantic Ocean on the northern side and the Pacific Ocean on the western side. The country also has huge natural resources, such as one of the largest water reserves in the world, a vast biodiversity, and a wealth of natural resources including petroleum and a variety of minerals. Paradoxically, throughout its history, Colombia's favorable conditions have not liberated the country from poverty and social inequality, due to the orientation of its economy toward capitalism and globalization.

The majority of Colombia's inhabitants are *mestizos*, resulting from the mixture between Spaniards and indigenous people. However, some indigenous groups as well as Black minority communities brought to the country from Africa survived the extinction and racial mixture of the colonial period. After the wars for independence from the Spanish monarchy beginning in 1819, the country constituted itself as a republic. During the rest of the 19th century, and a good part of the 20th century, the country suffered from constant and successive internal wars and bloody partisan quarrels. In the end, the confrontations were a response to the conflicts for the search for power and control of the land. This in turn, by means of violence, consolidated the social structure inherited from the colonial era, which was characterized by inequality and the exploitation of a large poor majority by a privileged minority.

Violence has been the backdrop of the national stage and the instrument by which many rural farmers were and continue to be displaced from their lands. This took place especially in the regions considered economically strategic and productive. The violence acquired especially cruel characteristics toward the middle of the 20th century. Around that same time, organizations of armed peasants arose in resistance to these oppressive conditions, and have by now formed the strongest guerilla group in the country, called: Fuerzas Armadas Revolucionarias de Colombia (FARC; Revolutionary Armed Forces of Columbia). This guerilla movement adopted a Marxist ideology in the 1960s, in the international context of the "cold war"; beginning in that same decade, other armed insurgent movements developed. Of those, currently in existence is the Ejército de Liberación Nacional (ELN; National Liberation Army), whose initial ideology was influenced by the Cuban revolution.

Faced with these insurgent forces, the Colombian state responded with repressive actions by means of its armed forces. These repressive

actions included the so called "Dirty War," which has included violations of human rights, legislative acts that curtailed civil liberties, and the
persecution of legitimate civilian organizations and dissident political
parties. In addition, since the 1980s Columbians have witnessed the active participation of another illegal armed group, the so-called *paramili-
tares*. This group is financed by private wealthy sectors, and operates
with the acquiescence and even complicity of the state's security organizations. The *paramilitaries* have assumed a good portion of the duties of
the "dirty war," not only against the insurgents, but also against civilians, leftist political organizations, human rights activists, and all others
whom they consider to be sympathizers or collaborators with the guerillas or supporters of leftist ideologies.

Another aspect of the distorted social conditions and the violence
that the country has tolerated during the last three decades is the scourge
of drug trafficking. The country has turned into the world's central location of this illegal business. In addition, the country is the primary pro-
ducer of substances like cocaine and heroin, which are in great demand
and are well paid for by consumers in Europe and the United States.

In sum, there are multiple factors that contribute to the dynamic of
violence in Colombia. First is the ancestral and privileged domination of
the land and the natural resources by the country's wealthy minority.
Second is the adherence to a neo-capitalist economic model that imposes
great inequality, concentration of wealth, and increased poverty. Third,
there is only a pseudodemocracy, with no groundwork laid for the development of a genuine democracy. This is the result of the control of the
state by a dominant class with a history of intolerance, expressed
through the two traditional political parties. A fourth factor contributing
to violence in Colombia consists of the weak institutions, corroded by
corruption and at the service of economically powerful sectors of society.
A fifth factor is the existing drug-dealing mafias who strengthen themselves through a business that generates enormous returns and in which
other illicit activities, like arms trading, are included. Sixth, insurgent
organizations (guerillas) have a long trajectory and their military and
financial capacity has increased, particularly so for one of the guerrilla
organizations, FARC. A seventh factor is the growing presence of other
armed organizations of "self-defense." These armed insurgent groups
were initially supported by the State's public armed forces and govern-

ment sectors through the omission, acquiescence or complicity in the subversive strategy of "dirty war." They are also financed by wealthy people, various economic groups, drug-traffickers, and even by multinational corporations.

All of these factors play key roles in the deteriorating Colombian armed conflict that is mainly directed, with extreme cruelty, toward the defenseless civilian population. As noted in a recent study: "Different sources have proven that the paramilitary model is the main factor in the humanitarian deterioration, and it has become increasingly clear that the violence is extending throughout the country with the consent and sponsorship, and the action or absence of action of the political authorities, and/or of the Colombian military, both at the national and regional levels" (Human Rights Commission of Columbia, 2000).

The most worrisome aspects of the country's current human rights situation are the increase in massacres, the forced displacement of people due to the conflict, and in general the armed actions against the civilian population. (See Map 5.1.) This situation is described in the report that was presented by the High Commissioner of the United Nations, Mary Robinson, on March of 2001. In that report, she gave an account of the increments in violations to the right of life by means of extrajudicial executions, selective homicides, and the taking of hostages. In the year 2000 there were 584 massacres, 800 people vanished, 318,000 people were displaced, and of the 30,000 violent deaths, 3,600 were related to political violence.

The humanitarian crisis, the result of a combination of these diverse factors contributing to the violence, has had as an immediate consequence the phenomenon of forced displacement. This phenomenon in Colombia reached a level in which an estimated 2 million people were forcibly displaced during the last 15 years of the 20th century. Of those 2 million, 580,000 were displaced during the last 2 years (Colombian Judges Commission and Center for Investigations and Popular Education, 2000.

Within this complex situation of violence that is hitting the country, internal displacement and exile, which in themselves imply a form of violence, are above all, the results of other grave forms of violence like: threats, harassment, assaults, murder or disappearance of family

MAP 5.1   COLOMBIA

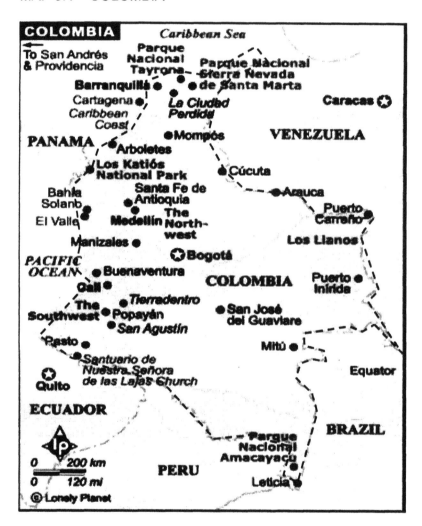

members or close ones, kidnapping, massacres and combat. People have suffered these to the point where they finally opt for internal displacement or exile. Internal displacement and exile are extreme resources to which people turn to free themselves from other harm to which they are exposed in contexts of social and political violence.

Mental Health and Psychosocial Implications

The effects of violence in the zones where Corporación AVRE works can be observed at the individual level, as well as the familial, community, and organizational levels. We understand these different levels to be interdependent, so that, for example, individual expressions of distress affect the individual's relationships with his or her family and community. Stated differently, when people have been affected by violence, the expression of their emotional distress is seen both in their individual subjectivity, and in their family and community life. In addition, to the extent that violent events contribute to the deterioration of the social fabric (e.g., if widespread distrust impedes communication among people and leads to isolation, or if meetings become dangerous activities, or if leadership activities are persecuted), people see their options for personal development limited and their possibilities for satisfying their need for social participation frustrated.

Through our therapeutic and psychosocial work with victims, we have observed that the particular manifestations of the impact of the violence, at the individual level, are related to the specific type of violent act that predominantly affects the person at any given time. For example, threats of violence create distrust, fear, isolative behaviors, fight or flight responses, and eventually symptoms of anxiety and depression. In the family members of murder victims, we found expressions of bereavement, frequently of a complicated nature. In the family members of people who have been "disappeared", there are usually complicated characteristics of suspended or "frozen" bereavement. For survivors of massacres or murders, we have frequently observed symptoms of trauma. With regard to the effects on the families, communities, and organizations, our observations have made it clear that one of the objectives of those who engage in political violence is to damage the social fabric, destroy organizations, and isolate people. According to Elena Martín of Corporación AVRE (Martín, 1998), "Sociopolitical violence gravely attacks the social fabric by generating intimidation, fear and distrust. This leads people to become isolated, and makes them more emotionally vulnerable."

The people of Colombia are living in a context of great uncertainty due to the fighting between different factions over the control of territories, city sectors, or entire cities. In addition, community, social, and political organizations have been forced to limit their activities and even suppress them, depending on the position vis-à-vis such organizations taken by the armed group that has assumed power in the region.

Specific Considerations About the Concepts of Mental Health and Disease

We should make clear that for the Corporación, the effects of violence imply an important degree of emotional suffering. However, this suffering does not always trigger a pathological mental disorder such as those listed in psychiatric nosologies. The terms *anxiety, fear, distrust, isolation* and other behavioral changes as well as sleeping disorders, among many other similar terms, all imply emotional suffering and in that sense imply psychological damage. However, when they happen as reactions to violent acts, they are not necessarily classified as pathology, but as normal responses to abnormal situations.

On the other hand, other extreme symptoms of psychopathology may be found if the victim suffered from a previous mental disorder that has been aggravated by violent events, or because violent events may unleash extreme, maladaptive changes. In such cases, we consider it important to diagnose the mental disorder, and to provide psychiatric or psychological treatment. However, the treatment must be offered from a psychosocial perspective, that is, without losing sight of the role that political violence played in unleashing or aggravating the symptoms. In addition, it is essential to utilize community resources in the healing process, and to repair the social fabric of which the individual forms a part. Equally important are legal and political actions aimed at overcoming impunity through truth and justice, and holistic reparations to the the victims, their families, and their communities (UNHRC, 1977).

Within a clinical–psychiatric framework, the most common diagnoses resulting from exposure to violence (including displacement) that Corporación AVRE has documented among the people and communities within which it works are, in order of their frequency: adjustment disorder with disturbance of mood, mourning (bereavement), acute stress disorder, and post-traumatic stress disorder (PTSD).

In cases of PTSD, the cross-cultural validity of which has been questioned, the diagnostic criteria of the DSM IV have been met. According to our observations, the post-traumatic symptomatology in victims of violence is related to situations in which the person has been exposed to terrifying events, and has suffered or witnessed the suffering of others due to acts of extreme cruelty. For example, PTSD has been documented among the survivors of massacres, those who witness the torture and execution of others, and the family members of murder victims upon finding their loved ones with signs of having been tortured prior to being killed.

Population of Focus

The Corporation's interventions are directed toward people affected by sociopolitical violence. These victims include men, women, children, and people involved with organizations that work for the defense of human rights or that provide aide to the victims violence. The Corporation also provides aid to organizations through activities that strengthen them and through workshops designed to prevent emotional exhaustion. Among people who have been affected directly by violence, the vast majority are of rural origin; however, the violence has also been directed at community and labor leaders and their families from urban areas. Women are the largest demographic group served by the Corporación

The population served by Corporación AVRE can be considered part of "western culture," but with regional variations in some groups determined by ancestry (e.g., people of African background), or by other factors such as rural background or the amount of time spent living in an urban environment. It is important to take these regional/cultural variations into account when doing psychosocial work with individuals or communities, for example when, in the wake of violent events, one is trying to identify personal or community resources, particular ways of experiencing and expressing grief, or the specific needs for assistance and reparation of particular communities.

INTERVENTION

In this chapter, we do not describe specific cases of people internally displaced or forced into exile. Instead, we present a holistic model of intervention designed for victims of the various types of political violence that exist in Colombia. In particular, our focus is on describing an important component of this intervention model, which involves training people from communities affected by violence, as well as people who work in organizations that work with victims of violence, so that trainees are able to work as *Popular (paraprofessional) Therapists (PTs)* and as *Multipliers of Psychosocial Attention, Mental Health, and Human Rights (MPAs)*.

Corporación AVRE team has offered psychosocial assistance activities to victims of violence since 1992. Our work places a strong emphasis on facilitating the emotional recovery of those affected by violence, an emphasis that is often overlooked or set aside by organizations working in emergency situations caused by violence. AVRE's work has developed on a national level, starting with its headquarters in Bogotá, through monthly visits to some of the zones most powerfully struck by political violence. In the last few years we have maintained permanent work activities in the counties of: Córdoba and Sucre, and the region of Magdalena Medio, especially the city of Barrancabermeja and more recently the city of Medellín. In addition, interventions have been developed in other places, mainly in the county of Valle.

The determination of both permanent and short-term zones of intervention depends on the necessities of the affected organizations or communities. These necessities emerge from the systematic violations of human, civil, and political rights related to the armed conflict. The Corporation tries to help based on the availability of time, financial resources, and personnel. However, due to the context of violence in the country, existing needs for psychosocial intervention overwhelm the capacity of all available organizations that provide humanitarian assistance, and that work to meet the material and emotional needs of victims of the violence.

Theory and Rationale

The work of Corporación AVRE is conceived of as psychosocial work for the mental health of victims of sociopolitical violence, and as the construction of an infrastructure to promote peace within a democratic culture. Corporación AVRE was formed by a group of psychiatrists with an orientation toward social psychiatry. During the development of their work, guidelines were developed to guide interventions aimed at promoting emotional recovery from the effects of violence. Within these guidelines it was agreed that emotional recuperation from the effects of violence depends on more than access to psychotherapeutic intervention; it also requires other activities focused on repairing the social fabric and the overcoming of impunity, on developing an understanding of the social context in which violence occurs, and on the identification and utilization of the resources that exist within people and communities, as well as the development of new resources. To achieve these ends, the Corporación works using three modalities that are interrelated and mutually reinforcing.

First Modality: Procedures and Actions for Strengthening Organizations

This modality is the key axis that coordinates the local, regional, national and international levels, and transversely the other two work modalities, clinical and training. It is guided by a framework that emphasizes a focus on, and commitment to, the rights of all victims of violence, and the attainment of peace through democratic practice and culture. Its strategies are the following (Salazar, 2001):

- To implement and extend its operative work by participating in networks and coordinated activities.
- To provide workshops and psychosocial projects aimed at strengthening group and organizational processes.
- To participate in inter-institutional and interdisciplinary projects.

- To participate in group work, investigations, humanitarian commissions and human rights monitoring, communication, and lobbying with state programs and organizations.
- To provide support to associations and strategic alliances that improve the impact, visibility, and institutional sustainability of the Corporation's efforts

Second Modality: Clinical Therapy

This modality consists of support for emotional recuperation that is provided by the Corporation's psychiatrists and psychologists, through individual, family, or group interventions (i.e., therapeutic workshops). These activities are conducted in conjunction with other organizations that work in different zones, or directly with people from communities affected by violence. These clinical services are not provided in an isolated manner, but in relation to the other two modalities. In other words, clinical work is conceptualized as one aspect of the larger group of activities that are implemented in coordination with other organizations, and/or directly with specific communities, as part of the overall intervention process. The clinical therapy modality is extended and reinforced through the pedagogical or training activities of the third modality, described next.

Third Modality: Training

This modality consists of carrying out training activities aimed at providing capacitacion in various areas. including mental health, human rights, protection strategies, and dealing with bereavement and fear. In addition, beginning in 1999, a new component was added which involves training Popular Therapists (PT) and Multipliers of Psychosocial Action, Mental Health, and Human Rights (MPA). We refer to these in detail in our discussion of the Corporation's psychosocial intervention efforts.

Training Popular Therapists and Multipliers
of Psychosocial Action, Mental Health,
and Human Rights.

Theoretical Frame

This process integrates the institutional strategies in order to create an intervention designed to facilitate and promote the integral healing of victims of violence. It also strengthens the communities to which victims of violence belong, as well as the organizations that work with them, and represents an integral part of the Corporation's overall efforts (Martín, 2001).

Within the proposal's design, careful consideration was given to the importance of pedagogic activities as instruments through which to help people recognize the emotional impact of violence and the importance of providing support to victims of violence in order to help them attenuate the impact of violence and overcome its effects. All this was done while attempting to promote the Corporation in its other modalities. At the same time, we also recognized the need to creatively develop training activities that would not be overly academic (a tendency of the professional staff within the organization). This was important in view of the varying levels of formal education among the participants in the training, which ranged from basic to intermediate. We recognized that the training needed to be accessible to all the participants if they were to be able to subsequently apply what they had learned in their communities.

General Objective

Our general objective was to train local community members in either of two complementary roles, entitled Popular Therapists (PTs) and Multipliers of Psychosocial Actions (MPAs). The PTs and MPAs should be capable of recognizing the impact that violence has on the mental health of individuals, as well as on the social fabric. They should also be able to engage in activities aimed at reversing these adverse effects, activities of a therapeutic or psychosocial nature that fit within the framework of coordinated and complimentary institutional activities.

Specific Objectives

1. *The Training of Popular Therapists.* The first objective concerns the formation of local agents, called *Popular Therapists (PTs)*, capable of performing individual as well as group crisis interventions with a psychosocial emphasis. The goals of this work include reducing emotional suffering and preventing the development of psychological disorders, as well as strengthening people individually and collectively so that they can participate in the process of repairing and reconstructing the social fabric. The training aims at the development of the following abilities:

- Recognize and analyze the sociopolitical context.
- Evaluate of the nature and magnitude of the emotional conditions presented by individuals and group, identifying strengths and weaknesses in each circumstance.
- Possess basic therapeutic abilities such as active listening, conveying empathy, and using helping techniques in a spontaneous and genuine manner to facilitate the expression of feelings by the individuals or groups being assisted.
- Recognize one's own emotions in the face of difficult circumstances, and ask for help when it is needed.
- Perform special crisis intervention techniques with individuals or groups.
- Be able to diagnose, and to mobilize those external resources that will lead to a favorable outcome of the intervention.

We hoped to organize the training process around three sets of themes, the first set applying to the training of both PTs and MPAs, and the second and third sets applying specifically to the training of PTs or MPS, respectively. Themes for the training of both the PTs and MPAs include:

- Mental health and human rights in a sociopolitical violence context
- Alternatives from a psychosocial perspective
- The impact of violence on the individual and collective levels
- General aspects of social and family groups and support networks

- Project elaboration

Specific themes for Popular Therapists:

- Individual interviews
- Individual interventions
- Group evaluation and intervention
- Fear and bereavement interventions

2. The Training of Multipliers of Psychosocial Actions. The second objective concerns the training of local agents, called *multiplier of psychosocial actions (MPAs)*, who are capable of performing psychosocial interventions through pedagogic group interventions in the areas of mental health, sociopolitical violence, and human rights. The work of the MPAs is grounded in a perspective that emphasizes working through networks, with the primary objectives of facilitating the mending and reconstruction of the social fabric and of increasing citizen participation. This is accomplished through the development of the following abilities:

- To recognize and analyze the sociopolitical and human rights contexts
- Basic therapeutic abilities (listening, empathy, spontaneity)
- To plan and implement pedagogic activities in different modalities
- To diagnose and to mobilize external resources that will enhance the likelihood of effective interventions
- To carry out psychosocial interventions, enhance the dynamics of organizational processes, and foster network-based activities

In addition to the common themes listed above for the training of both the PTs and the MPAs, training for the MPAs would also be organized around the following specific themes:

- Group processes and techniques
- Reconstruction of the social fabric
- Emphasis on identity, culture, adaptation, social roles, and gender

- Strategies for overcoming violence
- The domestic and international human rights crises
- Nonviolent problem resolution, nonviolent civil resistance initiatives
- Protection and self-defense with an emphasis on processes for obtaining peace
- Effects of impunity and alternatives for overcoming it
- Reparation and reconciliation

Summary of Training Objectives

Based on these principles and guidelines, the training process aims to develop, from a psychosocial perspective, the capacity to reflect on the impact that sociopolitical violence and human rights violations have on mental health. Through the Popular Therapist (PT) and the Multiplier of Psychosocial Actions (MPA) models, we expected that participants would readily acquire a specific set of concepts and abilities.

The main difference between the PTs and the MPAs centers on the orientation of their jobs once the training is done. The PTs develop abilities to identify the effects of the emotional impact of violence on people. They also provide individual and group assistance, and identify cases that need more specialized help. They have as primary objectives the attenuation of emotional suffering, the prevention of psychological distress, the strengthening of individuals and groups, and participation in the healing and reconstruction processes of the social fabric.

The MPAs develop abilities that allow them to perform pedagogical activities that permit the diffusion of knowledge regarding the effects of sociopolitical violence and human rights violations on the mental health of the affected communities. Their main objective is to cradle the construction and reconstruction of the social fabric from a group work perspective and encourage civic participation in this process.

Even though the two models have different emphases, they are closely related and have a common conceptualization of mental health. They both are predicated on the idea that mental health is not only dependant on the individual's characteristics and emotional experiences, but also on the social, economic, and political contexts of the individual's life. Likewise, individuals are elements of a social fabric whose integrity depends greatly on its development and well being.

This training process represents an important development of the Corporation's general mission. The process links pedagogical activities to therapeutic activities and to psychosocial actions aimed at reconstructing the social fabric; all this is done through the intervention activities of the PTs and the MPAs. While the training process helps empower the communities with regard to their psychosocial work, it also helps communities identify their own needs and resources, and provides them with the technical tools needed to address these needs. This way, the training process becomes a creative way of ensuring that psychosocial work projects are proposed and are carried out by the communities themselves. When this is achieved, the Corporación AVREs professional roles will be limited to supervision or support in the initial stages of these projects and interventions, with the Corporation becoming less and less necessary as the communities attain an ever greater degree of empowerment.

Work with Community-Based Organizations

This component of Corporación AVRE's work is directed at organizations working for the defense of human rights and with victims of violence, in the zones in which the Corporation has a presence. People from communities affected by violence, which are also being assisted by local non-governmental organizations (NGOs), are also a focus of this process. This aspect of our work was the result of an institutional recognition of the need to obtain a greater degree of impact for the psychosocial activities of the Corporation. We also recognized the importance of attaining greater sustainability of our efforts, through the adoption of our activities by local communities and the NGO's serving them. In this way, the organization's efforts would continue to flourish even after AVRE reduced or ended its presence in particular zones.

The participants in this process are people belonging to local organizations (Community-based NGOs, as well as social and religious organizations), with which AVRE has a thematic affinity and with which AVRE may have worked previously. These are organizations that work for the defense of human rights, and help victims of political violence, from a variety of different perspectives. Our aim is to introduce and reinforce a psychosocial focus into the projects of these organizations.

Some minimal criteria were established as "conditions of admittance" to the process. These criteria included: membership in a local NGO, and having within of the organization an interest related to the specific theme of training (in health, organizational development, or community education).

Implementation

Process

The initial proposal was that of a collectively developed pilot study that was developed and implemented over a period of approximately a year and a half in three cities in the country. Barrancabermeja, Montería, and Sincelejo are the capitals of the previously mentioned states where the organization's work is being developed. The pilot study was implemented through workshops lasting 8 hours each. The goal of the workshops was to train the first groups of Popular Therapists and Multipliers of Psychosocial Actions in accordance with the guidelines described above. The workshops were designed by the team of professionals from AVRE together with students from the Department of Social Work at the Universidad Nacional de Colombia. Once the initial implementation of the workshops had been completed, they were evaluated and modified according to feedback received from workshop participants, and with new insights from the Corporation's team.

Workshops 1 through 4, called General Workshops, included both the PTs and the MPAs. After these initial four workshops, the PT and the MPA groups were separated for the subsequent four workshops, which were tailored to the specific training needs of each group. *A central component of the training experience is the development by each participant of community-based psychosocial project that calls upon the particular set of knowledge and skills that participants acquire over the course of the training.* At the conclusion of the training process, a final General Workshop was conducted, in which the participants in the training presented work projects based on what they learned during the process. The culmination of the training process is an activity shared among the PTs and MPAs that we call a "Psychosocial Fair." The guests at the Psychosocial Fair include members representing the participants' organizations, along with other local organizations, as well as members of the participants' families and communities. The PTs and MPAs present their work projects, after which a graduation ceremony is performed, which includes the awarding of certificates based on their completion of the training. The importance of this activity lies primarily in the possibility of raising awareness among other sectors of the communities; in addition, for the participants, the event generates approval, visibility, recognition, and commitment by their communities.

In the general phase of the training process (Workshops 1 to 4 and the final workshop), the people who are trained as PTs and MPAs work together. These workshops are facilitated by a psychologist from the Corporation, and ideally should include a maximum of 30 participants. The workshops are intended to stimulate the active participation and contribution of participants, through small group activities as well as other activities conducted with the group as a whole. In each of the activities, we begin with the ideas and experiences that the participants have regarding whatever theme is being discussed. These ideas and experiences are organized and summarized by the facilitator, who helps stimulate and organize the discussion. Participants' own ideas and experiences are then integrated with materials related to the topic at hand that have been prepared prior to the workshop, to be handed out to the participants. With these materials and the ideas of the facilitator him or herself, the group works with the similarities and differences among the various points of view, questions are addressed, confusing points clarified, and conclusions drawn.

In each workshop written material is given to the participants. This didactic written material presents the topics that are discussed and the guidelines for the exercises that are utilized.

The experiential grasp of the concepts and the identification and development of the abilities that the PTs and MPAs will require in order to carry out their work are achieved through activities such as brainstorming, drawing, responding to questionnaires, role playing, dramatizations, and illustrative examples. All these exercises should relate to participants' own lived experiences, or to situations to which they have been exposed directly.

In the "profile-specific phase" of the process (workshops 5 through 8), the large group that participated in the first four general workshops is now divided into two groups, one of PTs and the other of MPAs. Each group now engages in the specific activities related to their own particular training. The methodology in these workshops is similar to that already described for the general workshops.

In the follow-up stage, after the aforementioned workshops, the participants' knowledge and abilities regarding how they developed the projects, at the community or individual level, are observed and evaluated. Their ability to integrate and articulate these same abilities and knowledge at the institutional or community level is of special concern. The difficulties that the PTs and the MPAs might face are identified and they are helped to overcome them. The workshops at this level focus on providing follow-up to their community-based projects, reinforcing the material learned during the training, and addressing the ways in which participants were able to work with key variables that are salient throughout the entire process, such as gender, culture, age, and ethnicity.

The pilot study was completed by the end of the year 2000 in two of the three cities, Barrancabermeja and Monteria. In the third city, Sincelejo, the process was finished in April of 2001. Of the 172 people from these three zones who started the training, 81 completed it (45 PT and 36 MPA). Of these 81 individuals, 56 were women and 25 were men, and the average age was 28.

Projects Developed as
a Result of the Pilot Study

As a result of the pilot study, the participants presented their own work projects with the support of the organizations with which they were affiliated. These projects were supported, followed up, and evaluated by Corporation AVRE Corporation over the course of one year.

TABLE 7.1.   PT and MPA Projects in the Cordoba Region

Project Title	Type of Group	Project Description: 1. Objectives 2. Coverage and duration 3. Main activities
Proposal for conflict resolution and group development.	2 MPAs	1. To strengthen the unity, mutual acceptance, and reconciliation of the group to achieve harmony and co-existence. 2. 20 teenagers, for 6 months. 3. Group workshops on group formation, identity and coexistence.
Psychosocial attention to families displaced from their homes, neighborhoods, and communities.	2 PTs 1 MPA	1. Support and follow-up to re-establish emotional well-being. 2. 20 families, for 6 months. 3. Family visits, parent workshops, integration activities.
Psychosocial support for children of displaced families from Robinson Pitallua, Paz del Rio.	2 MPAs	1. Help children cope effectively with their reality through psychotherapeutic support. 2. 90 children, for 9 months. 3. Integrative workshops for children's families, play and art activities.
Psychosocial attention to families who were victims of sociopolitical violence.	4 PTs 2 MPAs	1. Diminish the aftermath of violence in displaced people by providing them with psychological support. 2. 30 families, for 6 months. 3. Home visits, workshops with parents and children.
Psychosocial attention for the emotional recuperation of children displaced from the Del Diamante trails.	2 PTs	1. Emotional recuperation of displaced children. 2. 50 children, for 6 months. 3. Organizational analysis of follow-ups, workshops with support givers, group support, support to the children's families, evaluation.
Psychosocial attention for 53 mothers displaced by violence in the neighborhood of Canta Claro.	2 PTs 2 MPAs	1. Diminish the psychosocial impact of violence in groups of displaced mothers. 2. 53 women, for 11 months. 3. Survey of the displaced mothers, training workshops, home visits, and therapeutic support.

In the city of Monteria, in the state of Cordoba, the participants presented eleven projects. Of these, seven were implemented during 2001; they involved 197 people and 117 families. The population and geographic coverage of these projects is summarzied in Table 7.1 (Salazar, 2001).

To illustrate the effectiveness of these projects we analyze the activities and achievements of one of them entitled: "Proposal for Conflict Resolution and Group Development," whose objective was "to strengthen the unity, acceptance, and reconciliation of the group in order to achieve harmony and co-existence."

Two of the trained MPAs started this project with a group of 20 teenagers from a community of displaced people from Monteria. The teenagers were located in an urban sector experiencing dire socioeconomic conditions and were at a high risk of becoming involved with violent youth gangs (some of the youth had already joined gangs).

The project developed over a 6-month period, from April to September of 2001, during which five training workshops were held:

- **Workshop 1**: "Presentation of the Project and Activities for Getting Acquainted." The objective was the integration of the working group and the socialization of the project. The project was fully explained to the group, and the group's acceptance of, and commitment to, the development of the proposal was achieved.
- **Workshop 2**: "Reflection on Life, Building Dreams." The objective was to analyze the value of life and to awaken an interest in setting goals. A greater degree of group cohesion was achieved in this workshop, and enhanced the group's motivation for achieving success at both the individual and community levels.
- **Workshop 3**: "Groups: Their Structures, Characteristics, Functions, and Types." The objective was to examine and analyze the forms of socialization that one finds in communities as expressed through the groups that comprise them. In this workshop, participants achieved a greater degree of recognition of the value of group work, and of the need to improve the quality of community activities. A greater degree of communication among group members was also achieved in this workshop.

- **Workshop 4**: "Conflict resolution." The objective of this workshop was to provide the participants with the tools to identify, manage and resolve conflicts. Participants learned that there are benefits to dealing with problems through attitudes and actions other than those that lead to violence.
- **Workshop 5**: "Presentation of Group Participants' Proposal for Community Projects." For the fifth workshop, the young participants pre sented proposals for applying in their own communities the concepts and tools they had learned in the previous workshops. Their proposals were submitted to the group for discussion and improvement.

Table 7.2 summarizes the projects that were developed in the region of Sucre.

TABLE 7.2. PT and MPA Projects in the Sucre Region

Project Title	Type of Group	Project Description: 1. Objectives 2. Coverage and duration 3. Main activities
Training in psychosocial assistance to 3 groups of women from the counties of San Martin and Buena Vista.	1 MPA	1. Train and sensitize a base of community groups to attenuate the psychosocial impact that the presence of displaced people has on communities. 2. 60 women for 6 months 3. Training workshops, community exchanges, interaction campaigns, visits to institutions.
Psychosocial intervention for displaced widows aimed at attenuating their emotional suffering.	1 PT	1. Provide emotional support to a group of displaced widows that will allow them to over come and manage their fear and grief as well as repair the social fabric. 2. 10 widows for 6 months. 3. Group workshops, citizen participation workshops, family integration.

Psychosocial interventions for 10 families victimized by sociopolitical violence in the Montes de Maria, located in Sincelejo.	2 PT	1. To facilitate the emotional recovery process of 10 families victimized by sociopolitical violence and survivors of massacres. 2. 10 families for 6 months. 3. Visiting families for emotional support, cultural events aimed at rescuing traditional practices and beliefs, workshops designed to facilitated the participation of organizations and communities.
Psychosocial intervention for children displaced by sociopolitical violence.	2 PT and 2 MPA	1. Provide children with emotional support. 2. 75 children for 1 year. 3. Training workshops with teachers, the creation of a participation credential, organizing recreational programs.
Psychosocial and emotional recuperation for 42 displaced single mothers in Altos del Rosario.	4 MPA and 1 PT	1. Attenuate the emotional impact of displacement and other life stressors through the reconstruction of the social fabric. 2. 42 women for 6 months. 3. Emotional support visits, workshops, events designed to promote social integration.
Psychosocial intervention for 117 families of the Indigenous group from Calle Larga.	1 MP	1. To train the community about the impact of political violence. 2. 117 families for 6 months. 3. Group sensitization workshops, conflict resolution, family visits.

In addition to these six initial projects, a seventh one entitled "The Effects of Psychosocial Intervention in a Displaced Community in Chengue," was created during the follow-up process. This project was a result of the crisis intervention that Corporation AVRE made in this community and was implemented in the neighborhood of Ovejas. To give the reader a better sense of our work, a detailed summary of this project is found below in Table 7. 3. Three people developed it, one of them an MPA and the other two PTs. The target population consisted of 56 displaced survivors of a massacre living in Chengue. The activities included in the table were carried out during a six-month period in 2001.

TABLE 7.3. Chengue Community Project Description.

Activity	Purpose	Accomplishments	Difficulties
Workshop on psychosocial diagnosis and individual interviews	To determine the emotional impact of the violence in the community.	An accurate psychosocial diagnosis for the planning and implementation of concrete actions.	Group tensions. Tensions within the target community.
Therapeutic workshops	To support emotional recovery.	Emotional strengthening of the group.	Fear of threats. The interest of some individuals in tangible (i.e., material) assistance.
Individual therapy	To support individual recovery.	Contribution to individual psychological healing.	Inconsistency. Stigmatization by some people.
Informational workshops focused on self-esteem, communication, and group dynamics	To provide knowledge and tools that facilitate the restructure of the social fabric.	The strengthening of group cohesion. Empowerment in the process of negotiation.	Threats of seizure of property in the community of Ovejas. The death of people in Ovejas. Interruptions in the intervention due to other community meetings. Lack of continuous participation of some people.

To give the reader a further sense of our work, we provide in Table 7.4 a summary of a project entitled "Psychosocial Assistance for 30 Displaced Single Mothers in the Community of Altos del Rosario." Four MPAs and one PT developed the project.

TABLE 7.4. Altos del Rosario Community Project Description

Activity	Purpose	Accomplishments
Psychosocial diagnosis	To learn about the socio-economic, cultural and emotional situation of the target population.	Group selection and consolidation; Leader selection for the project.
Project presentation	To sensitize the group about the importance of emotional healing.	Appropriation of the project by the women participants.
Community organization workshop	To provide conceptual tools regarding community organization to improve the quality of life in the community.	Group cohesion and organization.
Therapeutic workshop and working with children	To socialize the experience and recognize the before and after effects.	Collective recognition of the participants' reality; The discovery of their artistic expression.
Occupational therapy	To teach manual skills that will allow them to utilize their spare time and improve their earnings.	Creation of decorative plates, mirrors, and gift bags.
Self-esteem and values workshop	To provide conceptual tools that will allow participants to value and recognize themselves as women with rights.	The recognition of identity and a sense of belonging; The expression of their emotions.
Participation in the Psychosocial Fair	To present and socialize the psychosocial activities developed with the group.	Becoming familiar with the experiences of other groups.
Individual visits	To analyze the difficulties and perspectives of the work.	Analysis of the project's progress; Corrections to the process and its continuation thereafter.
Evaluation and follow-up visit	To evaluate the process of psychosocial support in the group.	An acknowledgement of the psychosocial work.

Analysis of Projects Carried Out in This Zone

Objectives and Activities. The objectives lay within the realm of psychosocial assistance with an emphasis on emotional recovery and the reconstruction of the social fabric. The activities consisted of workshops designed to facilitate emotional support, and other workshops aimed at providing psychosocial training. In three of the projects, occupational therapy activities, such as the elaboration of crafts, were included, while two projects focused on human rights training.

Beneficiaries of the Projects

There was diversity among the communities and individual participants who benefited from the projects. Five of the seven projects provided direct attention to victims of violence. Of these, four were conducted with displaced communities and one with women whose family members had been assassinated or disappeared. Two other projects worked toward the strengthening of vulnerable and high-risk communities; one of them was a group of women from community organizations and the other was an indigenous community. We estimated that there were 295 people that benefited from these projects. Of this total, 122 were women in projects specifically for women, 75 were children in child-focused activities, and the remaining 98 were a mixture of adults and children in mixed groups.

Context of the Projects

Of the seven projects, three were carried out in marginal neighborhoods of the city of Sincelejo, one in Ovejas and another in Corozal, and in the two smaller communities Calle Larga and San Martin. Some of the participants had to commute from rural zones. In Sincelejo, especially in the more marginal neighborhoods, there is a high degree of control by illegal armed groups or paramilitaries. There are murders of people who are accused of being "helpers of the guerillas" or who engage in delinquent behavior. In addition, these communities lack access to basic services, display high levels of poverty, and a majority of their members are victims of displacement due to violence.

Projects From the Barrancabermeja Area

We will not give details of the proposed projects in Barrancabermeja because the intensification of violence and drastic changes in the socio-political context, as well as a crisis in one of the organizations where the formative process was developed, have impeded the implementation of the projects.

That which occurred in this zone illustrates the major threats and difficulties that psychosocial projects face: the intensification of armed conflict, the violent control of communities by armed groups, and the eventual internal crises affecting community organizations. In the other areas, the PTs and the MPAs faced the same difficulties, but to a lower degree of intensity, and thus they were able to overcome these obstacles and carry out their work.

EVALUATION

Method

For all of the projects developed by the PTs and MPAs, follow-up activities by the staff of Corporation AVRE were carried out. A combined qualitative/quantitative evaluation was done to assess the development and impact of the projects, as well as the difficulties that trainees encountered in the process of implementing their projects.. The follow-up activities also served to reinforce, in a practical way, the knowledge and abilities of the trainees. To illustrate how the follow-up and evaluation were done we mention some aspects of what was done with the projects in the region of Sucre.

The PT and MPA pilot training program in Sucre ended in April of 2001. The total number of PT and MPA graduates was 15. The objectives of the follow-up of the projects were to support their implementation, assess their development, reinforce the PTs' and MPAs' abilities, and analyze the impact of the projects on the target communities.

Follow-up activities included the following: meetings with organization directors to present the projects and affirm the institutional support that was required; provision of general assessments to evaluate the development of each project's activities, accomplishments and difficulties; and assessment "in the field" of specific project activities, such as training, therapeutic, and psychosocial workshops. We planned the follow-up to be done throughout the year by means of monthly meetings.

Negotiations With Organizations

Throughout the process we remained in close contact with those organizations that had members participating in our training. The objective was to sensitize the organizations to the importance of the participants' projects, in that way obtaining their conceptual, methodological, logistic, and financial support.

General and Project-Specific Assessment Strategies

Assessment efforts entailed evaluating the progress of the projects with respect to their proposed timelines, the difficulties that arose with regard to the various project activities, and the extent to which specific project goals had been achieved. Where indicated, necessary adjustments were made within each of the projects in response to this assessment. The follow-up also allowed the PTs and MPAs to reinforce their abilities and evaluate the impact and development of their projects.

Assessment and follow-up "in the field" consisted of providing support for the PTs' and MPAs' activities, evaluations with the target communities, and participant observation. These on-site visits helped us to evaluate how the PTs and MPAs were applying their abilities and resources, analyze the impact of each project, and provide support for the interventions. However, due to a variety of difficulties, some due to the contexts in which projects were implemented, these fieldwork visits were not carried out for all projects.

We made an effort to link several of the MPAs and PTs to the various activities that Corporation was involved with in the zone. This allowed them to reinforce experientially their abilities related to psychosocial intervention, and to become acquainted with the work of other groups. The work that they did in these interventions was not just as observers, but also as co-leaders of the workshops.

Workshops were held periodically to evaluate the progress, achievements, and difficulties encountered by each project. For the general evaluation of each project the methodology was to have each trainee reflect on the following points:

1. Description of the well-being of the people that had been served by the project (compared to their well-being at the beginning of the project);
2. Factors that facilitated the project;
3. Factors that made the project more difficult;
4. Different situational factors that affect the projects in various ways.

Preliminary Results

We now present the summary of the evaluation workshop of the previously described project developed in the displaced community of Chengue.

Description of the people following the implementation of the project:

- Emotionally recuperated.
- People felt empowered at the individual and group levels.
- Group members had developed negotiation skills, with leadership capabilities evident in some individuals.
- Greater solidarity among participants.
- Greater knowledge of their rights and the mechanisms for defending them.
- Motivation to continue their organized work with the legal system.
- Interest in multiplying what they learned.

Aspects that made project development easier:

- The facilitators (PTs and MPAs).
- Institutional support from a credible local organization (the Dioceses) to carry out the project.
- AVRE's evaluation
- Solidarity among participants

Aspects that made project development difficult:

- The armed conflict in the zone.
- The Dioceses' unplanned activities, which interfered with the activity timeline of the project.
- Attrition from the group by some members.
- The addition of new members later in the group's development who didn't have the knowledge acquired earlier in the group
- The lack of support of some local organizations and from the Mayor's office.
- Low academic level of the participants.
- Conflicts with the activities of other institutions and organizations.

An additional result of the follow-up process was the proposal by the PTs and MPAs to create new organizations. Two group evaluations were conducted to explore the theme of developing an organization of the PTs and MPAs. This was a positive result, for which the placement of capable people in the zone contribute to the psychosocial focus. However, we must make clear that this initiative arose as a result of the weak support that the PTs and MPAs received from their host organizations. Due to the precariousness of this support, the work of several projects ended up being the solitary efforts of the trainees in charge of the projects, without the support of their home organizations. However, this lack of institutional support was a stark contrast with mutual support that the PTs and MPAs provided to each other during several of the projects.

New Training Programs

Taking into account the evaluation of the pilot study, and incorporating the changes that were deemed necessary, we initiated new training programs in the cities of Barrancabermeja, Medellin and Monteria. Two modifications to the: e revised training procedures consisted of the intensification of the training process (to complete the training in nine months or less), and avoiding the training interruptions that had occurred previously at the end of the year, a major factor contributing to trainees abandoning the training.

The experience of the training process has constituted an important contribution to the integral attention to victims of violence. This is so in part because these victims are participants in the development of knowledge and abilities that allow them to confront the direct and indirect effects of violence in a context of armed conflict and grave human crisis. In addition, their intervention activities are an important factor in expanding the reach of psychosocial actions well beyond what would be possible if we relied solely on the work of the small number of available mental health professionals.

Another point worth mentioning about the focus of the training is that it is done as an activity that integrates interventions aimed at emotional support with attention to the reconstruction of social fabric, the quest for overcoming impunity, and people's recognition of themselves as subjects with rights.

CHALLENGES AND LESSONS LEARNED

Upon completion of the initial training process (the pilot program described thus far), we set as a central challenge to reduce participant attrition. The high rate of attrition (55.5%) was related primarily to a lack of adequate selection criteria when identifying potential trainees, and to the conditions of violence in the zones where the projects were implemented.

Another challenge lay in the need to achieve a greater commitment by the supporting organizations (from which trainees were selected to participate in the program). Greater assistance was needed from these host organizations in the process of training as well as during the follow-up of the projects in the communities.

Trying to get community-based psychosocial projects to function effectively in the midst of an armed conflict is a very hard thing to do. During the follow-up of the PT and MPA projects, it was necessary to reevaluate the risks of the planned activities. This raised questions about the sustainability of psychosocial projects in situations, such as Colombia's, that tend to worsen quickly in ways that heavily impact local organizations.

From the pilot study it was clear that it is necessary to both make more flexible and speed up the development of the process, so that nine training workshops are completed within 1 year (that is, without interruption by the New Year). It may also be necessary to adjust the frequency of the workshops, taking into account specific contextual factors in each zone, again with the aim of completing the training with 9 months, and possibly less.

In addition, it is crucial that the initial selection of participants be fine-tuned and that a greater degree of commitment be assured from the participating organizations, both during the training process and during the implementation of all subsequent projects carried out by project participants.

Finally, it is noteworthy that the projects developed by participants in the pilot program received considerable acceptance by the target communities. This suggests that the Popular Therapists and Multipliers of Psychosocial Actions had begun the important process of addressing the impact of violence on mental health and the social fabric.

SUMMARY

In this chapter we have presented an experience that is a part of the set of activities that comprise the psychosocial work of Corporation AVRE in Colombia. Our focus was on one of the components of our training program, in which we trained Popular Therapists and Multipliers of Psychosocial Actions, Mental Health, and Human Rights, in order to extend the reach of our psychosocial interventions by training local community members who could in turn reach a much greater number of people than could be reached solely by our team of mental health professionals. These trained community members were able to achieve considerable acceptance by their local communities of the projects they developed, and in the process helped their communities attain greater autonomy. We described the first stage of development of this training process, carried out as a pilot study. Through this pilot process, the training design was more fully developed, adjustments were made, and an evaluation was carried out. The project is now ready for a subsequent phase of implementation.

REFERENCES

Colombian Judges Commission and Center for Investigations and Popular Education (2000). *Dos años del gobierno Pastrana: Agravamiento de la Crisis Humanitaria.* Presented as part of the agenda for the Colombian overcoming of the human rights crisis seminar. Bogotá, Colombia.

Human Rights Commission of Colombia (2000, October). *Algunas propuestas desde la sociedad civil para la humanizacion del conflicto armado.*

Martin, E. (1998). *Violencia Sociopolitica y Trabajo Psychosocial.* Bogotá, Colombia: Corporación AVRE.

Martín, E. (2001). Evaluacion de la experiencia piloto del Proceso de Formacion de Terapeutas Populares y Multiplicadores de acciones Psicosociales, Salud Mental y Derechos Humanos (Internal document). Bogota, Colombia: Corporación AVRE.

Salazar, M. (2001, January-June). *AVRE Corporation semester report.* Bogota, Colombia: Corporación AVRE, p. 23.

United Nations Human Rights Commission (1977). According to what was established in the meeting of the Principles for the protection and the promotion of human rights through the fight against impunity. E/CN.4/Sub.2/1977/20/Rev.1 of the United Nations Commission of Human Rights.

8

Bosnian and Kosovar Refugees in the United States: Family Interventions in a Services Framework

Stevan Weine, Suzanne Feetham, Yasmina Kulauzovic,
Sanela Besic, Alma Lezic, Aida Mujagic,
Jasmina Muzurovic, Dzemila Spahovic, Merita Zhubi,
John Rolland, and Ivan Pavkovic[1]

This chapter describes an evolving program of family-focused interventions and services research with refugee families from Bosnia-Herzegovina and Kosova in Chicago. This program has been conducted by a group of university scholars and community associates, including Americans, Bosnians, and Kosovars, who are engaged in a multidisciplinary approach to inquiry concerning service utilization, while helping refugees and the organizations that help refugees. A

[1]From the Project on Genocide, Psychiatry and Witnessing; Department of Psychiatry and the Health Research and Policy Centers, University of Illinois at Chicago. The work described in this chapter has been supported by the National Institute of Mental Health (K01 MH02048-01 and RO1 MH59573-01).

central focus of the work has involved multifamily support and education interventions named CAFES (Coffee and Family Education and Support) that are based on the conceptual framework of *Prevention and Access Interventions for Families*. Preliminary evaluation analyses support the feasibility and psychosocial benefits of the interventions and distinguish characteristics of families based on their level of engagement with the interventions. Family interventions of this type are an underutilized but necessary means for addressing the suffering and difficulties of refugee communities. A mental health services approach focusing on issues of prevention and access provides a promising intellectual framework for building innovative, family-focused interventions and for learning more about how to help refugee families.

BACKGROUND

Trauma Focused Interventions in Refugee Mental Health

Refugees of political violence, such as the large number that have come to the United States from South-East Asia over the past several decades, are exposed to multiple different types of extreme conditions that irrevocably change their lives (Leopold & Harrell-Bond, 1994; Westermeyer, 1986). These are likely to include exposure to traumatic events of state sponsored violence and oppression, internment in refugee camps, displacement to a third county, family loss and prolonged separation, low socioeconomic status, unemployment and cultural transition (Kinzie, Fredrickson, Ben, Fleck, & Karls, 1984; Mollica, Wyshak, & Lavelle, 1987). This chapter concentrates on family-focused interventions with two recent groups of refugees: those persons who survived ethnic cleansing and siege in Bosnia-Herzegovina and Kosova before coming to the United States (Judah, 2000; Weine, 1999).

American psychiatry has predominately approached the problem of traumatization from political violence from the clinical perspective of the individually oriented focus of the diagnosis of Post-traumatic Stress Disorder (PTSD) (van der Veer, 1992). Multiple studies conducted on different refugee populations have demonstrated high severity and prevalence of PTSD (De Girolamo & McFarlane, 1996; Jaranson & Bamford, 1987; Williams, 1986). Similar to the epidemiological studies on refugees, the mental health interventions most often discussed in relation to refugees have tended to focus on the individual and the presence of trauma-related mental health symptoms, especially traumatic stress symptoms (Mollica, Wyshak, & Lavelle, 1990; Smajkic et al., 2001; Weine, Vojvoda et al., 1998). Trauma treatment interventions discussed in the clinical 0literature on refugees include crisis intervention, individual-focused supportive or exploratory psychotherapy, cognitive and behavioral therapies, group psychotherapy, psychopharmacology, creative arts therapies, rehabilitation, play therapy, and marital and family therapies (van der Veer, 1992). The treatments described are most often provided in specialized refugee mental health clinics, torture rehabilitation centers, community mental health clinics, primary care clinics, or multiservice agencies.

Research has demonstrated that, in addition to PTSD, refugees have considerable prevalence rates of other kinds of trauma-related mental health problems, including depression and somatic symptoms (Moore & Boehnlein, 1991). Refugee trauma also is known to effect marriages and families (Agger & Jensen, 1996; Sluzki, 1979), as well as community and society (Weine, 1999). For refugees living in exile, there is the related problem of being in cultural transition (Marsella, Bornemann, Ekblad, & Orley, 1994). Further multidisciplinary and mixed method investigations are needed to fully characterize these other trauma and displacement related mental health problems that are a part of the broader picture of refugee trauma and distress.

What also is needed is the further development of interventions and programs that will work for refugees in the social contexts in which they live. Utilizing a mental health services approach for refugees can help toward this goal because this approach is primarily concerned with how to make available services that fit with the "real world" conditions of refugees' lives and how to increase the ability of services to address the needs and concerns of various refugee groups. Mental health services approaches address such matters as the challenges to implementing interventions, the obstacles to accessing interventions, the impact of contextual influences (social, economic, cultural, and political), and how to best meet a community's needs. A services approach can help to improve a community's capacity for delivering mental health services to refugees who are suffering trauma-related mental health consequences, but who do not have access to or decline to utilize mental health care.

Bosnian Refugees and the Underutilization of Mental Health Services

Between 1992 and 1996, more than one million Bosnians became refugees as a consequence of ethnic cleansing, siege, or war by extreme ethnic nationalists. Approximately 200,000 Bosnians have been resettled in the United States, with about 30,000 in Chicago (Weine, 1998). Free mental health services in a non-institutional, friendly setting with bicultural workers have been offered to Bosnian refugees in the Chicagoland area. However, a generous estimate (made by a consortium of community persons and professionals in 1999) was that, at most, 2000 of the 30,000 (an estimated 7.5%) Bosnian refugees in Chicago have received some mental health services through one of several refugee mental health programs in the area, as well as through primary care, community mental health, and clerical counseling programs (Weine, 1998). Does this represent an underutilization of refugee mental health services among Bosnians in Chicago?

Several small studies (e.g., Weine, Vojvoda et al., 1998; Weine et al., 2000) reporting high rates of PTSD and depression among community samples of Bosnians suggest that it is fair to presume that in the remaining population of Bosnian refugees in Chicago, there is substantial distress that is not being treated with mental health interventions. This would be consistent with reports concerning other nonclinical refugee populations that have demonstrated high rates of psychiatric symptoms (Garcia-Peltoniemi, 1991). It further can be presumed that a subset of those persons suffering the mental health consequences of trauma who do not receive appropriate services are likely to be at increased risk for the development of increasingly severe, chronic, or disabling conditions—with ensuing familial, educational, economic, and social disruptions. For this reason, it is necessary to consider why some refugees might be underutilizing existing mental health services and how this failure to access services can be addressed.

Traumatic stress theory predicts that traumatized refugees will avoid traumatic reminders, suggesting that refugees' failure to access mental health services could be a manifestation of psychopathology. However, it would be inadequate to reduce this issue to a matter of individual psychopathology, when there are other, possibly more fitting, conceptual explanations.

An ecological perspective would posit that the act of not seeking mental health treatment, instead of being an expression of psychopathological processes, could instead reflect the workings of family, community, and/or cultural systems that are attempting to maintain an equilibrium of basic sociocultural processes (Klein & White, 1996). In other words, the ecological perspective would consider the possibility that those persons who are suffering, but not seeking mental health services, could be finding some support through other avenues—such as the family, peers, ethnic community, religion, employment, or through physical health care. It would also posit that existing frameworks of mental health treatment (which often are pathologically and individually focused) might clash with the belief structures of these social resources—especially those of the family or religion—in ways that present obstacles to obtaining mental health care (Sue & Sue, 1999). This perspective suggests the need to design family-focused interventions that aim to diminish such obstacles, and perhaps also enhance existing family and community supports.

Presently, the mental health literature on refugees lacks studies that systematically examine nonservice recipients to investigate what might constitute obstacles to mental health care seeking among these refugees, and what alternative resources might they be utilizing. This is not so different from the traumatic stress literature in general, where a few mental health service studies concerning survivors of other forms of violence and trauma suggest an underutilization of formal mental health services (Lindy, Grace, & Green, 1981; Rosenheck & Fontana, 1996). Likewise, in the mental health services literature, several studies of general populations have demonstrated that ethnic minorities tend to underutilize health care and mental health care services (Lin & Lin, 1978; Szapocznik et al., 1988).

Studies of Bosnian refugees comparing mental health service "help seekers" versus "non-help seekers" found significant differences between the two groups in multiple realms indicating that those who did not seek services had substantial trauma-related symptoms (although less so than those who did present for care), but did not identify themselves as being especially distressed or dysfunctional (Weine et al., 2000). For example, they would say: "I'm not crazy," in effect, associating seeking mental health services, even for trauma, with the stigma of being chronically mentally ill. Thus, it appeared that symptomatic nonpresenters had a very different set of attitudes about trauma and mental health services than did presenters, and those attitudes could be associated with barriers to them or their family members seeking mental health services.

Refugee Families and Interventions

Family is clearly at the center of both Bosnian and Kosovar cultures, as has been well documented (Bringa, 1995; Malcolm, 1994, 1998; Weine, 1999). For those Bosnians and Kosovars who became refugees, and whose homes and communities were destroyed, the family is the most important remaining social institution. Even prior to 1992, both Bosnian and Kosovar families in the former Yugoslavia experienced several generations of massive social pressures—including experiences of poverty, migration, urbanization, war, and ethnic nationalism. Despite these adversities, family still plays a significant role in shaping the lives of Bosnians and Kosovars, including their experience as refugees. Of course, these claims are true not only for Bosnians and Kosovars, given that the family is universally claimed to be the primary micro-social institution of human life in all cultures (Castells, 1997).

Qualitative investigations with Bosnians indicate that refugees may experience a disconnect from traditional, clinic-based mental health services for refugees because of the lack of emphasis upon the family and its strengths (Weine, Ware, Knafl, & Feetham, 2002). Although "family" is often a professed value in the field of refugee mental health, neither the field's service activities, nor its research and writings, actually define, conceptualize, or operationalize a family approach to refugee mental health services in substantial or meaningful ways. Little professional attention is paid to understanding mental health services from a family centered point of view or to making those services more family oriented. For example, a study of Bosnian refugee health providers found limited involvement of families in mental health treatment, and little explicit concern about families among providers (Weine, Kuc, Dzudza, Razzano, & Pavkovic, 2001). Westermeyer (1991) noted a general bias against family focused interventions for refugees, due to the increased complications for therapists already challenged by language and cultural differences.

In the research literature, little attention has been paid to how refugee families adjust and recover over time and how the family influences service use and treatment outcomes. We are unaware of any published reports on family focused intervention programs with refugees, although family-focused interventions have been described (although not evaluated) in unpublished accounts of refugees resettled in Australia (Aroche, unpublished manuscript, 2001) and refugees in Africa (N. Barron, personal communication, November 2000).

The small family therapy literature on refugees consists of clinical reports and theoretical discussions that tend to focus on problematic interpersonal aspects of the survivor experience, such as family disruptions, traumatic remembrances, and intergenerational conflict. For instance, Chambon (1989) emphasized the importance of helping families choose how they want to address memories of traumatic events, and Chambon (1989) and McGoldrick, Giordana, and Pearce (1996) emphasized the interactions of family with culture and ethnicity. The idea of cultural transitions has been addressed by Sluzki (1979) and DiNicola (1997), among others. Sluzki's (1979) case study explored a family's silence after torture, and the role of family therapy in helping the family to find the words to express their traumas. Danieli (1996), Bar On (1996), and Volkan, Ast, and Greer (2002) have addressed the intergenerational transmission of traumatic memories. Simon (1983) studied Soviet and Vietnamese refugees, and looked at intergenerational conflict between mothers and daughters amongst Soviet and Vietnamese refugees. Ben-Porath (1987) addressed the problem of different rates of acculturation in the family and loss of family members. Weine, Vojvoda, Hartman, and Hyman (1997) published a case study in which changes in individuals' symptoms were related to disruptions in family communication and structure in the context of cultural and intergenerational processes. Westermeyer and Wahmanhold (1996) identified family factors that contribute to pathogenesis: trauma to or loss of parents, child neglect and abuse, intergenerational conflict, parental acculturation failure, parental psychiatric disorder, role reversal, partial families, and solo parents. Agger and Jensen (1996) discussed the destruction or confusion of ordinary family roles, especially between the generations. A theme expressed by many of these authors is that refugee families may tend to not let outsiders know of family problems, because they feel that these are best dealt with inside the family.

Some of the family problems identified by these authors fit with our observations of Bosnian and Kosovar families. However, because we did not want to be limited to a pathological framework, we sought to approach these types of issues from a family strengths perspective focusing on the family and its particular values, meanings, needs, and resources, as articulated by McCubbin and McCubbin (1996), Rolland (1994), and Walsh (1998). In order to think more contextually about these matters, we also turned to a family ecological perspective, which explains how families adapt to changes in the environment through the unique role of the family as a social unit, and its complex interactions with other units and levels of the human ecosystem (Bubolz & Sontag, 1993). Lastly, because we were concerned with developing interventions, we turned to the growing literature on innovative community and family focused interventions with other marginalized populations (McKay, Gonzalez, Stone, Ryland, & Kohner, 1995; Szapocanik et al., 1988; Tolan & McKay, 1996). This literature emphasizes the importance of the family's engagement with services, which may be facilitated by reassuring the family that the work will focus on mutually agreed upon problems and goals (Holder et al., 1998; Szapocznik et al., 1988).

A Services View of Interventions

In consideration of the aforementioned problems, and based on a review of the existing literature and 10 years of clinical, community, research experience, three central questions emerge concerning refugee families' mental health needs. First, by what means can services address the fact that massive numbers of refugee families have members at high risk for

PTSD, depression, and other mental health problems? Second, how can access interventions be created to reach those families whose members are suffering, but for whom the obstacles toward receiving mental health services are too great? Third, how can preventive interventions be created that build on the inherent strengths of refugee families and facilitate their adjustment and recovery?

These are the kinds of issues that have been raised in multiple recent dialogues of governmental and nongovernmental organizations involved in providing psychosocial assistance to refugees, including Kosovars in Kosova and in exile in countries such as the United States (Waldman, 1999). However, by and large, serious attempts to address these questions with innovative, practical solutions are scarce—the result being that individual, psychopathologic, or psychotherapeutic oriented clinical approaches are being utilized to address profound services, public health, family, and scientific challenges (Weine et al., in press). Unfortunately, clinic based refugee mental health programs, like traditional mental health services overall, can be critiqued for being structured in a "waiting" framework—in which the patients are responsible for presenting to the clinic. A small subset of refugees will present for clinical mental health treatment, and may accept the patient role, but what of the many who do not? Those who fail to present may not have the social networks or the shared set of help-seeking behaviors that would serve to channel their distress into becoming service recipients. Several contemporary theoretical frameworks of mental health services can help to explain the challenges that refugee families face with respect to accessing services.

The *social network approach* to mental health services looks at the role of community social networks in accessing or implementing effective services. Social networks are "a specific set of linkages among a defined set of persons, with the additional property that the characteristics of the linkages as a whole may be used to interpret the social behavior of the persons involved" (Pescosolido, Boyer, & Lubell, 1999, p. 448). These networks emanate out from the family, and include both lay and professional systems, bringing both cultures to bear upon one another. Pescosolido, Gardner, and Lobell (1998) emphasized that what is critical in enhancing the effectiveness of service delivery is understanding the interaction between the social networks of communities, on the one hand, and clinical organizations and providers, on the other hand. For example, she notes that the presence within a social network of an "authoritative layman," who is knowledgeable about mental health, has been shown to facilitate the accessing of mental health care among those in that network. Pescosolido (1986) conducted a network study of immigrants and found that the expansion of social networks beyond the family correlates with higher seeking of medical practitioners. The importance of the relationship between health providers and the families of consumers is also demonstrated by research on treatment programs that include family components (e.g., family support groups) and evidence improved outcomes (Gottlieb, 1981). As summarized in Campbell and Patterson's (1995) review, a great deal of research concerning multiple health problems has shown that when the family is involved in treatment, program effectiveness is improved.

Help-seeking theory provides another perspective for understanding the processes by which persons seek mental health services. The concept of "help seeking pathways" is used to describe, "the sequence of contacts with individuals and organizations prompted by the distressed person's efforts, and those of his or her significant others, to seek help, as well as the help that is supplied to such efforts" (Rogler & Cortes, 1993, p. 555). Several critical phases in the help-seeking process are described, including: problem recognition; the decision to seek help; and the decision to select specific services. This process is impacted by multiple factors, such as: predisposing factors (e.g., age, gender, beliefs), enabling factors (e.g., facilities, barriers, social pressure), and illness profile factors (e.g., objective conditions and subjective appraisal). Rogler and Cortes (1993) made the fundamental claim that the help-seeking pathway starts in the family, "the quintessential primary group." The family context, including beliefs, structure, and functioning, is likely to impact upon the family's sensitivity to, interpretation of, and rules with respect to a family member's psychological distress, and their decisions to seek help.

This leads to a consideration of preventive interventions. Preventive interventions aim to improve patterns of health related behaviors through supporting functional patterns of behavior and changing problematic behaviors through changing relationship networks, teaching new knowledge and skills, and changing attitudes (Elliot & Tolan, 1999). Populations targeted for preventive interventions are usually at-risk populations who have been exposed to a set of traumatic and stressful life events and who, consequently, are at risk for poor mental health or behavioral outcomes. Williams (1989, 1996) has called for the development of preventive interventions to address mental health problems in refugees and torture survivors. A number of preventive interventions for refugee youth have been conducted through the schools, whereas those for adults have utilized the mass media (Lum, 1985; Owan, 1985) and mutual assistance associations (Barger & Truong, 1978; Vinh, 1981). Preventive interventions have also been utilized and studied in other vulnerable urban populations. For example, Szapocznik (1988) addressed the problems of underutilization and difficulty engaging immigrant families by devising and testing a strategic structural systems approach to engage otherwise difficult to engage cases. A number of researchers have developed and tested preventive interventions for urban families with children at high risk for delinquent behavior (McKay et al., 1995; Tolan & McKay, 1996; Szapocanik et al., 1989).

When speaking of preventive interventions for refugee families, we do not mean prevention either in the sense of preventing the acts of violence, which of course is an important human rights and political issue, or preventing the occurrence of trauma-related distress, which we sadly recognize as inevitable for many. Delineating the prevention foci of interventions with refugee families requires elaborating a new conceptual framework.

Conceptual Framework: A Prevention and Access Intervention for Families (PAIF)

A services framework of *Prevention and Access Interventions for Families (PAIF)* of refugees was developed to facilitate services innovations, including the CAFES intervention, in the field of refugee mental health (Weine, 1998). This framework offers an alternative to mainstream clinical mental health approaches that emphasize the individual and do not address either the family as the unit of interest or the specific circumstances of families that are recovering from trauma, adjusting to the circumstances of forced-migration, and facing cultural transition.

Traditional clinical approaches also do not address the family as an important potential catalyst for help seeking and service utilization for vulnerable family members. The PAIF framework can help to reconceptualize and develop mental health service interventions in ways that better draw upon families as resources, and that help families see mental health services as potential resources. PAIF facilitates rethinking refugees' interactions with mental health services, particularly around issues of access and prevention, in a more family-oriented way.

The PAIF framework is based on knowledge derived from 7 years of engagement in clinical, research, advocacy, ethnographic, and theoretical work concerning Bosnian refugee families (see Weine et al., 1995–2002). It also is grounded in the aforementioned theory and research on social networks, help-seeking and preventive interventions, as well as theory and research on families, resilience and adversity.

The PAIF framework rests on the following assumptions:

1. The family is the primary social unit for refugees. The family mediates refugees' connections to other families, to community groups and organizations, to the resettlement social service system, to schools, and to mental health and health service systems (see Figure 8.1).

2. The family, as a system, is critically important for guiding and supporting its members' approaches to a wide range of choices that have a major influence on their adjustment, recovery, and health.

3. Traumatization and displacement in refugee families can overwhelm and undo the inherent strengths that reside in families. This is primarily because the family's existing values, knowledge, and behaviors may not fit well with the demands of their present and future lives, or with potential resources external to the family, including those of other families, as well as community and service organizations.

4. Through support and education aimed at helping refugee families adapt to meet the demands of their new situations, family-focused services interventions can help refugee families take the appropriate steps toward adjustment, acculturation and recovery.

The family-focused services interventions informed by the PAIF framework encompass both prevention and access dimensions. It is important to emphasize that the PAIF conceptual framework specifically does not focus directly on treating individuals' symptoms of PTSD or depression, but focuses, rather, on family level phenomena—such as family beliefs, knowledge, attitudes, behaviors, social networks, communication, and service utilization—as a way to promote adjustment and recovery in refugee families.

PAIF'S Prevention Foci of Intervention With Refugees

The first critical issue for a preventive intervention is determining that individuals and families are at risk for negative psychosocial outcomes because of their exposure to some stressor(s), such as the extreme conditions of war and war-related traumas. Of course, in the case of refugees, we cannot change an individual's past trauma exposure, but we may be able to change how they and their families understand and manage trauma-related mental health consequences. This may include a focus upon PTSD and depression, but also may involve targeting other important domains—such as employment, parenting, and youth issues such as school functioning, drug and alcohol use, and other high-risk behaviors—that impact mental health and adjustment. Based on the aforementioned mental health services theories, as well as family strength and family ecological theories, we hypothesized that a family-focused preventive intervention would help change refugee families' social networks; knowledge and attitudes about mental health; and family communication and problem solving. Thus, we considered these to be the prevention foci of the intervention we developed for refugee families. Specifically, the intervention aimed to: expand participant families' social networks; improve family members' knowledge and attitudes concerning trauma mental health; and enhance family processes (e.g., resiliency, problem solving, and communication).

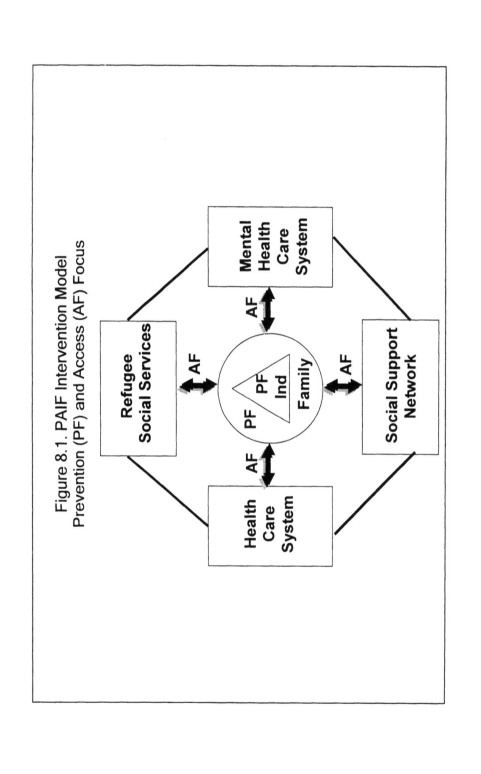

Figure 8.1. PAIF Intervention Model Prevention (PF) and Access (AF) Focus

PAIF's Access Foci of Intervention With Refugees

Some refugee families have members that are suffering from mental health consequences of political violence, including PTSD and/or depression. For these families, preventive interventions may not be enough, and access to mental health services may be needed. However, in vulnerable populations, focusing on the need for mental health treatment in lieu of prevention efforts, can end up weakening families, by adding to their sense of shame, guilt, blame, inadequacy and isolation, or deterring families from accessing helpful resources and creating more obstacles to recovery. Thus, it makes sense first to help strengthen families by providing them with knowledge, skills, and support. Conducting prevention work focused on strengthening families provides a perch from which access to services for vulnerable individuals becomes achievable, with knowledgeable and strengthened families working in collaboration with service providers. This approach also may help improve common problems with adherence to clinical treatments that are to be expected.

Access includes access to mental health services. Some of the obstacles to accessing mental health services have been articulated through prior research and clinical work with refugees. These include problems in the areas of attitudes (stigma, fear, shame, avoidance), information (lack of knowledge about treatments and their benefits), and trust (lack of connection with persons who can vouch for appropriateness of services). Therefore, the access foci and goals of the intervention described in this chapter were: (1) to connect participant families with persons who can endorse the value of services; (2) to provide the families with new knowledge and information regarding trauma mental health and other services; (3) to give families an opportunity to talk together about issues of trauma mental health and services; (4) to assist families in connecting with service providers.

Most refugee families may not need clinical mental health services, but do face obstacles to accessing other types of services. Refugees, and those who work with them, report difficulties in their relationships with a range of service organizations including schools, employers, social service agencies, health care agencies, immigration authorities, law enforcement, and financial services. Refugees' experiences with helping professionals and service agencies in their countries of origin are often vastly different from what they are presented with in the country of resettlement. As a consequence, refugees and those who work with them often have difficulty clarifying their expectations of and obligations to one another. Along these lines, a couple of themes can be discerned. First, refugees often report that they don't have access to information about their rights or what services are available to them. Second, refugees may have difficulty establishing an adequate level of trust with service providers. These types of difficulties concerning access also can be the foci of access interventions with refugee families.

Two programs for refugees in the United States that were developed and implemented based on the PAIF framework are now described.

INTERVENTION

CAFES: A PAIF With Bosnian Refugees in Chicago

Despite the availability of community based mental health services for Bosnian refugees in Chicago, the vast majority of refugees choose not to seek mental health services. Based on the PAIF services framework for refugees, CAFES was developed to target those families who have members who are suffering but have not sought mental health services. CAFES is a multifamily education and support intervention that was provided for Bosnian refugees in Chicago from 1999 to 2002 through funding by the National Institute of Mental Health.

CAFES is a time-limited intervention, which lasts a total of 15 weeks. The intervention consists of nine family group sessions, with approximately seven families per group. The multifamily group meetings serve three primary functions: *Networking*: Linking the family with other families and with organizations, so as to expand the families' social networks and to create linkages between community and service networks; *Educative*: Building families' knowledge and skills that they can use to strengthen themselves; *Supportive*: Facilitating family-group cohesion and creating an atmosphere of mutual interest and concern. CAFES groups do not focus on the telling of trauma stories or the processing of traumatic memories, because Bosnian families have repeatedly informed us that they would avoid trauma-focused groups.

CAFES groups are run by Bosnian refugees who are not health professionals but were trained and supervised by a multidisciplinary professional team. The intervention is manualized and group meetings take place in a community setting. It was decided not to allow younger adolescents and children to attend the groups, and instead to provide childcare in an adjacent space so that this would not be a barrier to participation.

There are four phases to the CAFES group:

I. Joining (Pre-engagement and CAFES Meeting 1)

Because refugee families tend to be isolated from other refugee families, the overall goal of this phase of the intervention is to facilitate families forming supportive relationships with other families. The pre-engagement contacts with the family (primarily by home visits) involve emphasizing the importance of strengthening families; assessing barriers to participation and developing a plan to address them; and inviting the family to the first group meeting. The critical element of the engagement process is identifying and problem solving around barriers to initial and ongoing participation in the intervention. Another primary goal is to establish rapport with the caretaker most likely to mobilize the family's participation in the program. All adult and older adolescent family members' participation is emphasized.

The goals of the first group meeting are to: generate enthusiasm around helping to strengthen families; outline the goals and structure of the CAFES program; teach families about families in transition; help families to introduce themselves as a family to the group; help families to make the commitment to return for the next group meeting. The CAFES facilitators give a brief didactic talk on *Families in Transition*. The facilitators then engage the families in a discussion of the question: "Why is a strong family so important to doing well in adjustment after survival and displacement?" In response, families have told us: *"Our family is our greatest strength"; "Our strength comes from each other"; "I could not have survived all of this if I didn't have my family. My family is the reason I'm alive today."* The facilitators then emphasize, in positive terms, the importance of the family (and its strengths) as a resource for family members and other families, and the CAFES groups as a place for families to get additional help, and to help one another.

II. Defining the Family (CAFES Meetings 2, 3, and 4)

The experience of enduring trauma and displacement often disrupts family members from their prewar developmental paths, and can render them overwhelmed and disconnected from who they once were as a family. The family cannot be the same as it once was, but it can be redefined as family members evolve. The goal of this phase is to empower families by assisting them in clarifying and updating their sense of the family as a system, the family's place in the life cycle, and the family's beliefs.

There are three sessions in this phase which all introduce key framing ideas taken from John Rolland's (1994) family systems-illness framework. Session two presents the *Family as a System* and emphasizes helping families to view themselves and the problems confronting them through a systems-oriented lens that provides an organizing framework that fosters empowerment and effectiveness. Session three, the *Family in the Life Cycle*, provides the framework of individual and family life cycles within which families are asked to locate themselves and their recent experiences of trauma and displacement. Session four focuses on *Family Beliefs*, which help to shape the families' ways of coping and understandings of health, illness, disability; and transition (Wright et al., 1996). For example, some families have addressed coping by saying, *"I don't talk about the war with my children. I don't want them to remember the war. Having a better life here is what's most important now."*

III. Working Together in the Family (CAFES Meetings 5, 6, and 7)

This phase is designed to help families to more effectively identify, communicate, and manage distress and problems in the family. This phase of the intervention is divided into three sessions, each devoted to a specific area of family functioning.

Session five focuses on *Strengthening Family Identity*. The overall dilemma that refugee families face concerns how they integrate aspects of their prior identities with their current realities in ways that are supportive to both the family as a whole and to its individual members. For example, participant families have expressed, *"We are Bosniaks and our children must not forget that. They will also become American and will live like Americans, but they are Bosniak first."* In this session, the facilitators engage the families in a collage making exercise and discussion that focuses on family identity.

Sessions six and seven concentrate on *Family Communication*. The content of these sessions is based on the premise that families know how to communicate, but the experiences of trauma and displacement may overwhelm their existing communicative capacities. The work of these sessions focuses on addressing the challenges to family communication presented by traumatic memories and cultural transition. For example, one family member shared, *"I don't like to talk about my own pain about the war because I don't want to burden my family. They have enough to worry about."* The aim of these sessions is not to teach families one set way for communicating, but to help them to identify and frame communication dilemmas and obstacles, and to familiarize themselves with a range of possible helpful options. Overall, these three sessions are intended to bolster the families' ability to make better use of its own interpersonal resources to deal with the challenges and vulnerabilities of its members.

IV. Using Resources Outside of the Family (CAFES Meetings 8 and 9)

Families can benefit from learning how to access and use external resources, which can include health and mental health care, social services, community resources, and of course, other families. A special focus in these sessions is mental health, given that there are neither the informal or formal social networks, nor the information or assumptions regarding mental health, which can reliably serve to link refugee families with mental health services. Thus, the overall aim for the last phase of the CAFES intervention is to set goals and make plans for the family's and its members' continued involvement with other families and with service organizations.

Toward these ends, session eight, *Families to Organizations*, focuses on utilizing services and session nine, *Families to Families*, focuses on families using other families. The CAFES facilitators help families discuss the importance of learning to utilize and negotiate with organizations, particularly for mental health services, and also the importance of forming family-to-family supportive relationship networks. The last sessions also are intended to put some closure on the CAFES groups, by reviewing families' experiences and accomplishments in the group, and by helping families plan how to continue to make use of what they learned in the group. Ongoing contact between families is encouraged.

TAFES: A PAIF With Kosovar Refugees in Chicago

The PAIF framework also provided the conceptual framework for the development and implementation of the Kosovar TAFES (Tea and Family Education and Support) program. In 1999—after more than a million Kosovars were forced from Kosova by the ethnic cleansing carried out by Serbian forces—around 20,000 Kosovars came to the United States as refugees (Judah, 2000; Malcolm, 1998). New Kosovar arrivals to Chicago, beginning in the summer of 1999, were facing the simultaneous multiple challenges of displacement, resettlement, and traumatization—made more difficult given the extreme rapidity of their becoming refugees and the immediate possibility of return. Kosovars were facing many additional obstacles that made their resettlement process quite difficult, including geographic disbursement, unfamiliarity with institutionally based health, mental health and social services, and large extended families. Similar to our work with Bosnians, preliminary ethnographic investigation and clinical experiences indicated that efforts to help Kosovars should be focused on the Kosovar family.

As with the CAFES experience, TAFES centered on a time-limited multifamily group intervention, but with modifications (Weine, 1999). The intervention consisted of six multiple family group sessions, which lasted a total of 8 weeks, with up to six families per group. As with CAFES, there were four phases of the TAFES intervention:

1. Joining (Family home visits and TAFES meeting 1)
2. Defining the Family and its Needs and Obligations (TAFES meetings 2 and 3)
3. Using Resources Outside of the Family (TAFES meeting 4)
4. Working Together in the Family (TAFES meetings 5 and 6).

Several structural and content changes were made for the TAFES intervention and manifested in a new TAFES group intervention manual.

In response to the sense of urgency that Kosovars felt, the TAFES intervention was designed to have fewer sessions over less time (i.e., the CAFES design included 9 sessions over 16 weeks, while the TAFES included 6 sessions over 8 weeks). Fewer families (6 per group) were invited, because families were generally larger and higher rates of participation were anticipated. The multifamily groups focused more on issues of family cohesiveness, adjustment, and choices in the face of recent calamitous life events and life-transitions, than on the bicultural questions of family identity that frequently came up with Bosnians (now several years into their displacement). The central questions that were discussed with Kosovar families were: Where is our family now? Should we stay or should we return? How do we adjust to work life in America? How do we speak with our children about all that has happened? How do we get help for sadness, fear, sleep problems? These were the highest priority questions that had emerged from the ethnographic and empirical investigations conducted prior to and concurrent with the development of TAFES. When Kosovars were identified as needing clinical psychiatric services, our team either provided those services (through a psychiatrist and nurse from a collaborating organization who were part of the TAFES team), or assisted the person in being seen by an appropriate service provider.

CHALLENGES AND LESSONS LEARNED

To build family-focused interventions for refugees is a complex and multifaceted endeavor that requires an approach that is interdisciplinary, collaborative, and culturally sensitive. A broad intellectual context — encompassing such concerns as ethnic nationalism, colonization, traumatization, immigration, cultural transition, poverty, ethnicity, gender, and development — is needed to expand the focus of intervention beyond traumatic events per se to address these other issues impinging upon families, only indirectly related to trauma, but nonetheless important.

We have come to feel strongly that a family-focused conceptual model is needed to support the development, implementation and evaluation of family oriented interventions. That conceptual model itself must be subject to modification to fit the particular set of families being targeted (i.e., oriented to how they define family) and the particular social niches of the community, and flexible enough to address important emerging issues.

In addition, the delivery of services to refugee families is very likely to involve non-health professionals, who must be adequately trained and supervised. Effective service delivery also requires collaboration among resettlement, health, mental health, and educational service organizations. Clients must be identified and referred for appropriate services, including mental health services. Lastly, an evaluation of the process of adaptation and of the outcome of the services must be conducted, and the results of the work must be disseminated so that they may inform the work of colleagues elsewhere.

The process of implementing CAFES and TAFES has not been without difficulties. One constant challenge we have encountered concerns the engagement of families — many of whom are very busy or may not trust other families or service providers.

Another source of difficulty we've encountered in our groups concerns gender. Families from Bosnia-Herzegovina and Kosova can be highly (although not equivalently) patriarchal, with rigid gender roles and expectations, especially in relation to the gender attitudes of American providers (Fox & McBride-Murry, 2000). The experience of being refugees in America presents a serious challenge to the patriarchal structure of refugee families, due to such factors as the father's inability to economically provide for the family, the mother's entering the workforce, women's greater access to education, exposure to feminist thinking, and women's greater independence (Castells, 1997). Differences in ideology and philosophy between family members and group facilitators must be negotiated in order to find effective ways to talk with families. For example, with Kosovar families, we found ourselves having to make necessary adjustments (e.g., not visiting Kosovar women and children without permission of the men) and choosing to address gender issues in other ways (e.g., encouraging women to speak up in multifamily groups).

Another problem area concerned conflicts within or between families. When families did not get along (either for reasons that were interpersonal, political, or sociological) with other families in the group, groups had to be reconfigured. Overall, the implementation of family interventions requires tremendous flexibility and willingness to compromise, especially when core cultural values are at stake for both families and providers.

EVALUATION

The family-focused interventions described in this chapter are being scientifically evaluated using methods developed and implemented over the past 7 years doing services focused research concerning Bosnian and Kosovar refugees. Guided by the PAIF conceptual framework, CAFES uses standardized and investigator designed measures to determine whether the intervention: (1) increases social support and expands the social networks of participant families; (2) improves knowledge and attitudes concerning trauma mental health among families; (3) enhances family processes; (4) increases service utilization. It was hypothesized that participation in the CAFES intervention would lead to improvements in these four realms. The CAFES intervention research design was as follows: Persons were randomly assigned to receive either the intervention or the control condition (which did not receive the CAFES intervention, but was given information about treatment available in the community). Longitudinal assessments occurred every 6 months for 18 months in order to document effects over time (post-intervention). In the TAFES intervention for Kosovar refugee families, neither control group, nor randomized assignment, nor repeated longitudinal follow-up were possible (Weine, Raijna et al., 2001). However, follow-up assessments were conducted and analyses compared families who engaged and with families who did not engage. In this chapter we are able to report on preliminary findings that indicate the intervention's feasibility.

The CAFES groups are still running and follow-up assessments are still being conducted. At the time of this writing, the CAFES program has had contact with more than 200 families, of which more than 100 were assigned to control groups and over 100 assigned to intervention groups. Approximately three out of every five families assigned to interventions groups actually engaged in the CAFES groups. The demographic characteristics that distinguish families who engaged in CAFES groups are older age, more marital disruption, and older age of first child. The experience of these families in the United States is characterized by: being newer arrivals to the United States; having lower rates of employment; having lower monthly family income; exhibiting lower rates of English speaking; and reporting higher rates of PTSD and depression. As far as the effectiveness of the CAFES intervention is concerned, preliminary analysis of the data set indicates that the CAFES intervention is associated with improvements in psychiatric service utilization, knowledge and attitudes concerning trauma related mental health, family communication, mental health service utilization, and symptoms of depression.

The TAFES program had contact with 61 Kosovar refugee families of which 42 families (69%) engaged in TAFES groups. The TAFES intervention was able to engage a wide range of persons including those who were working and more highly educated. Several characteristics were associated with those who engaged, including: higher age of parents; lower monthly family income; higher number of children; and higher age of first child. All families were new arrivals to the United States. The uncontrolled post-intervention assessments demonstrated increases in social support and psychiatric service utilization, both of which were associated with engagement in the TAFES group. Engagers also showed time changes in scale scores assessing trauma mental health knowledge, trauma mental health attitudes, and family hardiness (Weine, Raijna et al., 2001).

These preliminary results of the CAFES and TAFES interventions are generally consistent with a claim found in the family literature—that the results of family interventions are, "promising but not conclusive" (Campbell & Patterson, 1995). In particular, the findings in the area of change in knowledge and attitude and service utilization is consistent with the claim that family psychoeducation has been shown to be most effective.

As we await the complete analysis of the outcome data, the three questions for family intervention research posed in Gillis and Davis's (1992) review article seem very pertinent to family interventions after refugee trauma: Which outcomes are we best able to influence? What types of interventions are most effective for what types of families? What types of interventions are most effective for what types of clinical problems? It follows that, in research on family-focused interventions with refugees, the intervention must be targeted to the specific needs and strengths of a sub-population of refugee families and the study measures must be closely integrated with the factors that the intervention intends to change. Qualitative investigations can also be very helpful in research with families and family focused interventions. Currently we are conducting qualitative investigations of CAFES implementation, TAFES implementation, CAFES engagement, and Bosnian adolescents and their families.

Services research concerning refugee families has a long way to go. The systems that provide and fund mental health services are largely oriented in other directions (e.g., individual, psychopathological, psychodynamic). The agencies providing services are often competitive and resistant to linkages into a broader network. The concepts and methodologies for addressing the complex issues involved in family-focused services research are not yet accepted as part of the refugee mental health field. However, when we see refugee families providing necessary strength and meaning to family members, and when we see that services can better facilitate those efforts, we believe that this is a struggle worth undertaking.

REFERENCES

Agger, I., & Jensen, S. (1996). *Trauma and recovery under state terrorism.* London: Zed Books.

Barger, W. K., & Truong, T. V. (1978). Community action work among the Vietnamese. *Human Organization, 37,* 95-100.

Bar-On, D. (1996). Attempting to overcome the intergenerational transmission of trauma. In R. J. Apfel & B. Simon (Eds.), *Minefields in their hearts: The mental health of children in war and communal violence* (pp. 165-188). New Haven and London: Yale University Press.

Ben-Porath, Y. S. (1987). *Issues in the psychosocial adjustment of refugees.* (Contract No. 278-85-0024 CH) Rockville, MD: National Institute of Mental Health.

Bringa, T. (1995). *Being Muslim the Bosnian way.* Princeton and Chichester: Princeton University Press.

Bubolz, M. M., & Sontag, M. S. (1993). Human ecology theory. In P. G. Boss, W. M. Doherty, R. Larossa, W. R. Schumm, & S. K. Steinmetz (Eds.), *Sourcebook of family theories and methods: A contextual approach* (pp. 419-448). New York: Plenum.

Campbell, T. L., & Patterson, J. M. (1995). The effectiveness of family interventions in the treatment of physical illness. *Journal of Marital and Family Therapy, 21*(4), 545-583.

Castells, M. (1997). *The power of identity.* Padstow, Cornwall, Great Britain: T. J. International Limited.

Chambon, A. (1989). Refugee families' experiences: Three family themes – family disruption, violent trauma, and acculturation. *Journal of Strategic and Systemic Therapies, 8,* 3-13.

Danieli, Y. (Ed.). (1998). *Intergenerational handbook of multigenerational legacies of trauma.* New York and London: Plenum Press.

Danieli, Y., Rodley, N., & Wesaeth, L. (Eds.). (1996). *International responses to traumatic stress: Humanitarian, human rights, justice, peace and development contributions, collaborative actions, and future initiatives.* Amityville, NY: Baywood Publishing.

De Girolamo, G., & McFarlane, A. C. (1996). The epidemiology of PTSD: A comprehensive review of the international literature. In A. Marsella, M. J. Friedman, E. T. Gerrity, & R. M. Scurfield (Eds.), *Ethnocultural aspects of posttraumatic stress disorder* (pp. 33-85). Washington, DC: American Psychological Association.

DiNicola, V. (1997). *A stranger in the family.* New York and London: W. W. Norton & Company.

Elliott, D., & Tolan, P. H. (1999). Youth violence, prevention, intervention and social policy: An overview. In D. Flannery & R. Hoff (Eds.), *Youth violence: A volume in the psychiatric clinics of North America* (pp. 3-46). Washington, DC: American Psychiatric Association.

Fox, G. L., & McBride-Murry, V. (2000). Gender and families: Feminist perspectives and family research. *Journal of Marriage and the Family, 62,* 1160-1172.

Garcia-Peltoniemi, R. (1991). Epidemiological perspectives. In J. Westermeyer, C. Williams, & A. Nguyen (Eds.), *Mental health services for refugees.* Washington, DC: U.S. Government Printing Office.

Gillis, C. L., & Davis, L. L. (1992). Does family intervention make a difference? An integrative review and meta-analysis. In S. Feetham, S. Meister, C. Gilliss, & J. Bell (Eds.), *Nursing of families: Theories/research/education/practice* (pp. 259-265). Newport, CA: Sage Publications.

Gottlieb, B. (1981). Preventive interventions involving social networks and social support. In B. H. Gotlieb (Ed.), *Social support and social networks* (pp. 201-232). Beverly Hills: Sage.

Holder, B., Turner-Musa, J., Kimmel, P., Alleyne, S., Kobrin, S., Simmens, S., Druz, I., & Reiss, D. (1998). Engagement of African American families in research on chronic illness: A multisystem recruitment approach. *Family Process, 37*(2), 127-151.

Jaronson, J., & Bamford, P. (1987). *Program models for mental health treatment of refugees.* A report for the Refugee Assistance Program–Mental Health Technical Assistance Center. University of Minnesota. NIMH Contract # 278-85-0024 (CH).

Judah, T. (2000). *Kosovo: War and revenge.* New Haven and London: Yale University Press.

Kinzie J. D., Fredrickson, R. H., Ben, R., Fleck, J., & Karls, W. (1984). Postraumatic stress disorder among survivors of Cambodian concentration camps. *American Journal of Psychiatry, 141,* 645-650.

Klein, D. M., & White, J. M. (1996). *Family theories: An introduction.* Thousand Oaks, CA: Sage Publishers.

Leopold, M. B., & Harrell-Bond (1994). An overview of the world refugee crisis. In A. M. Marsella, T. Bornemann, S. Ekblad, & J. Orley (Eds.), *Amidst peril and pain.* Washington, DC: American Psychological Association.

Lin, T., & Lin, M. (1978). Service delivery issues in Asian-North American communities. *American Journal of Psychiatry, 135*(4), 454-56.

Lindy, J., Grace, M., & Green, B. (1981). Survivors: Outreach to a reluctant population. *American Journal of Orthopsychiatry, 51*(3), 468-478.

Lum, R. G. (1985). A community-based mental health service to Southeast Asian refugees. In T. C. Owan (Ed.), *Southeast Asian mental health: Treatment, prevention, services, training, and research* (pp. 283-306). Washington, DC: U.S. Government Printing Office.

Malcolm, N. (1998). *Kosovo: A short history.* New York: New York University Press.

Malcom, N. (1994). *Bosnia: A short history.* New York: New York University Press.

Marsella, A. M., Bornemann, T., Ekblad, S., & Orley, J. (Eds.). (1994). *Amidst peril and pain.* Washington DC: American Psychological Association.

McGoldrick, M., Giordana J., & Pearce, J. (Eds.). (1996). *Ethnicity and family therapy* (2nd ed.). New York: Guilford Press.

McCubbin, M. A., & McCubbin, H. T. (1996). Resiliency in families: A conceptual model of family adjustment and adaptation in response to stress and crises. In H. I. McCubbin, A. I. Thompson, & M. A. McCubbin (Eds.), *Family assessment: Resiliency, coping and adaptation–Inventories for research and practice* (pp. 1-64). Madison: University of Wisconsin Press.

McKay, M., Gonzalez, J., Stone S., Ryland, D., & Kohner, K. (1995). Multiple family therapy groups: A responsive intervention model for inner-city families. *Social Work with Groups, 18,* 41-56.

Mollica, R., Wyshak, G., & Lavelle, J. (1987). The psychosocial impact of war trauma and torture on Southeast Asian refugees. *American Journal of Psychiatry, 144,* 1567-1572.

Mollica, R., Wyshak, G., & Lavelle, J. (1990). Assessing symptom change in Southeast Asian refugee refugees of mass violence and torture. *American Journal of Psychiatry, 47,* 83-88.

Moore, L., & Boehnlein, J. (1991). Post traumatic stress disorder, depression, and somatic symptoms in U.S. Mien patients. *Journal of Nervous and Mental Diseases, 179,* 728-733.

Owan, T. C. (1985). Southeast Asian mental health: Transition from treatment services to prevention–A new direction. In T. C. Owan (Ed.), *Southeast Asian mental health: Treatment, prevention, services, training, and research* (pp. 141-167). Washington, DC: U.S. Government Printing Office.

Pescosolido, B. A., Gardner, C. B., & Lubell, K. M. (1998). How people get into mental health services: Stories of choice, coercion and 'muddling through' from 'first timers'. *Social Science and Medicine, 46,* 155-164.

Pescosolido, B. A., Boyer, C. A., & Lubell, K. M. (1999). The social dynamics of responding to mental health problems: Past, present and future challenges to understanding individuals' use of services. In C. S. Aneshensel & J. C. Phelan (Eds.), *Handbook of the sociology of mental health* (pp. 441-460). New York: Kluwer Academic/Plenum Publishers.

Pescosolido, B. A. (1986, August). Migration, medical care preferences and the lay referral system: A network theory of role assimilation. *American Sociological Review, 51,* 523-540.

Rogler, L. H., & Cortes, D. E. (1993). Help-seeking pathways: A unifying concept in mental health care. *American Journal of Psychiatry, 150,* 554-61.

Rolland, J. S. (1994). *Families, illness, and disability: An integrative treatment model.* New York: Basic Books.

Rosenheck, R., & Fontana, A. (1996). Ethnocultural variations in service use among veterans suffering from PTSD. In A. J. Marsella, M. J. Friedman, E. T. Gerrity, & R. Scurfield (Eds.) *Ethnocultural aspects of posttraumatic stress disorder* (pp. 483-504). Washington DC: American Psychological Association.

Simon, R. (1983). Refugee families' adjustment and aspirations: A comparison of Soviet Jewish and Vietnamese immigrants. *Ethnic and Racial Studies, 6,* 492-504.

Sluzki, C. E. (1979). Migration and family conflict. *Family Process, 18,* 379-389.

Smajkic, A., Weine, S., Bijedic, Z., Boskailo, E., Lewis, J., & Pavkovic, I. (2001). Sertraline, paroxetine and venlafaxine in refugee post traumatic stress disorder with depression symptoms. *Journal of Traumatic Stress.* 14(3), 445-452

Sue, D. W., & Sue, D. (1999). *Counseling the culturally different: Theory and practice* (3rd ed.). New York: Wiley.

Szapocznik, J., Perez-Vidal, A., Brickman, A. L., Foote, F. H., Santisteban, D., Hervis, O., & Kurtinex, W. (1988). Engaging adolescent drug abuses and their families in treatment: A strategic structural systems approach. *Journal of Consulting and Clinical Psychology, 56*(4), 552-557.

Szapocznik, J., Santisteban, D., Rio, A., Perez-Vidal, A., Santisteban, D., & Kurtines, W. (1989). Family effectiveness training: An intervention to prevent drug abuse and problem behaviors in Hispanic adolescents. *Hispanic Journal of Behavioral Sciences, 11*(1), 4-27.

Tolan, P. H., & McKay, M. (1996). Preventing serious antisocial behavior in inner-city children: An empirically based family prevention program. *Family Relations, 45,* 148-155.

van der Veer, G. (1992). *Counseling and therapy with refugees.* Chichester: Wiley.

Vinh, H. T. (1981). Indochinese mutual assistance associations. *Journal of Refugee Resettlement, 1,* 49-52.

Volkan, V., Ast, G., & Greer, W. (2002). *The Third Reich in the unconscious.* New York: Brunner-Routledge.

Waldman, R. (1999). *Psychosocial effects of complex emergencies: Symposium report.* Washington, DC: The American Red Cross.

Walsh, F. (1998). *Strengthening family resilience.* New York and London: Guilford Press.

Weine, S. M. (1998). A Prevention and Access intervention for survivor families. National Institute of Mental Health (RO1 MH59573-01).

Weine, S. M. (1999). *When history is a nightmare: Lives and memories of ethnic cleansing in Bosnia-Herzegovina.* New Brunswick and London: Rutgers University Press.

Weine, S. M. (2001). From war zone to contact zone: Culture and refugee mental health services. *Medical Student Journal of the American Medical Association, 285,* 1214.

Weine, S. M., Becker, D. F., McGlashan, T. H., Laub, D., Lazrove, S., Vojvoda, D., & Hyman, L. (1995). Psychiatric consequences of ethnic cleansing: Clinical assessments and trauma testimonies of newly resettled Bosnian refugees. *American Journal of Psychiatry, 152*(4), 536-542.

Weine, S. M., Becker, D., McGlashan, T., Vojvoda, D., Hartman, S., & Robbins, J. (1995). Adolescent survivors of "ethnic cleansing": Notes on the first year in America. *Journal of the Academy of Child and Adolescent Psychiatry, 34,*(9), 1153-1159.

Weine, S. M., Danieli, Y., Silove, D., van Ommeren, M., Fairbank, J., & Saul, J. (in press). Guidelines for international training in mental health and psychosocial interventions for trauma exposed populations in clinical and community settings. *Psychiatry.*

Weine, S. M., Kuc, E., Dzudza, E., Razzano, L., & Pavkovic, I. (2001). PTSD among Bosnian refugees: A survey of providers' knowledge, attitudes and service patterns. *Journal of Community Mental Health 37*(3), 261-271.

Weine, S. M., Kulenovic, T., Dzubur, A., Pavkovic, I., & Gibbons, R. (1998). Testimony psychotherapy in Bosnian refugees: A pilot study. *American Journal of Psychiatry, 155,* 1720-1726.

Weine, S. M., Raijna, D., Kulauzovic, Y., Zhubi, M., Huseni, D., Delisi, M., Feetham, S., Campbell, R. T., Mermelstein, R., & Pavkovic, I. (2001). *The TAFES multi-family group intervention for Kosovar refugees: A descriptive study.* Poster presentation at the Third Annual Summer Institute of the Family Research Consortium III, sponsored by the National Institute of Mental Health. Lake Tahoe, California.

Weine, S. M., Razzano, L., Miller, K., Brkic, N., Ramic, A., Smajkic, A., Bijedic, Z., Boskailo, E., Mermelstein, R., & Pavkovic, I. (2000). Profiling the trauma related symptoms of Bosnian refugees who have not sought mental health services. *Journal of Nervous and Mental Diseases, 188*(7), 416-421.

Weine, S. M., Vojvoda, D., Becker, D., McGlashan, T., Hodzic, E., Laub, D., Hyman, L., Sawyer, M., & Lazrove, S. (1998). PTSD symptoms on Bosnian refugees one year after resettlement. *American Journal of Psychiatry, 155*(4), 562-564.

Weine, S. M., Vojvoda, D., Hartman, S., & Hyman, L. (1997). A family survives genocide. *Psychiatry, 60,* 24-39.

Weine, S. M., Ware, N., Knafl, K., & Feetham, S. (2002). Family beliefs adaptation and ethnographic evidence in services research with refugee families. Plenary Paper presented at the 15th International Conference on Services

Research: Evidence in Mental Health Services Research: What Types, How Much, and Then What? Washington, D.C.

Westermeyer, J. (1986) Indochinese refugees in community and clinic: A report from Asia and the United States. In C. L. Williams & J. Westermeyer (Eds.), *Refugee mental health in resettlement countries* (pp. 113-130). Washington: Hemisphere.

Westermeyer, J. (1991). Frameworks of mental health services. In J. Westermeyer, C. L. Williams, & A. N. Nguyen (Eds.), *Mental health services for refugees*. Washington, DC: U.S. Government Printing Office.

Westermeyer, J., & Wahmanhold, K. (1996). Refugee children. In R. J. Apfel and B. Simon (Eds.), *Minefields in their hearts: The mental health of children in war and communal violence* (pp. 75-103). New Haven and London: Yale University Press.

Williams, C. L. (1986). Mental health assessment of refugees. In C. Williams & J. Westermeyer (Eds.), *Refugee mental health in resettlement countries* (pp. 175-187). Washington, DC: Hemisphere.

Williams, C. L. (1989). Prevention programs for refugees: An interface for mental health and public health. *Journal of Primary Prevention, 10,* 167-186.

Williams, C. L. (1996). Toward the development of preventive interventions for youth traumatized by war and refugee flight. In R. J. Apfel & B. Simon (Eds.), *Minefields in their hearts: The mental health of children in war and communal violence* (pp. 201-217). New Haven and London: Yale University Press.

Wright, L., Watson, W., & Bell, J. (1996). *Beliefs: The heart of healing in families and illness.* New York: Basic Books.

9

Hmong Refugees in the United States: A Community-Based Advocacy and Learning Intervention

Jessica Goodkind, Panfua Hang, and Mee Yang

As a country founded by individuals seeking religious and political refuge, the United States has accepted more refugees than any other country (Idelson, 1995). Upon resettlement, most refugees struggle to adjust psychologically, physically, socially, and economically to their new communities. The adjustment of Hmong refugees has been particularly challenging (e.g., Rumbaut, 1989; Yang & Murphy, 1993). We developed the Refugee Well-Being Project at Michigan State University[1] to promote the well-being and empowerment of Hmong refugees. It was rooted in

[1]The Refugee Well-Being Project was funded by the National Institute of Mental Health (Grant # F31 MH 12789). The authors wish to acknowledge the contributions to this research made by Cris Sullivan, Deborah Bybee, Kou Lee, Pao Yang, Yer Yang, Xue Vue, Noerung Hang, Kyle Pund, Nancy Vue, and all of the Hmong residents and undergraduate students who participated in this project.

an ecological perspective, focusing on improving the community's responsiveness to the needs of refugees and emphasizing adaptation as a mutual process by both the refugees and their environments. For a period of 6 months, Hmong adults and undergraduate students participated together in the intervention, which had two major elements: an educational component, which involved cultural exchange, opportunities to address community issues collectively, and one-on-one learning opportunities for Hmong adults, and an advocacy component which involved undergraduates advocating for and transferring advocacy skills to Hmong families to increase their access to resources in their communities. An evaluation with both quantitative and qualitative components revealed that participants' quality of life, satisfaction with resources, English proficiency, and knowledge for the United States citizenship test increased and their levels of distress decreased over the course of the intervention.

BACKGROUND

Sociopolitical Context

Before the late 1970s, the majority of immigrants and refugees who resettled in the United States were of European descent. However, the Immigration and Nationality Act of 1965 removed discriminatory country-by-country quotas that favored Europeans and Canadians. Subsequently, one of the largest groups of refugees to resettle in the United States were Southeast Asians, who began arriving in large numbers in the 1970s and 1980s, as a result of the Vietnam conflict and the Pol Pot regime in Cambodia. One of the many groups among this influx was the Hmong people, a minority ethnic group from the mountains of Laos. Their resettlement in the United States since the 1970s follows a long history of persecution and suffering as an ethnic minority in several countries. Originally from China, many fled Chinese efforts of forced assimilation and migrated to the mountains of Laos and Vietnam about 150 years ago. As a result of their recruitment by the CIA to fight against the North Vietnamese and their communist allies in Laos during the Vietnam Conflict, many Hmong were forced to flee from Laos to Thailand between 1975 and 1990, where they spent up to 20 years in refugee camps. Between 1975 and 1996, the United States accepted many of these Hmong refugees for resettlement. Approximately 250,000 Hmong currently live in the United States, and, during the 1990s, the number of Hmong in the United States was increasing faster than the population of any other Asian group (Yang & Murphy, 1993).

In order to promote the well-being of Hmong refugees, it is essential to understand some of the important aspects of Hmong culture and its strengths. Hmong culture is a collectivist, clan-based culture (Scott, 1982), which, as opposed to American and other Western cultures that emphasize autonomy, privacy, and individual initiative, is based on a "we" orientation and the importance of group solidarity, duties and obligations, and a collective identity. More than any other immigrant group, the Hmong have succeeded in preserving many aspects of their culture, interdependency, and sense of ethnic community (Fadiman, 1997). This emphasis on clan and community is an important strength of the Hmong community, which commonly results in an incredibly extensive and strong support system (Dunnigan, 1982; Hutchison, 1991).

Despite these strengths, the Hmong have been particularly challenged in their adjustment to life in the United States. Numerous factors have contributed to their difficulties: significant language and cultural differences, limited previous education (which puts any individual or group at a disadvantage in the United States), limited transferable occupational skills, and the particular context into which they were relocated (most Hmong arrived here in the 1980s in the midst of a severe economic recession with high unemployment). As a result of these factors, the Hmong have experienced a large gap between the abilities they possess and the needs they must fulfill here (Scott, 1982). In fact, statistics from the U.S. Department of Commerce indicate that the quality of life for the Hmong community is precarious. In 1990, the median household income for the Hmong was $14,300, 67% of households received public assistance, 87% of Hmong lived in rental units, 86% did not have a high school degree, and 60% were linguistically isolated (Hein, 1995). It is also important to understand that many Hmong families are faced with limited income and other resources in the context of having many people to support. In a representative study of 355 Hmong households, Rumbaut (1989) found that they had an average of nine people per household. The large gap between their skills and needs and the time Hmong refugees have spent in refugee camps (anywhere from a few months to 20 years) have resulted in many Hmong refugees feeling particularly powerless in the United States. Many have lost a sense of control over their lives. This is contradictory to Hmong people's usual experiences of being active in their communities and in decision-making processes, and has exacerbated their distress (e.g., Westermeyer, Vang, & Lyfong, 1983; Westermeyer, Vang, & Neider, 1983).

Mental Health and Psychosocial Implications

The adverse mental health consequences related to becoming a refugee (i.e., the trauma of war, violence, escape, and resettlement), particularly for the Hmong and other Southeast Asian refugees, have been extensively documented (e.g., Carlson & Rosser-Hogan, 1991; Rumbaut, 1991; Westermeyer, Neider, & Callies, 1989). Many of these studies have focused particularly on psychiatric symptoms such as depression, somatization, phobia, anxiety, hostility, and paranoia (e.g., Carlson & Rosser-Hogan, 1991; Westermeyer et al., 1989). Westermeyer and colleagues found that there was a large subgroup of Hmong adults who continued to experience many of these symptoms even after 8 years in the United States.

However, other researchers have measured psychological well-being of Hmong refugees using the Psychological Well-Being Scale (Rumbaut, 1991), which is an adapted version of the General Well-Being Index (Dupuy, 1974) that assesses frequency of affective symptoms of well-being and distress. According to Rumbaut (1985), the Psychological Well-Being Scale measures emotional and somatic distress and overall demoralization, rather than depression or other clinical disorders. The measure also includes a happiness subscale. Taken together, these scales are "reliable measures of general and persistent affective states as reported by the person" (Rumbaut, 1989, p. 155). In a broad study of refugee adjustment, Hmong refugees' rates of distress/demoralization were three times higher than that of other Americans (Rumbaut, 1991). Furthermore, their average levels of distress/demoralization were significantly higher and their average happiness levels significantly lower than Vietnamese, Cambodian, Laotian, and Chinese-Vietnamese refugees (Ying & Akutsu, 1997).

Rumbaut (1991) has also widely assessed refugees' psychological well-being in terms of life satisfaction, which he describes as a cognitive rather than affective appraisal of well-being. Compared to other Southeast Asian refugee groups (Khmer, Chinese-Vietnamese, and Vietnamese), the Hmong were the least satisfied with their lives and were the only group whose life satisfaction decreased over time (Rumbaut, 1989). Rumbaut (1991) emphasized that distress and life satisfaction are not opposite dimensions of a single scale, but rather measure very different psychological processes. Thus, it seems important to consider definitions of psychological well-being that include both affective and cognitive components, and which use measures that have been developed to assess a wider range of people's experiences rather than only clinical populations. Furthermore, including life satisfaction and happiness measures provides opportunities to present research findings that are not solely deficit-focused.

Given the traumatic circumstances most Southeast Asian refugees have had to endure prior to their resettlement in the United States and their high rates of demoralization and distress, it is important to consider the prevention of further distress. Ying and Akutsu (1997) pointed out that refugees' existing distress will be exacerbated and that refugees may be more likely to develop clinical psychiatric symptoms and disorders if their adjustment in their country of resettlement is difficult. Rumbaut (1991) argued that refugees are at particular risk for psychological distress because of their marginal position and relative powerlessness. It is difficult for them to deal with the extensive changes (usually undesired) they have endured and to try to achieve their life goals in a new, foreign environment. Thus it is important for refugees to feel they have influence and control in their new environments. Recent research has documented that much of refugees' distress in their countries of resettlement is due to what Miller (1999) termed exile-related stressors—that is, daily economic concerns about survival in a new country, racism and discrimination, loss of community and social support, and loss of meaningful social roles—rather than solely to past traumas (e.g., Gorst-Unsworth & Goldenberg, 1998; Lavik, Hauff, Skrondal, & Solberg, 1996; Pernice &

Brook, 1996; Silove et al., 1997). Taken together, these findings highlight the potential for amelioration of distress through attention to refugees' postmigration experiences in their communities.

When considering a move away from traditional individual, trauma-focused interventions, it is also important to note that distressed refugees often do not use mental health clinics—both because they are not necessarily responsive to the needs of refugees and ethnic minorities and because of the common stigma of seeking psychological help (Sue & Morishima, 1982). In addition, research has shown that therapy and/or drugs alone are not effective without also addressing the social and economic needs of refugees (e.g., Kinzie & Fleck, 1987; Pejovic, Jovanovic, & Djurdic, 1997)Furthermore, individual interventions can be culturally inappropriate and even disempowering, particularly for refugees with collectively oriented cultures (e.g., Strawn, 1994). Finally, they may pathologize individuals (Ryan, 1976) and fail to utilize resources and strengths in their communities (Rappaport, 1981).

INTERVENTION

Theory and Rationale

An ecological and strengths-based perspective guided the design of the Refugee Well-Being Project. An ecological perspective on refugee well-being is based on several important principles. First, it is essential to attend to the culture and histories of individuals, their particular context, and the fit between the two (Kelly, 1968). An ecological perspective also emphasizes structural forces and the mobilization of community resources for disenfranchised populations that lack adequate access (Levine & Perkins, 1987). This is particularly important given the structural barriers such as prejudice and racism (e.g., Benson, 1990; Goode, 1990) and lack of economic opportunity and support (e.g., Bach & Argiros, 1991) which many refugees face. Third, an ecological paradigm suggests that it is important to consider adaptation in understanding human behavior because environments constrain and facilitate different behaviors (Kelly, 1968). This principle is particularly relevant to refugees, who are forced to adapt to new, very different environments, and also emphasizes that adaptation can occur not only by changes in individuals, but through changes in the environment as well. Thus, an intervention should not focus solely on refugees adjusting to their existing environment, but also on changing the environment if it is unfair or constraining. Finally, an ecological perspective directs us to create collaborative, culturally appropriate interventions that do not rely solely on outside "experts" but instead involve individuals and groups in solving their own problems (Rappaport, 1977; Trickett, 1996).

A strengths-based perspective emphasizes the importance of focusing on the strengths that individuals and communities already possess or that can be developed and the creation of settings that allow them to contribute their culture and knowledge to their broader communities and to develop skills and knowledge that they want (Dunst, Trivette, & Thompson, 1990). In sum, an ecological, strengths-based perspective suggests a focus on addressing social issues from a multilevel perspective that locates problems and solutions beyond the individual and on designing interventions with particular attention to a specific group, their context, and the mobilization of community resources.

Components and Goals

Based on an ecological perspective, the Refugee Well-Being Project was developed with two major elements: an advocacy component, based on the Community Advocacy model (Sullivan & Bybee, 1999), which involved the mobilization of resources with and for Hmong families, and an innovative group learning component, called learning circles, which involved cultural exchange, focus on community issues, and one-on-one learning opportunities for Hmong adults. The fundamental goals of the intervention were to promote the well-being of Hmong refugees by creating opportunities for individual and collective empowerment and by improving the community's responsiveness to their needs. Specifically, the program was intended to provide opportunities for Hmong participants to contribute their knowledge, skills, and abilities to their communities, acquire new skills and knowledge, direct their own learning, participate in and understand democratic processes in their communities, raise their critical consciousness, overcome feelings of powerlessness, and increase their access to community resources.

In order to accomplish these goals, trained undergraduate students worked with Hmong adults and their families in numerous ways for a period of 6 months. Undergraduates participated in the learning circles, including facilitating and sharing their experiences during the cultural exchange and working one-on-one with Hmong adults on whatever each adult wanted to learn (e.g., learning English or preparing for the U.S. citizenship exam). Undergraduates also worked individually with Hmong families as their advocates to help ensure their access to resources and opportunities in the community in areas such as employment, health care, housing, or education. These efforts also involved the undergraduates transferring their advocacy skills to the Hmong families by showing the families how to do things rather than doing things for them and by documenting the steps that they took together to mobilize resources so that the families would know how to obtain resources they needed in the future when the students were no longer there.

Rationale for Advocacy Component

The advocacy component of the intervention was based on the Community Advocacy model, which has been successfully applied to women and children who have experienced domestic violence (Sullivan & Bybee, 1999) and to juvenile offenders (Davidson, Redner, Blakely, Mitchell, & Emshoff, 1987). These advocacy projects are predicated on the belief that access to community resources is fundamental to promoting the well-being of disenfranchised individuals and groups. Refugees and immigrants who resettle in the United States often struggle to access the resources they need from their communities. They also face numerous barriers, including language and cultural differences and lack of knowledge of the system. Refugees may not be aware of their rights and responsibilities with respect to the community and community resources. In particular, the needs of Asian refugees are often ignored because service providers believe they prefer to seek and receive help exclusively from members of their own communities (Lee, 1986; Starret, Mindell, & Wright, 1983).

Rationale for Learning
Component

Newcomers to the United States often need to acquire new skills and knowledge, such as English proficiency, knowledge about political, social, and economic processes, literacy, and job skills. This type of learning is termed *instrumental learning* and is an important aspect of empowering individuals because it enables them to acquire the skills and knowledge they need to participate in their communities (Zimmerman, 1995). Learning English is also important because English proficiency is an essential resource for the economic and social adaptation of immigrants and refugees (Rumbaut, 1989) and is negatively related to depression, anxiety, and other mental health problems in Hmong refugees (Rumbaut, 1989; Westermeyer, Neider, & Callies, 1989). However, learning can further empower disenfranchised individuals by raising their consciousness, increasing their understanding of their oppression and the structural forces affecting them, and providing mechanisms through which they can work collectively for social justice. This type of learning is also referred to as *popular education* (Cunningham, 1992) or *transformative learning* (Cunningham, 1998), and places individuals and their experiences in the center of their own learning, as subjects (rather than objects) of their learning (Freire, 1998). The popular education perspective argues that individuals are shaped by their context, including their social location, and therefore it focuses on transforming social structures in order to achieve a more just society.

The work of Jane Addams is fundamental to an understanding of adult/popular education for refugees and immigrants and the educational component of the intervention. Jane Addams formed one of the first settlement houses in Chicago, because she felt that all community members must share responsibility for immigrants' well-being. Her actions were predicated on several beliefs, including the interdependence of all human beings and the importance of education as the basis of social change and the vehicle through which immigrants could contribute their unique abilities, skills, and vision to their communities. She believed that education must begin from the experiences of the learners but must also help learners to see their place in the larger world (Addams, 1964). It is important to note that popular education and Freire and Addams' approaches to learning are intimately linked to the processes of community participation, empowerment, and access to resources. They recognize education as a social as well as individual act (Cunningham, 1998) and they problematize a sole focus on individual learning without accompanying change in social structures or mobilization of resources.

Rationale for Combining Advocacy and Learning Components

The learning and advocacy components of the intervention were two inextricable parts of one holistic intervention. The intervention was centered around the group learning circles. Undergraduates and Hmong participants met in the learning circles for almost 1 month before beginning advocacy together, and often they would discuss their advocacy efforts during the learning circles to share ideas and resources with other group members, to address an unfair institution or system collectively, and/or to get the input or translation assistance of the group facilitators. The intervention was designed by the first author after her work on an advocacy intervention for women who experienced domestic violence (see Sullivan & Bybee, 1999), through which she realized that refugee families faced many of the same struggles accessing resources and being ignored by systems that were supposed to assist them, but with an awareness that an individual advocacy intervention would be ineffective because it would not build on the strengths of the Hmong community, would not provide opportunities for collective validation and action, and would not address the learning needs of Hmong refugees. Furthermore, the most important need expressed by Hmong women in the community was for opportunities to learn English and study for the U.S. Citizenship exam. Thus, by combining the advocacy and learning components, the intervention had the potential to incorporate the strengths, needs, and wants of the Hmong community. In addition, the intervention as a whole addressed the multiple aspects of the empowerment process (Parsons, Gutierrez, & Cox, 1998): (1) Building skills and knowledge for critical thinking and action (e.g., awareness of oppression, English proficiency, citizenship knowledge, advocacy skills); (2) changing attitudes and beliefs (e.g., value of own culture and knowledge, self-efficacy, ability to make change); (3) validation through collective experiences; and (4) securing real increases in resources and power through action and mobilization of community resources.

The Refugee Well-Being Project was designed to enable Hmong participants to take greater control over their lives by providing mechanisms through which they could define and solve their own problems, rather than rely on outside "experts." Gaventa (1995) pointed out both external barriers (e.g., lack of organization, lack of voice in community, limited funds to influence politics) and internal barriers (e.g., lack of critical consciousness, lack of understanding of possibilities for social change), which exclude many disenfranchised people from meaningful participation in their communities. Thus, effective participation and real gains in power require both community organizing in order to bring a group together and to establish a power-base, as well as popular education in order to enable individuals to transform how they think about themselves and their place in the world (Gordon, 1998). This project addressed both of these components by offering opportunities for transformative learning in the learning circles and for community organization through both cultural exchange and the mobilization of community resources. This project was based on the premise that "participation means that there has to be real surrender of power by the 'experts'" (Ashworth, 1997, p. 102). In this intervention, Hmong participants directed their own advocacy and controlled their own learning. No one involved in the intervention was an "expert." Rather, Hmong participants and undergraduate students learned from each other—including sharing cultural knowledge, skills, language, and information about resources. Thus, the learning and advocacy components of this intervention were specifically designed to promote the empowerment and well-being of Hmong refugees.

Implementation

Setting

The Refugee Well-Being Project was fully based in the communities of the Hmong participants. The learning circles occurred at the community centers of two public housing developments where many of the participants lived. In addition, the advocates were trained to focus on developing resources and planning activities within the Hmong families' natural environments. Thus, the project was not only convenient and accessible for Hmong participants, but also created a safe and familiar environment in which to learn and work together.

Hmong Participants

Twenty-eight Hmong adults (26 women, 2 men) from 27 families participated in the project. They were an average of 41 years old (range 22 to 77), most (79%) were married (4 were widowed, 1 was single, and 1 was legally separated), and they had an average of six children (range 0 to 11). Fifty-four percent were employed, 82% had no previous education, none of the participants had a high school degree from the United States (one woman graduated from high school in Laos), and 33% were not literate in any language. They had been in the United States an average of 12 years (range 6 months to 22 years) and resettled here at the average age of 29 (range 16 to 66). Fourteen were residents of public housing, 10 owned their own homes, and 4 rented apartments or houses. The majority of the Hmong participants were among the second wave of Hmong refugees to arrive in the United States (Yang & Murphy, 1993), possessing less education and other resources and being less equipped for life here than those who came in the first wave. Within the local Hmong community, they were among those struggling the most—many living in public housing, and most having no previous education and very low levels of English proficiency despite not being recent newcomers. Originally, the intervention was open to the participation of all Hmong adults in the community. However, much greater interest was expressed by Hmong women, and, therefore, the project was predominantly an intervention with refugee women.

Recruitment of Hmong Participants

Individuals' backgrounds are very important to most Hmong people and the mutual exchange of this information is an essential part of establishing trust. Thus, non-Hmong individuals need to be able to form a connection with Hmong people when they first meet. Even within the

Hmong community, it is important when meeting other Hmong to know their clan name and who their parents are. The first author, a Caucasian woman, worked with Hmong people in a refugee camp in Thailand for 2 years and was involved with Hmong residents in the Lansing community for several years—conducting research and teaching English. The knowledge acquired and relationships established were important in recruiting participants and creating a successful intervention. However, it was also essential to be working in collaboration with Hmong community members. Therefore, potential participants were either contacted by the first author accompanied by one of the Hmong co-facilitators of the project or solely by one of the Hmong co-facilitators (the second and third authors). All Hmong families living in the three public housing developments in the city were contacted first, by visits to their homes in which the first author and either the second or third author would describe the project and invite adults in the household to participate. There were a total of 25 Hmong families in the housing developments and 13 (52%) chose to participate. When it was determined that extra space was available, the project was opened up to other Hmong families in the community (based on the network of the authors and spreading the word throughout the Hmong community). Initially, some Hmong families were hesitant, and often called their friends or family to determine what others knew about the project and its facilitators. However, within the first week that the project began, interested Hmong adults were showing up spontaneously at the learning circles and a waiting list was created.

Undergraduate Participants

This project was implemented with the use of 27 trained paraprofessionals, who were undergraduate students at Michigan State University. Of the 27 students, there were 21 women and 6 men, 19 European Americans, 3 Latino/as, 2 Asian/Asian Americans, 2 Arab Americans, and 1 African American/Native American. All but one were juniors and seniors. Students made a two-semester commitment to the project, earned eight course credits, and received 48 hours of training over a period of 12 weeks. The training began 2 months before the commencement of the 6-month intervention and was based on a manualized curriculum (see Goodkind, 2000) adapted from the Advocate Training Manual of the Community Advocacy Project (Sullivan, 1998). Students received weekly grades based on their comprehension of the material, which included readings and units on adult education and social change, refugee learning, specifics of the experiences and culture of Hmong refugees, the special needs of refugee children, oppression and diversity, and collective action and the immigrant experience. Students also participated in discussions, role plays, class exercises, community projects, and thought papers to prepare them for their work with a family. In addition, students learned how to be effective advocates and about the importance of community resources and community responsiveness in meeting the needs of refugees, as well as how to use empathy, values clarification, and problem-solving skills. Another important component of training involved helping undergraduates identify and make connections with community resources and networks, so that they could successfully link the Hmong families they worked with to needed resources or recognize when further efforts were necessary to mobilize resources that were not currently available. Undergraduates were also trained how to instruct their family and their family's natural advocates (e.g., family and friends) in the methods of advocacy from the beginning of the intervention, through their mutual discussion and efforts as well as the family's observations of the undergraduates' advocacy strategies. Training continued during the first month of the learning circles. For the final 5 months of the intervention, weekly supervision replaced training. Undergraduates met for supervision once a week in small groups (6–8 students) to review the progress of their advocacy and discuss their experiences in the learning circles.

The use of paraprofessional undergraduates provided several advantages, including lower cost to the community and less stigma for participants. In addition, the undergraduate students had important opportunities to learn from and with the Hmong families, to develop advocacy and teaching skills, to engage in experiential learning that allowed them to apply what they learned in the classroom, to develop critical awareness and work toward a more just society, to earn course credit for work in the community, and to acquire good experience for graduate school or a career in human services. Although a detailed discussion is beyond the scope of this chapter, interviews with the undergraduate advocates upon completion of the project revealed that the benefits they accrued were numerous and widespread.

Project Facilitators/Coordinators

The ·project was co-facilitated by the three authors (1 White American woman and 2 Hmong American women). As discussed previously, the first author had worked extensively with Hmong people in Thailand and the United States for 7 years and she spoke and understood some Hmong. The second and third authors were bicultural and bilingual, one of whom was first generation born in the United States, and the other of whom was born in Laos, spent time in a refugee camp in Thailand, and resettled in the United States when she was 14 years old. This project was conceived and developed by the first author, in close consultation with Hmong adults in the community. The second and third authors were initially hired to help recruit participants, to translate during cultural exchange time, to be available during one-on-one learning time to translate concepts, and to facilitate communication between advocates and Hmong participants in or outside of the learning circles. However, their roles quickly expanded and they became co-leaders and facilitators of the learning circles and the project in general. They helped lead and participate in cultural exchanges, and they were both teachers and learners (as was everyone in the learning circles). Many Hmong participants confided in them if they were concerned about an aspect of the project, and thus they were able to facilitate communication and understanding between Hmong participants, undergraduates, and the first author. In addition, they often accompanied Hmong participants and their advocates on trips to the doctor, the bank, or other places where translation or explanation might be required. Most importantly, they were truly leaders and facilitators of the learning circles and were an integral and essential aspect of the entire project. It would not have succeeded without their knowledge, expertise, hard work, and interpersonal skills. However, they were careful not to allow undergraduates and Hmong participants to become too dependent on them, because we wanted to keep the focus on advocates transferring skills to their families and on encouraging participants to practice their English as much as was feasible.

Components of the Intervention

Learning Circles

The learning circles were based on a model created by the Jane Addams School for Democracy in Minneapolis and have their theoretical foundation in the principles of popular education and transformative learning, as discussed previously. In addition, given the collective orientation of Hmong culture, the learning circles were important because they provided a group setting in which Hmong refugees could learn and collectively address community issues. Participants met in learning circles twice weekly at one of the housing development community centers[2] for 6 months. Each meeting was 2 hours in length and was composed of equal numbers of Hmong participants and undergraduate students.

The learning circles involved two components: cultural exchange and one-on-one learning. Cultural exchange occurred for the first 30 to 45 minutes of each meeting and was facilitated together by an undergraduate and a Hmong participant. Initially, as the three project coordinators, we also facilitated some of the discussions. In order to enable all participants to share in the discussion, regardless of English or Hmong language ability, two of the project coordinators translated Hmong to English and English to Hmong throughout the cultural exchange discussions. The purpose of the cultural exchange was to provide a forum for Hmong participants and undergraduate students to learn from each other, share ideas, develop plans for collective action, and realize the important contributions they were capable of making. Discussion topics (primarily chosen by participants and undergraduates) included: the presidential election and process (as the intervention was occurring during the 2000 presidential election), the Bill of Rights and a comparison of

---

[2]Participants had the option of joining morning learning circles or evening learning circles. This accommodated people who worked either 1st or 2nd shift. Also, the morning and evening learning circles were held at different housing developments (to ensure that locations were accessible), and transportation was provided for participants who needed it. Twelve Hmong adults (10 women, 2 men) and 11 undergraduates participated in the morning learning circles and 16 Hmong women and 16 undergraduates participated in the evening learning circles.

rights in Laos and the United States, holidays celebrated by different group members (e.g., Thanksgiving, Hmong New Year, Valentine's Day, Passover), ideas about how to raise children in the United States, health beliefs, stereotyping, and genetic cloning. In addition, numerous guest speakers were invited to the learning circles, including a city clerk who brought a voting machine and demonstrated its use, an union organizer who discussed workplace issues and workers' rights, two representatives from a Hmong woman's organization in Detroit, and a Hmong youth leader who focused on issues kids face in school. Finally, group members took several field trips, including visits to the Capitol building to see the state legislature, the state museum, and a speech by President Bill Clinton.

The second component of the learning circles was one-on-one learning. For the remaining 1¼ to 1½ hours of the meeting time, undergraduates and Hmong participants worked in pairs and focused on whatever each Hmong adult wanted to learn (e.g., speaking, reading, and writing English, studying for the U.S. citizenship exam, learning to complete employment applications and practice interviews, writing checks, or any area of learning each chose). This aspect of the one-on-one learning was very important and different from most other learning situations. Vella (1994) called this "participation of the learners in naming what is to be learned" (p. 3), and stated that it is essential for effective adult learning. Hmong participants were actively engaged in their own learning processes and received individual attention, which provided them with control over their own learning and more concentrated learning time. It is also important to note that the undergraduates were also engaged in learning, as they learned about the culture, experiences, and knowledge of Hmong participants. Materials, such as citizenship study guides and English as a Second Language (ESL) materials (picture and word cards, workbooks), were available to facilitate learning.

As the project developed, the learning circles took shape in unexpected ways. This was intentional—based on the assumption that by creating the space for Hmong adults and undergraduate students to learn together and develop relationships, they would make the learning circles into places and experiences that were fun, welcoming, and beneficial. For instance, many Hmong and undergraduate participants brought snacks to learning circles, prepared and brought food to celebrate holidays together, tried on each other's traditional clothes, took pictures, and planned field trips together. Exchanges were not only material, but emotional as well. There were commonly discussions of pregnancies, illnesses, friends and family, and other signs of mutual support.

Advocacy

Once relationships began to form between individual Hmong participants and undergraduate students, each undergraduate was matched with a participating Hmong adult, with whom they had been working during the learning circles, to serve as an advocate for that person and her family. Rather than deciding who would work together, we let relationships between the Hmong participants and undergraduates develop naturally, and people tended to gravitate toward someone who matched their personality and style of learning. It is important to note that relationships between Hmong participants and undergraduate paraprofessionals formed during the learning circles, *before* sending the students into the homes of Hmong families to do advocacy. As discussed in more detail previously, forming a connection with a Hmong individual is essential to developing a good relationship. In addition, the continuation of the learning circles during the advocacy component was essential because these biweekly meetings provided a forum for Hmong adults and undergraduates to share advocacy successes and struggles with each other and to access a translator to facilitate communication when necessary. The intervention was not only an intervention with individuals, but also with the Hmong community as a whole. This is an important distinction because some of the strengths of Hmong culture are its collective orientation and the high level of mutual support within the Hmong community. These aspects of community life were important to preserve within this intervention and were important components of its success.

Each advocate spent an additional 4 to 6 hours each week (outside of the learning circles) with the Hmong adult and her family to provide advocacy on any issues the family wanted to address. Advocacy continued for 5 months, with some undergraduates mainly working with the adult participant and some undergraduates working closely with both the Hmong adult and her children. The undergraduates first worked with the families to identify the specific issues each family wanted to

focus on during the 5 months of advocacy. Often these discussions occurred during learning circles, so that translators could assist with communication. Once an unmet need was identified, the advocate and family proceeded through the four phases of advocacy they had learned during their training: assessment, implementation, monitoring, and secondary implementation.

During assessment, the unmet needs of the family, such as employment, education, health care, transportation, or material goods, were
identified. Next, the advocate and family attempted to identify any and
all resources in the community that might meet this need. Once these
potential resources were identified, implementation began. In this phase,
the advocate and family worked together to generate and/or mobilize
community resources to satisfy the need. Monitoring was the important
next step of advocacy, in which the advocate and family evaluated the
effectiveness of the resources mobilized in meeting the family's needs. If
it was decided that the particular need had not been adequately addressed, then the undergraduate and family began secondary implementation to mobilize additional resources or adjusted current efforts to further satisfy the need. Because most families had multiple unmet needs,
the advocate and family were most often engaged simultaneously in
several phases of the advocacy process, in order to address the various
needs the family had identified.

In addition, undergraduates continually worked hard to transfer advocacy skills to the Hmong participants and their families. Undergraduates made sure that they helped Hmong participants do things for themselves, rather than the undergraduates doing things for them. They often
demonstrated or modeled certain actions with their families, and then
encouraged the families to take the lead. They would role play what the
undergraduate and the adult(s) or children in the family would say in
various situations (including how to say things in English), and they
would clarify how involved each of them would be in the advocacy process. For instance, if they were going to meet a resource provider, they
would agree beforehand who would do what and would never assume
that their family wanted them to talk on their behalf. Advocates also
helped Hmong participants identify other family members who could
communicate well in English if they were not able to themselves.
Undergraduates made it clear to their family from the beginning that

they were going to be working together for a 20-week time period. As the intervention progressed, undergraduates encouraged their families to perform many of the advocacy tasks on their own, so that transfer of advocacy skills did not only involve talking to the family about how to execute self-advocacy, but also first-hand experience for the family. During the last four weeks of the intervention, the undergraduates tried to provide their families with all of the information they had been using together, so that the family and their significant others would have an alternative to passive acceptance of unfulfilled needs.

An example of one participant's experiences follows, although it is important to note that the intervention process was different for each participant, because the learning and advocacy were directed by the Hmong individual and her family, rather than by what the undergraduate thought the participant might want or need.

Case Illustration [3]

Mai, a 31-year-old Hmong woman with four children, came to the United States in 1989. She and her family lived in the housing development where the morning learning circles were held, which fit well into her schedule because she worked 2nd shift (2:30 pm to 11:00 pm) baking donuts at a local bakery chain. She joined the project with one main goal—to study for the U.S. citizenship test. From the first day, Mai was very intent and dedicated to studying, and in fact sometimes wanted to study her citizenship materials before cultural exchange time was completed. However, Mai and her advocate Sara did participate in cultural exchange and facilitated several interesting discussions.

Mai and Sara started to work with each other immediately during the first learning circle meeting and became attached very quickly. After the first month of working together during learning circles, Sara and Mai were "officially" matched together and Sara began her assessment with Mai by spending time getting to know Mai and her children and husband by doing things with them such as shopping and cooking. Initially, Mai did not express many unmet needs besides U.S. citizenship. Thus,

---

[3]Names and identifying information have been changed to protect the participants' privacy.

Sara focused on helping Mai fill out her citizenship application, creating flashcards of the 100 citizenship questions for Mai, and spending extra time studying with her each week. Throughout the 6 months Sara and Mai spent together, however, several other needs emerged.

The first need to arise was that Mai and her family's green cards were expiring and they were not sure what to do. They hoped to become citizens before renewing them, but Sara helped them contact the Immigration and Naturalization Service, determined that they did need to renew their cards, and accompanied them to Detroit to do so. Soon after that and about halfway through the project, Mai's husband was laid off and Sara was able to help him file for unemployment. Around the same time, Mai developed a severely swollen neck and Sara learned that Mai did not have any health insurance. Sara found a free health clinic where Mai could be tested and treated and was also able to help Mai sign up for health insurance through the county. Another salient issue for Mai was the stress she endured at work. She and many of the other women in the project, who worked at the same bakery, were required to work many hours of overtime and were on their feet constantly. Mai frequently hurt her hands or back lifting heavy trays of donuts and shared with the group that she had miscarried during her last pregnancy due to the stress and strain of her job. We invited a union organizer to talk to the group about workers' rights and although Mai and the other women were wary about trying to organize a union at their workplace, they felt that they understood more about their rights and that there were people who cared about their predicaments.

Sara was extremely effective at not only locating resources for Mai and her family, but also in transferring the advocacy skills she had learned to Mai and her children. When Mai's oldest daughter needed a physical exam for school, she talked to Sara, who helped her find places to call and encouraged her to make the calls herself. Mai explained this transfer of skills in an interview:

Like, for example, she [Sara] take me to renew my green card, and so, show us how to do it, and then what to do, and then . . . I learned more because of that.

Sara's enthusiasm and interest was effusive and she took outside initiative to find articles on Hmong culture to read and to share with Mai and her oldest daughter. By the end of the 6 months, Mai felt that she could continue to study for the citizenship test on her own. However, she invited Sara to Hmong New Year to celebrate with her family and she made plans to continue to spend time with Sara—teaching Sara how to garden and doing fun things together with Sara and the children. At the final graduation ceremony, Mai brought Hmong clothes and asked Sara to wear them, which is a very high compliment. Mai and her husband (with whom she shared her learning materials) passed the U.S. citizenship test several months later.

Ending the Project

The Refugee Well-Being Project was designed as a small pilot project. In consideration of this, as well as the nature of undergraduate students' schedules, the project was conceived of as having a clear ending point. Another purpose of this structure was to try to avoid Hmong participants becoming overly dependent on their advocates—rather the focus was intentionally on the undergraduates transferring advocacy skills to the Hmong participants and their families. Thus, after 8 months of work with the undergraduates and 6 months of the Hmong participants and undergraduates working together, the project officially ended. Several plans were made to attempt to lessen the difficulty of an abrupt ending. First, the undergraduates were trained to continually work on transferring their advocacy skills to their families, and this was particularly emphasized during the last month of the project. In addition, the ending date of the project was made clear to all participants from the beginning. As this date approached, undergraduates created separate "termination packets" for their adult and any children with whom they had worked closely. These packets contained pictures, letters, stories, quotes, suggestions for fun activities in the community, and other creative material. The packets were also very important because they included community resources in areas that each pair had worked on together or that the Hmong family might need in the future. Finally, a graduation ceremony and celebration was planned collaboratively and held at a park. Everyone cooked food, brought their families and friends (including lots of children). Graduation certificates were presented to all Hmong participants and undergraduates (since everyone learned together), undergraduates gave their families the termination packets, and many photos were taken. Some undergraduates and Hmong participants maintained their relationships with each other after the project ended, whereas others did not. In addition, due to the interest of many Hmong participants and undergraduate students, smaller learning circles have continued to be held twice a week. Although the advocacy component has ended, these groups meet to study and talk and the undergraduates are participating without receiving course credit.

CHALLENGES AND LESSONS LEARNED

Overall, the Refugee Well-Being Project was quite successful. In addition to the positive impacts on participants discussed subsequently, the project's success was evident by the fact that all participants continued to attend throughout the 6 months. However, it is important to recognize that there were numerous challenges throughout the process. One of the most salient was the language difference. Despite the excellent translation provided by the co-facilitators, many participants often felt frustrated with their inability to communicate with each other. This frustration subsided in some regards, as everyone learned that relationships can develop across language barriers and learned more English (or Hmong in some cases), but as relationships grew stronger, participants' inability to fully express themselves to each other was also highlighted. The short length of time of the project was also difficult for many participants. As the ending date approached, many of the Hmong participants began mentioning it during learning circle discussions and expressed their concern and disappointment. On the other hand, another challenge of this project was that it required a large time commitment from Hmong participants and undergraduate students, all of whom had many competing responsibilities including children, work, and classes. Finally, despite the explicit attention devoted to avoiding dependency and the extensive steps discussed previously that undergraduates took to transfer their advocacy skills to the Hmong participants, their families, and other natural advocates (e.g., extended family members and friends), there was a constant tension evident because many Hmong participants' limited English proficiency made it difficult for them to access resources in the community without the assistance of their undergraduate or an interpreter.

EVALUATION

Method

To assess the impact of the intervention, a comprehensive, multimethod strategy was implemented, including a within-group longitudinal design with four data collection points over a period of 9 months and in-depth qualitative recruitment and post-intervention interviews with participants. This design allowed for a thorough exploration of the processes at work in the intervention.

Recruitment Interviews

The initial recruitment interviews were conducted in participants' homes by the first author with either the second or third author interpreting. They were designed to learn about participants and what they were interested in learning and obtaining from their participation in the project, as well as to begin to form relationships with the participants by listening to their flight and resettlement stories and to what their current lives in the United States were like.

Quantitative Interviews

Four quantitative interviews were completed to measure the impact of the intervention on five specific hypothesized outcomes. These interviews occurred at 3-month intervals (pre-intervention, midpoint of the intervention, immediately following the conclusion of the project, and 3 months after the project ended). The interviews were conducted in Hmong in participants' homes by trained bilingual interviewers who were not a part of the learning circles. The interviews took an average of 90 minutes and contained the following measures:

Outcomes

• *English proficiency* was measured by the Basic English Skills Test (BEST), which is a standardized measure of English as a Second Language ability, designed to assess English communication, fluency, pronunciation, and listening comprehension for adults at the survival and pre-employment skills level. It has an established internal consistency of .91 (Kenyon & Stansfield, 1989).

• *Citizenship knowledge* was measured by 10 questions from the Immigration and Naturalization Service's list of 100 questions applicants for citizenship need to know to pass the United States' citizenship exam (average Cronbach's α = .87).

• *Access to resources* was measured by adapted versions of the "Satisfaction with Resources" scale (Sullivan et al., 1992) and the "Difficulty Obtaining Resources" scale (Sullivan & Bybee, 1999). For the first scale, Hmong participants were asked to rate, on a 7-point scale, how satisfied they were about the resources they had in 11 specific domains (e.g., education, health care, housing, employment). The latter scale asked participants to rate, on a 4-point scale, how difficult it had been or would be in the future to obtain resources they needed in 14 specific life domains (e.g. transportation, employment, material goods, and services). Average Cronbach's α's for these scales were .70 and .79, respectively.

• *Psychological well-being* was measured using modified versions of the distress and happiness subscales of Rumbaut's (1985) Psychological Well-Being Scale. Each subscale consisted of six items measured on a 4-point scale with possible responses of never, a little, sometimes, and a lot. The distress scale included questions such as: In the last month, how often have you felt under strain, stress, and pressure? How often have you felt you had so many problems that you wondered if anything was worthwhile? The happiness subscale included items such as: How often have you felt happy, satisfied, or pleased with your present life? How often have you felt cheerful and lighthearted? Average Cronbach's α's for these scales were .70 and .49, respectively.

•   *Quality of life* was measured by the Satisfaction with Life Areas (SLA) scale (Ossorio, 1979), which has been employed in several studies of Hmong and other Southeast Asian refugee groups (e.g., Rumbaut, 1989, 1991). Respondents rated their satisfaction with nine areas of everyday life (work, money, home life, children, neighborhood, social contacts, health, religion, and leisure) on a 7-point scale ranging from *very dissatisfied* to *very satisfied* (average Cronbach's α = .66).

Descriptive statistics for all outcome variables are shown in Table 9.1.

Paired Qualitative Interviews

Because this was a new project involving refugees from a nondominant culture, it was important to understand the experiences of the Hmong participants in the intervention, as well as how their participation may have impacted their lives. Thus, it seemed essential to allow participants to speak in their own words. Often, the voices of refugees are not heard, particularly because of language differences. In addition, we wanted to understand the experiences of the undergraduates and, most importantly, provide opportunities for Hmong participants and their advocates to share with each other what they learned. Fundamentally, it was important that the evaluation methods we used were consistent with the principles of the intervention—which was intended to be emancipatory, participant-focused, and reciprocal. Therefore, in addition to the primarily fixed-response interviews, each Hmong participant and her advocate were interviewed together at the end of the project. The first author and either the second or third author participated in each interview and these interviews were conducted in Hmong and English, tape recorded and transcribed. The interviews lasted approximately 1 to 1.5 hours and were semistructured with 10 open-ended questions about the most important things each advocate and Hmong participant had learned from each other and taught each other, the best and most

Table 9.1. Descriptive Statistics on Outcome Measures

Outcome Scales	Mean (Standard Deviation) Range			
	Pre	Midpoint	Post	Follow-up
English Proficiency	38.96	44.12	45.00	54.19
	(23.07)	(22.89)	(23.95)	(22.61)
	0 – 73	0 – 79	0 – 78	0 – 80
Citizenship Knowledge	.43	2.79	3.10	3.05
	(1.16)	(3.17)	(3.31)	(2.42)
	0 – 5	0 – 8	0 – 9	0 – 7
Satisfaction with Resources	3.18	3.55	4.08	3.22
	(.84)	(.84)	(.86)	(.94)
	1.44 – 4.40	2.22 – 5.20	1.40 – 5.38	1.70 – 4.78
Difficulty Obtaining Resources	2.91	3.02	2.84	3.10
	(.59)	(.61)	(.50)	(.52)
	1.70 – 4.00	1.50 – 3.86	1.64 – 3.70	2.14 – 3.86
Quality of Life	3.62	3.83	4.25	3.93
	(.73)	(.99)	(.53)	(.82)
	1.78 – 4.78	2.22 – 5.67	3.00 – 5.11	2.56 – 5.56
Psychological Well-Being/Distress	1.92	1.36	1.29	1.66
	(.68)	(.75)	(.53)	(.64)
	.33 – 3.00	.33 – 2.83	.33 – 2.33	.33 – 3.00
Psychological Well-Being/Happiness	1.57	1.50	1.55	1.76
	(.61)	(.56)	(.30)	(.45)
	.50 – 2.83	.33 – 2.50	1.00 – 2.00	.67 – 2.67

difficult things about working together, what their expectations of the project were and whether the project had met them, as well as opportunities to add other thoughts or ideas.

Participant Observation

In order to augment the interview data collected, the first author recorded field notes throughout the project—after each learning circle, during supervisions with the undergraduate advocates, and following interviews. These notes were used to help explain and understand the quantitative findings (e.g., growth curves) and qualitative data, and to document the fidelity of the intervention (e.g., amount of time each advocate spent with her family, what each advocate and participant accomplished). Field notes were also important in order to record the process of this new intervention.

Evaluation Challenges

Designing and implementing the evaluation of this project was challenging for many reasons. First of all, a true experimental design might have been an ideal way to test the efficacy of the intervention, but was not feasible given several constraints. After extensive discussion with many people in the Hmong community, it was decided that it would be culturally inappropriate to offer some Hmong people the opportunity to participate in the project while excluding others, especially given Hmong culture's collective orientation which places concern for community well-being above that of individuals. Furthermore, it seemed likely that Hmong participants who were assigned to the experimental group but had relatives in the control group would be likely to either not participate at all or to share the intervention with their relatives.

A second difficulty involved the translation of the quantitative interview protocol. Initially, the interview was constructed in English and translated into Hmong. However, it was extremely difficult to find interviewers who were fluent in both English and Hmong and who could also read Hmong. Therefore, it was necessary to print the interview in English and review it as a group (co-facilitators and interviewers) during interviewer training to ensure that all interviewers would translate the questions consistently. Another limitation of the quantitative interviews was uncertainty about the applicability and translatability of many of the measures. Furthermore, many participants had limited education and were not accustomed to forced-choice questions. (We used picture re- sponse cards and simplified response choices for some scales to address this issue.) Finally, many Hmong participants felt nervous about being "tested" during the English and citizenship sections of the interview, despite assurances that the project was being tested, not them. In fact, participants seemed more comfortable speaking English to the advo- cates, other native English speakers, and the co-facilitators of the project than to the Hmong interviewers. Despite these challenges, however, a comprehensive evaluation strategy with multiple methods compensated for many difficulties and provided much valuable information.

Results

The quantitative data was analyzed using growth curve modeling, which is a technique related to regression that determines whether there was significant change over time on specified variables and whether indi- viduals followed consistent patterns of change over time (see Byrk & Raudenbush, 1992 for further discussion of this technique).

Outcomes

In order to measure whether the intervention was effective, growth curves for English proficiency, citizenship knowledge, satisfaction with resources, difficulty obtaining resources, quality of life, distress, and happiness were examined (see Table 9.2 for coefficients of significant models). English proficiency significantly increased throughout the in- tervention and continued to increase after the intervention ended. Hmong participants' satisfaction with resources increased significantly throughout the intervention, but decreased somewhat between the end of the intervention and the follow-up interview, which occurred 3 months later. However, participants' satisfaction with resources re- mained higher at the follow-up interview than it was pre-intervention.

Table 9.2. Growth Curve Models of Initial Level and Change on Outcome Variables (N = 27 individuals, 103 observations across 4 time points)

Coefficients for Each Outcome Variable

Parameter	English Proficiency	Citizenship Knowledge	Access to Resources	Quality of Life	Distress
Average (fixed) effects					
Intercept – initial level (B0)	38.65 ***	0.49	3.09 ***	3.57 ***	1.92 ***
Linear change (B1)	4.85 ***	2.44 *	.94 ***	0.53 *	0.73 **
Quadratic change (B2)	-----	-0.54 *	-0.29 ***	-0.13 *	0.22 **
Random Variance Estimates					
Intercept variance	471.46 ***	-----	0.35 ***	.18 ***	0.32 ***
Linear change variance	-----	12.04 ***	-----	-----	0.38 *
Quadratic change variance	-----	0.86 ***	-----	-----	0.03 *

*$p < .05$, **$p < .01$, *** $p < .001$.

Participants' quality of life significantly increased throughout the intervention, but decreased slightly after the intervention ended, although it remained above its initial level. Participants followed consistent patterns of change on all of these measures. Citizenship knowledge increased significantly throughout the intervention, but decreased slightly after the intervention ended (remaining much higher than its initial level). Distress decreased significantly throughout the intervention, but increased a small amount after the intervention ended (remaining lower than its initial level). However, although the overall effects of increased citizenship knowledge and decreased distress were significant, individuals did not follow consistent patterns of change. Unlike the other measures, there was individual variability in the growth curves of citizenship knowledge and distress. Attempts to account for this variability by examining individual and intervention characteristics (e.g., age, years in U.S., English ability, level of participation in the intervention) were unsuccessful. This could be because levels of participation in the intervention were consistent and high (participants attended an average of 32 of the 41 learning circles, with 75% of participants attending at least 28 learning circles), because we did not measure the variable that might explain the different patterns, or because with only 27 participants we did not have the power to delineate the effect. Difficulty obtaining resources and happiness did not change significantly over time; no adequate models for these outcomes could be constructed or presented. In sum, positive effects were demonstrated on most outcome measures, although some of these effects diminished after the intervention was completed (see Table 9.2).

Qualitative Findings

The paired interviews, which were conducted with Hmong participants and undergraduates at the end of the intervention, were transcribed and checked for accuracy. The first author completed a content analysis of these interviews and her field notes, in which she identified a comprehensive list of themes and grouped these themes into larger meta-themes. The interviews and field notes were extremely valuable in understanding the experience of the intervention for participants and the range of ways in which it impacted them. A full discussion of these findings is beyond the scope of this chapter. However, it is important to emphasize that we found validation and support for our quantitative findings. Participants talked about English and citizenship knowledge they had learned, resources they had been able to access, improvements in their quality of life, reductions in their distress, how their understanding of the ways in which society is structured had changed, and how they had taught undergraduates about their culture, values, and ways of life. In addition, unexpected and unmeasured impacts were revealed in our qualitative analyses, including that participants often experienced improved social support, formed more critical understandings about American and Hmong cultures and how to decide what aspects of each to preserve or adopt, developed strong relationships with the undergraduates with whom they worked, and gained self-efficacy and confidence in their abilities to accomplish their goals.

The accumulated effects demonstrated by the growth curves and the qualitative findings suggest that the intervention had a positive impact on participants and that empowering refugees by addressing resource and learning needs and valuing refugees' strengths may be important in reducing refugees' distress and improving their quality of life. It is important to note that without a control group, we cannot conclude that the effects we observed were definitely due to the intervention. For instance, there might be historical effects such as something else occurring in participants' lives or their community or a maturation effect of a natural trajectory of decreased distress over time as refugees are in the United States. However, the pattern of the growth curves of distress, quality of life, and satisfaction with resources, which showed positive effects that diminished after the project ended, suggest that these effects were due to the intervention. A measurement issue, such as participants giving increasingly positive responses because of the general interest taken in their lives, is another possibility, but it is difficult to imagine how participants could show improvements in English proficiency or citizenship knowledge if this were the case. Thus the patterns we observed, our qualitative findings, and our immersion in the community suggest that this intervention demonstrated promising results.

Implications

Our findings have several implications for policy and practice. First, it is important to recognize that refugees need assistance beyond the initial resettlement period. Most refugee organizations, policies, and programs focus on the first 6 months after refugees arrive in the United States. Although this is a crucial time period, it is evident from the participants in the Refugee Well-Being Project that the challenges of adjusting to a new place persist for many years for some people, particularly those who have limited education and English proficiency. Second, the success of this project lends support to the idea that attention to the psychological needs of refugees is important but inadequate if other needs are ignored. Holistic interventions that address material, social, and educational needs, as well as psychological needs and that build upon the strengths of participants are important.

The success of this intervention, as evidenced by its impact on participants and participants' high attendance rates at the learning circles was due not only to its holistic focus, but also to its community-based and culturally grounded nature. It is important to understand and account for the role culture plays in people's behavior and values, especially when designing an intervention designed to promote their well-being (Berry, 1998). Individuals are less likely to participate in community interventions and projects that are not culturally relevant or appropriate (Marin, 1993). In addition, interventions developed and implemented without cultural awareness often fail, and can even result in the disempowerment of individuals or communities that researchers intended to empower (Strawn, 1994).

The Refugee Well-Being Project was developed collaboratively with Hmong families, based on what was culturally relevant and appropriate and what they wanted and needed. Furthermore, the combination of the advocacy and learning components of the intervention was important because, in addition to addressing the particular needs of Hmong refugees (i.e., increased English proficiency, improved access to community resources), it was specifically structured to take into account the unique attributes of Hmong culture, particularly its collective orientation. Kim, Triandis, Kagitcibasi, Choi, and Yoon (1994) found that an individualist/collectivist model is an important model for understanding many cultural differences because it coherently summarizes fundamental differences between the rules, practices, and values of groups of people. Collectively oriented cultures value the well-being of the group above that of the individual, and this intervention was designed with that fundamental consideration in mind. By structuring the intervention around the learning circles, Hmong participants had a space to come together to learn, address issues and social problems collectively, and build on the skills and cultural strengths they had to contribute to their communities. Therefore, effective interventions must attend to the particular attributes of participants' cultures and be developed collaboratively with participants.

Another implication of our findings is that interventions such as the Refugee Well-Being Project need to be longer than 6 months. Many of the positive impacts the project demonstrated began to erode once it ended. Although this might suggest Hmong participants' dependency on the undergraduate students, our observations and the qualitative interviews suggest that the types of processes that were occurring, the skills and knowledge we were trying to help participants build, and the social change efforts we were engaged in together, require longer periods of time. Empowerment is a process that takes time and that must include real and enduring increases in power and resources (Speer & Hughey, 1995). We have seen some evidence that this has occurred in the Hmong community in Lansing, and that it has persisted even after the intervention ended. For instance, at least 10 participants and their spouses have become U.S. citizens due to their involvement in the project. This accomplishment has had radiating effects throughout the Hmong community. U.S. citizenship has been a widespread goal among many members of the Hmong community, because it secures certain resources, rights, and protections. Previously, many Hmong people in Lansing perceived this goal as unattainable. However, now there is a common sentiment that it is possible, because people have seen their cousins, friends, and neighbors pass the test. Furthermore, many of the Hmong participants have shared their knowledge and materials with others (e.g., flash cards to study for the test, the test questions and study guides, knowledge of how to fill out applications and mail them in, an understanding of how and where to complete the process, and confidence that it is possible). The same phenomenon has occurred with other resources as well (e.g., health insurance for uninsured adults, tutoring resources for children).

The strong social network that existed within the Hmong community in Lansing has thus been infused with more material resources and knowledge. A growing body of research demonstrates that increased access to resources improves individuals' quality of life, which in turn has long-term impacts on their future access to resources (e.g., Bybee & Sullivan, 2002; Hobfoll & Lilly, 1993; Diener & Fujita, 1995). We were not able to measure follow-up beyond 3 months but it is important to consider this aspect of sustainability as well. However, we believe that the full potential of the project was not achieved because it was implemented in a way that could not be sustained.

We envision an on-going project involving learning circles and advocacy, in which community members participate as long as they would like. Thus, it is important to consider how this type of endeavor could be sustained and institutionalized within refugees' communities. An on-going partnership between universities and refugee communities and organizations, in which undergraduates make a two-semester commitment and refugee community members participate as long as they want is our idea. As such a project grew and social and material resources within the community developed, coordination and ownership could be increasingly shifted to the refugee community. However, many refugee communities have so few resources that it takes time to reach this ultimate goal. Our project demonstrated that universities possess untapped resources that have great potential for improving the well-being of refugees and that undergraduates can be effective change agents and engage in relationships with refugees and their communities that are mutually beneficial. Therefore, we think this model has great potential on which to build more sustainable interventions.

Finally, we would like to address a tension that existed throughout the project: balancing efforts to eliminate refugees' distress through the reduction of individuals' barriers and problems versus elimination of the causes of the distress (Strawn, 1994). Particularly with refugees, who are usually survivors of numerous traumas and face multiple resettlement challenges, it is important to address their individual needs. However, a focus on larger social and system change, both in terms of the treatment of refugees in the United States and the dynamics that create ever-increasing numbers of refugees worldwide, also deserves attention. The Refugee Well-Being Project sought to reduce refugees' distress through attention to multiple levels of change. Although it was certainly a small step toward broader social change efforts, we hope by creating a space for learning to occur across different cultures, ages, experiences, languages, and races and providing opportunities for critical thought and collective action, that seeds of change have been planted.

SUMMARY

Newcomers to the United States bring with them unique perspectives, skills, and traditions, which have the potential to make great contributions to our country. Therefore, the impetus to understand the processes through which refugees can thrive in the United States and become integrated into their resettlement communities, while maintaining their own cultural identities, is strong. The Refugee Well-Being Project sought to clarify and facilitate some of these processes. Given that it was successful in empowering Hmong participants, reducing their distress, improving their quality of life, and increasing their skills, knowledge, and access to resources, the next step is to develop similar projects that reach more people, extend the length of time of the intervention, carefully adapt it to the needs and wants of other refugee groups, and, most importantly, create more ongoing engagement in refugee communities by building participants' and local organizations' capacities to develop sustainable resources and relationships.

REFERENCES

Addams, J. (1964). *Democracy and social ethics*. Cambridge, MA: Belknap Press of Harvard University Press.

Ashworth, P. D. (1997). The meaning of participation. *Journal of Phenomenological Psychology, 28*(1), 82-103.

Bach, R. L., & Argiros, R. (1991). Economic progress among Southeast Asian refugees in the United States. In H. Adelman (Ed.), *Refugee policy* (pp. 322-343). Toronto: York Lanes Press, Ltd.

Benson, J. E. (1990). Good neighbors: Ethnic relations in Garden City trailer courts. *Urban Anthropology, 19*(4), 361-386.

Berry, J. W. (1998). Acculturation and health: Theory and research. In S. S. Kazarian & D. R. Evans (Eds.), *Cultural clinical psychology: Theory, research, and practice* (pp. 39-57). New York: Oxford University Press.

Bybee, D. I., & Sullivan, C. M. (2002). The process through which an advocacy intervention resulted in positive change for battered women over time. *American Journal of Community Psychology, 30*(1), 103-132.

Byrk, A., & Raudenbush, S. (1992). *Hierarchical linear models.* Newbury Park, CA: Sage.

Carlson, E. B., & Rosser-Hogan, R. (1991). Trauma experiences, posttraumatic stress, dissociation, and depression in Cambodian refugees. *American Journal of Psychiatry, 148*(11), 1548-1551.

Cunningham, P. M. (1992). From Freire to feminism: The North American experience with critical pedagogy. *Adult Education Quarterly, 42*(3), 180-191.

Cunningham, P. M. (1998). The social dimension of transformative learning. *PAACE Journal of Lifelong Learning, 7,* 15-28.

Davidson, W. S., Redner, R., Blakely, C. H., Mitchell, C. M., & Emshoff, J. G. (1987). Diversion of juvenile offenders: An experimental comparison. *Journal of Consulting and Clinical Psychology, 55*(1), 68-75.

Diener, E., & Fujita, F. (1995). Resources, personal strivings, and subjective well-being: A nomothetic and idiographic approach. *Journal of Personality and Social Psychology, 68*(5), 926-935.

Dunnigan, T. (1982). Segmentary kinship in an urban society: The Hmong of St. Paul-Minneapolis. *Anthropological Quarterly, 1,* 126-134.

Dunst, C. J., Trivette, C. M., & Thompson, R. (1990). Supporting and strengthening family functioning: Toward a congruence between principles and practice. *Prevention in Human Services, 9*(1), 19-43.

Dupuy, H. J. (1974). Utility of the National Center for Health Statistics' General Well-Being Schedule in the assessment of self-representation of subjective well-being and distress. In *National Conference on Education in Alcohol, Drug Abuse, and Mental Health Programs.* National Center for Health Statistics. Washington, DC: U.S. Government Printing Office.

Fadiman, A. (1997). Heroes' welcome. *Civilization, 4*(40), 52-61.

Freire, P. (1998). The adult literacy process as cultural action for freedom. *Harvard Educational Review, 68*(4), 476-521.

Gaventa, J. (1995). Citizen knowledge, citizen competence and democracy building. *The Good Society (Journal of the Committee on the Political Economy of the Good Society), 5*(3), 28-35.

Goode, J. (1990). A wary welcome to the neighborhood: Community responses to immigrants. *Urban Anthropology, 19*(1-2), 125-153.

Goodkind, J. (2000). *MSU Refugee Well-Being Project Training Manual.* Michigan State University, East Lansing, Michigan.

Gordon, J. (1998). *The campaign for the Unpaid Wages Prohibition Act—Latino immigrants change New York wage law: The impact of non-voters on politics and the impact of political participation on non-voters.* A paper prepared for the Ford Foundation.

Gorst-Unsworth, C., & Goldenberg, E. (1998). Psychological sequelae of torture and organized violence suffered by refugees from Iraq: Trauma-related factors compared with social factors in exile. *British Journal of Psychiatry, 172,* 90-94.

Hein, J. (1995). *From Vietnam, Laos, and Cambodia: A refugee experience in the United States.* New York: Twayne.

Hobfoll, S. E., & Lilly, R. S. (1993). Resource conservation as a strategy for community psychology. *Journal of Community Psychology, 21*(2), 128-148.

Hutchison, R. (1991). *Acculturation in the Hmong community.* University of Wisconsin System Institute on Race and Ethnicity.

Idelson, H. (1995). Immigration: Bridging gap between actions and ideas. *CQ,* 1065-1071.

Kelly, J. G. (1968). Towards an ecological conception of preventive interventions. In J. W. Carter (Ed.), *Research contributions from psychology to community mental health.* New York: Behavioral Publications.

Kenyon, D., & Stansfield, C. W. (1989). *Basic English skills test manual.* Washington, DC: Center for Applied Linguistics.

Kim, U., Triandis, H. C., Kagitcibasi, C., Choi, S., & Yoon, G. (1994). *Individualism and collectivism: Theory, method, and applications.* Thousand Oaks, CA: Sage.

Kinzie, J. D., & Fleck, J. (1987). Psychotherapy with severely traumatized refugees. *American Journal of Psychotherapy, 41*(1), 82-94.

Lavik, N. J., Hauff, E., Skrondal, A., & Solberg, O. (1996). Mental disorder among refuges and the impact of persecution and exile: Some findings from an outpatient population. *British Journal of Psychiatry, 169,* 726-732.

Lee, J. A. (1986). Asian-American elderly: A neglected minority group. *Journal of Gerontological Social Work, 9*(4), 103-116.

Levine, M., & Perkins, D. V. (1987). *Principles of community psychology: Perspective and applications.* New York: Oxford University Press.

Marin, G. (1993). Defining culturally appropriate community interventions: Hispanics as a case study. *Journal of Community Psychology, 21,* 149-161.

Miller, K. (1999). Rethinking a familiar model: Psychotherapy and the mental health of refugees. *Journal of Contemporary Psychotherapy, 29*(4), 283-306.

Ossorio, P. G. (1979). *An assessment of mental health-related needs among the Indochinese refugees in the Denver metropolitan area.* Longmont, CO: Linguistic Research Institute.

Parsons, R. J., Gutierrez, L. M., & Cox, E. O. (1998). A model for empowerment practice. In L. M. Gutierrez, R. J. Parsons, & E. O. Cox. (Eds.), *Empowerment in social work practice: A sourcebook*. Pacific Grove, CA: Brooks/Cole.

Pejovic, M., Jovanovic, A., & Djurdic, S. (1997). Psychotherapy experience with patients treated for war psychotraumas. *Psychiatriki, 8*(2), 136-141.

Pernice, R., & Brook, J. (1996). Refugees' and immigrants' mental health: Association of demographic and post-migration factors. *Journal of Social Psychology, 136*, 511-519.

Rappaport, J. (1977). *Community psychology: Values, research, and action*. New York: Holt, Rinehart, & Winston.

Rappaport, J. (1981). In praise of paradox: A social policy of empowerment over prevention. *American Journal of Community Psychology, 9*(1), 1-25.

Rumbaut, R. G. (1985). Mental health and the refugee experience: A comparative study of Southeast Asian refugees. In T. C. Owan (Ed.), *Southeast Asian mental health: Treatment, preventions, services, training, and research* (DHHS Publication No. ADM 85-1399). Rockville, MD: National Institute of Mental Health.

Rumbaut, R. G. (1989). Portraits, patterns, and predictors of the refugee adaptation process: Results and reflections from the IHARP Panel Study. In D. W. Haines (Ed.), *Refugees as immigrants: Cambodians, Laotians, and Vietnamese in America* (pp.138-190). Totowa, NJ: Rowman & Littlefield.

Rumbaut, R. G. (1991). Migration, adaptation, and mental health: The experience of Southeast Asian refugees in the United States. In H. Adelman (Ed.), *Refugee policy: Canada and the United States* (pp. 381-424). Toronto: York Lanes Press Ltd.

Ryan, W. (1976). *Blaming the victim*. New York: Vintage Books.

Scott, G. M., Jr. (1982). The Hmong refugee community in San Diego: Theoretical and practical implications of its continuing ethnic solidarity. *Anthropological Quarterly, 55*(3), 146-160.

Silove, D., Sinnerbrink, I., Field, A., Manicavasagar, V., & Steel, Z. (1997). Anxiety, depression and PTSD in asylum-seekers: Associations with pre-migration trauma and post-migration stressors. *British Journal of Psychiatry, 170*, 351-357.

Speer, P. W., & Hughey, J. (1995). Community organizing: An ecological route to empowerment and power. *American Journal of Community Psychology, 23*, 729-748.

Starret, R. H., Mindell, C. H., & Wright, R. (1983). Influence of support systems on the use of social services of the Hispanic elderly. *Social Work Research and Abstracts, 19*(4), 35-40.

Strawn, C. (1994). Beyond the buzzword: Empowerment in community outreach and education. *Journal of Applied Behavioral Science, 30*, 159-174.

Sue, S., & Morishima, J. K. (1982). *The mental health of Asian Americans.* San Francisco: Jossey-Bass.

Sullivan, C. M. (1998). *Resilient child study advocate training manual.* Michigan State University, East Lansing, MI.

Sullivan, C. M., & Bybee, D. I. (1999). Reducing violence using community-based advocacy for women with abusive partners. *Journal of Consulting and Clinical Psychology, 67*(1), 43-53.

Sullivan, C. M., Tan, C., Basta, J., Rumptz, M., & Davidson, W. S. (1992). An advocacy intervention program for women with abusive partners: Initial evaluation. *American Journal of Community Psychology, 20*(3), 309-322.

Trickett, E. J. (1996). A future for community psychology: The contexts of diversity and the diversity of contexts. *American Journal of Community Psychology, 24,* 209-229.

Vella, J. (1994). *Learning to listen, learning to teach: The power of dialogue in educating adults.* San Francisco: Jossey-Bass.

Westermeyer, J., Neider, J., & Callies, A. (1989). Psychosocial adjustment of Hmong refugees during their first decade in the United States. *Journal of Nervous and Mental Disease, 177*(3), 132-139.

Westermeyer, J., Vang, T., & Lyfong, G. (1983). Hmong refugees in Minnesota: Characteristics and self perceptions. *Minnesota Medicine, 66,* 431-439.

Westermeyer, J., Vang, T., & Neider, J. (1983). Migration and mental health among Hmong refugees: Association of pre- and post-migration factors with self-rating scales. *Journal of Nervous and Mental Disease, 171*(2), 92-96.

Yang, P., & Murphy, N. (1993). *Hmong in the '90s: Stepping towards the future.* St. Paul, MN: Hmong American Partnership.

Ying, Y., & Akutsu, P. D. (1997). Psychological adjustment of Southeast Asian refugees: The contribution of sense of coherence. *Journal of Community Psychology, 25*(2), 125-139.

Zimmerman, M. A. (1995). Psychological empowerment: Issues and illustrations. *American Journal of Community Psychology, 23,* 581-599.

PART III

CRITICAL ISSUES

10

Evaluating Ecological Mental Health Interventions in Refugee Communities

Jon Hubbard and Kenneth E. Miller

As the preceding chapters have shown, considerable progress has been made in the design and implementation of ecological mental health projects with communities displaced by political violence. Innovative strategies have been developed to help refugee communities respond effectively to their own mental health needs, using methods that integrate local and Western knowledge, beliefs, and practices. The critical question now is whether these programs are achieving their goals of empowering communities and improving the mental health and psychosocial well-being of community members. That is, to what extent are ecological mental health interventions with refugees *effective*?

In order to answer this question, the editors of this volume asked the contributing authors to (1) describe the methods they used in evaluating their projects, (2) summarize their evaluation findings, and (3) discuss any challenges they encountered while carrying out their evaluations. For authors who were unable to evaluate their interventions, the editors asked that they discuss the obstacles they had encountered to conducting systematic evaluations. The emphasis on identifying challenges and obstacles to conducting evaluations was intended to generate a discussion of commonly encountered evaluation roadblocks, and to begin exploring a range of possible solutions to those roadblocks.

In reviewing the evaluation sections of the preceding chapters, we found that two themes were readily apparent. First, it is considerably easier to carry out systematic evaluations of ecological interventions in the comparatively safe and stable environments of resettlement countries such as the United States. In contrast to projects implemented in or near zones of ongoing violent conflict, interventions in the United States and other industrialized nations do not have to contend with the recurrent threat of violence and forced relocation; they have greater access to evaluation resources (materials, computers, consultants); and they typically have greater control over participation in their interventions, which allows for the development of more rigorous evaluation designs. Conversely, ecological interventions in or near conflict zones must contend with precisely the opposite conditions: ongoing vulnerability to further acts of violence that may result in repeated experiences of displacement, a lack of evaluation resources, and minimal control over who participates (and who does not) from week to week in the project. From an evaluation standpoint, such conditions are clearly far from ideal. In fact, they appear to be sufficiently formidable as to discourage program staff from attempting to carry out systematic evaluations of their projects—the second theme evident in our review of the evaluation sections of the chapters in this book. The authors in this volume are not alone; indeed, a review of other published accounts of ecological interventions with refugees in areas of ongoing conflict reveals a similar pattern: innovative program designs, compelling implementation strategies, and minimal discussion of actual outcome data (e.g., de Jong, 2002).

We appreciate the magnitude of the obstacles that program staff working in or near zones of conflict commonly encounter when trying to evaluate their interventions, and mean no disrespect in underscoring the lack of sound evaluation data. Indeed, we have encountered these same obstacles in our own work. We are concerned, however, about inadvertently creating what psychologist Robin Dawes (1994) has termed a "house of cards"—a substantial body of anecdotal evidence with little empirical data to support it. In the absence of sound evaluation findings, we cannot know the extent to which our interventions are truly effective.

We have no way of knowing which aspects of our programs are working well, and which components need to be altered or discarded. Confidence in the effectiveness of our interventions becomes more a matter of faith than knowledge, based more on subjective impression than organized assessment. This was precisely the situation with the highly funded Project DARE ("Dare to keep kids off drugs"), a U.S.-based project designed to prevent drug abuse and promote healthy psychosocial development among youth. Faith-based confidence in the DARE program was extremely high, and the program was implemented, at a cost of millions of dollars, in schools throughout the country. Unfortunately, a systematic evaluation of the DARE program in the state of Illinois showed it to have only minimal impact on students' drug use immediately after the intervention and *no impact at all* at 1 and 2 years post-intervention. In addition, the program had no effect on enhancing children's social skills (Enett et al., 1994). As it turned out, confidence in the DARE program was indeed something of a house of cards, one that cost a great deal of time and money while yielding few, if any, beneficial results.

Clearly, evaluations are essential if we wish to have well-founded confidence that our interventions are achieving their intended goals. Further, evaluations can help us identify problems with the design or implementation of our programs that may be diminishing their effectiveness. Finally, well conducted evaluations can help us answer a range of other interesting questions, such as: Who are we reaching with our programs? Who are we failing to reach, and why? What unanticipated effects are our programs having in the community, both positive and negative?

The goals of this chapter are twofold: (1) to describe the rationale and methods of two key types of program evaluation: process evaluations and outcome evaluations; and (2) to suggest strategies for carrying out process and outcome evaluations in refugee settings that are in or near situations of ongoing conflict. We recognize that organizations working with refugees in developing countries typically have limited budgets, work under chaotic and often stressful conditions, and may lack staff members with expertise in program evaluation. However, we believe that informative evaluations can be conducted using modest resources, that evaluation designs can be tailored to the demands of highly challenging settings, and that sound evaluations can be carried out with a minimum of evaluation expertise. Our hope is to both demystify the evaluation process, and to outline a set of evaluation strategies that can provide meaningful data yet still be implemented under the difficult circumstances in which ecological interventions with refugees are typically conducted.

PROCESS EVALUATIONS

Several years ago, one of us helped to evaluate the outcome (effectiveness) of an ecological mental health project for rural communities in a Latin American country that had been devastated by a widespread campaign of state-sponsored violent repression. For nearly 3 years, representatives of numerous villages had traveled to a central location in order to participate in week long trainings in the theory and methods of the mental health intervention. The expectation was that they would return to their villages and implement what they had learned, developing workshops designed to help community members, and children in particular, heal from the effects of the violence and subsequent displacement.

Unfortunately, it was impossible to evaluate the effectiveness of the participants' work in their own communities, for it turned out that no one had actually implemented the mental health activities they had learned in the trainings. This was quite a surprise for the staff of the organization that had provided the training, who had assumed that project trainees were actively putting into practice the knowledge and skills they had acquired. In a subsequent workshop held to explore the reasons for the trainees' failure to implement the mental health intervention in their home communities, the participants offered a list of significant obstacles they had encountered, including a lack of supervision and consultation by program staff, the lack of a written manual to which they could turn for descriptions of the various intervention techniques, and resistance from religiously conservative community members who regarded the intervention as subversive and had threatened to alert the army if the intervention was carried out. These and other data gathered during this *process evaluation* workshop provided invaluable information to the staff of the project, who were then better informed about the kinds of support trainees needed, and the kinds of challenges they faced upon returning to their home communities.

Process evaluations are designed to answer several key questions:

- To what extent has an intervention been implemented as planned?
- What factors are causing an intervention to be implemented differently than planned (or to not be implemented at all)? How might those factors be addressed?
- To what extent is an intervention reaching the intended (target) population?
- Who within the target population is *not* being reached by the intervention, and what are the obstacles to participation for these individuals (families, groups, communities)?

Evaluations that address the first two questions are sometimes referred to as implementation or fidelity evaluations, while those addressing the latter two questions are sometimes called efficiency evaluations (Dalton, Elias, & Wandersman, 2001; Miller, 1999). In this chapter, we use the term *process evaluation* to refer collectively to any evaluation that addresses any or all of these questions.

It is an axiom of program evaluation that an intervention is unlikely be effective if it is not implemented appropriately. In the example offered earlier, the intervention was not implemented at all. More commonly, however, interventions are not effective because they have been implemented poorly rather than not at all. For example, one of our colleagues was involved in a well designed community intervention designed to increase safe sex behavior among gay men in a large urban area of the United States. At the completion of the multisession group intervention, the program was found to have had little effect on increasing the participants' safe sex behavior. Although it would have been easy to conclude that the project was poorly designed and therefore ineffective, a closer examination revealed something quite different. It turned out that one of the group leaders was quite uncomfortable talking explicitly about the kinds of sexual behaviors that put gay men at risk for the transmission of HIV, the virus that causes AIDS. The group leader's discomfort led to an avoidance of the very sort of discussions that were to essential to the program's success. No wonder that the program showed few beneficial effects—it had not been implemented as designed.

This example illustrates an important point: Process evaluations can help us determine whether an intervention that is not effective suffers from a poor *program design*—in which case the intervention itself should be modified, or from problems of *program implementation,* in which case, obstacles·to effective implementation should be addressed (Dalton et al., 2001). There is another important point to be drawn from this example and that of the project in Latin America: until we can be reasonably certain that a program has been well implemented, it makes little sense to evaluate the outcome or effectiveness of the program. *The effectiveness of any intervention depends in part on the quality of its implementation.*

Strategies for Evaluating the Implementation of Ecological Interventions

The first and most obvious question asked by a process evaluation is whether an intervention was actually conducted. Although it may seem odd to even ask such a basic question, our earlier example of the mental health project that was *not* implemented by trained paraprofessionals in their home communities underscores the importance of ensuring that people are actually conducting the intervention. In our experience, the risk of non-implementation increases when paraprofessional staff are trained in a central location and expected to implement what they have learned in their home communities without regular supervision and consultation from project staff. Mental health work, especially with survivors of extreme violence and forced displacement, is inherently complex and challenging. A brief but intense period of training cannot substitute for ongoing guidance and consultation. Of course, support and supervision are needed whether paraprofessional staff are working in communities distant from the central training site, or in the same community in which the training is offered.

Let us assume that trained community members are receiving adequate support from more experienced project staff members, and are actively involved in implementing an ecological mental health intervention with other community members. The question now becomes one of assessing the fidelity of the project's implementation; that is, is the intervention being conducted as planned? If not, why not?

There are several ways of examining the issue of fidelity.

- **Co-facilitation.** Co-facilitation involves having trained community members co-lead the intervention with a more experienced staff member (who may also be a member of the target community), who can serve as a role model for the appropriate implementation of the intervention while also ensuring that activities are implemented as designed.

- **Observation.** Experienced staff members can observe directly the implementation of an intervention, noting areas of fidelity as well as obstacles to implementing the intervention as designed.

- **Post-session interviews with trained paraprofessionals.** Supervisory staff can regularly conduct interviews with trained paraprofessionals following each session of the intervention. In addition to ensuring that all of the planned activities were carried out (or to discovering why some activities were not implemented), regular interviews also provide time for providing paraprofessional staff with support and supervision.

- **Videotaping sessions or events.** Videotaping intervention sessions or specific intervention events provides an invaluable source of data regarding what actually happened during the implementation of project activities. For example, the process of videotaping the implementation by schoolteachers of the *Playing to Grow* intervention with Guatemalan refugee children in Mexican refugee camps provided the project staff with invaluable data regarding the kinds of activities that worked well and those that needed to be altered, and also helped staff identify areas in which the schoolteachers needed additional training (Miller & Billings, 1994;

Miller, Billings, & Farias, 1995). A major concern with video-taping is the extent to which participants feel comfortable being videotaped. In our experience, children are often more comfortable being videotaped than adults. It is also possible that cultural differences in what it means to allow oneself to be photographed or videotaped may shape a given community's openness to having the intervention (or parts of it) captured on video.

- **Focus groups with project participants.** Focus groups are a form of group interview, in which a small group of participants is asked to discuss a set of questions related to a particular topic (Dean, 1994; Krueger, 1994). Focus groups are ideal for conducting process evaluations, because it is relatively easy to ask participants in an intervention to talk about the activities that were conducted, and to comment on those activities they found most helpful and those they believe should be altered or dropped. Focus groups are efficient, as data are gathered from several people at once. Focus groups typically have about 8 to 10 people, and can run as long as participants are willing to continue discussing the questions at hand (we usually limit focus groups to a maximum of about 2 hours). The groups can take place in any community setting, such as a school room, a clinic, or a community member's home. *The most effective focus groups are those in which the facilitator is able to generate discussion among group members, rather than fostering dyadic interactions between each group member and the facilitator.* For those interested in learning more about focus groups, Richard Krueger (1994) and Debra Dean (1994) have written excellent guides.

- **Questionnaires.** Another approach to ensuring fidelity of implementation is to have paraprofessional staff (i.e., trained community members) complete brief questionnaires or checklists, indicating which of the planned activities were actually carried out, and which were not. Supervisory staff should then discuss with the paraprofessionals the reasons that specific activities were either not carried out, or were implemented differently than planned. It is also useful, although time and labor intensive, to have *project participants* complete **participant satisfaction questionnaires** at the conclusion of each meeting, or alternatively, at the midpoint and conclusion of the intervention. The questionnaires should ask participants to indicate their level of satisfaction with the specific intervention activities, and may also cover other areas such as satisfaction with the performance of the paraprofessional staff, the quality and appropriateness of the intervention materials, and so forth. For participants with limited reading skills, project staff can read the questionnaire items aloud and participants can indicate their responses using such answer choices as an empty circle ("not at all satisfied"), a partially filled circle ("somewhat satisfied"), or a completely filled circle ("very satisfied"). Methods of analyzing questionnaire data are discussed farther below.

Strategies for Assessing Who Is (and Who Is Not) Being Reached by an Intervention

We suggested earlier that process evaluations can also be used to assess the extent to which an intervention is reaching the target population. The importance of this type of process evaluation cannot be overstated. If the intervention is designed for a particular subgroup within a community (e.g., people experiencing persistent symptoms of psychological distress) but is reaching only people who are showing few signs of distress, it is unlikely to be effective and may represent a poor expenditure of limited resources. Similarly, if an intervention is designed to serve a community in its entirety but people don't participate in it, or participate only sporadically, the intervention is unlikely to show positive results. Although low participation rates may suggest a problem with the design of an intervention, they may also reflect factors that having nothing to do with the program's design. Such factors might include negative inaccurate perceptions of the project, a lack of trust between community members and the project's staff members, a lack of effective recruitment and ad-

vertisement efforts, or conflicts with other community or family com-
mitments. We return shortly to a discussion of obstacles to participation.

To assess the extent to which an intervention is reaching the target
population, it is necessary to answer a number of related questions:

- Who is the target population for the intervention?

- Who is actually participating in the intervention?

- What constitutes "participation"? (e.g., attendance at 75% of
  the meetings, activities, or sessions)

- What percentage of the target population can be realistically
  expected to participate in the intervention?

- Of those who could benefit from the intervention, who is *not*
  participating? What are the obstacles to their participation,
  and how these obstacles be overcome?

Who Is the Target Population for the Intervention?

This is a relatively straightforward question. Who do you want to
reach with your intervention? The whole community? Parents with
school age children? Widows? Adolescents? New or expectant mothers?
Unemployed men? Schoolteachers? Families? Individuals experiencing
high levels of war-related trauma?

Once you have designated the target population, it is ideal (although
not absolutely necessary) to try to assess the number of people or families in the community who comprise this target group. Obviously, if your
intervention targets the whole community, this is simple: The number of
people or families in the community is the same as the number in your
target group. However, because many interventions have components
that serve specific subgroups, it is helpful to know the size of those subgroups, as this allows you to estimate a proportion of the subgroup that
your intervention should reasonably be able to reach. For example, if you
are developing a project to assist children disabled by political violence,
and you estimate that there are roughly 100 such children in the com-

munity where you are working, you might aim to involve 50 of them with your intervention during the first year (the actual numbers you designate will depend on the resources available and the nature of your intervention). Having set a realistic goal of reaching 50 children, you have set the stage for a relatively straightforward evaluation to determine whether you have achieved your goal at the year's end.

Monitoring Participation: Who Is Actually Taking Part in the Intervention?

There are several strategies available to assess who is and is not participating in an intervention. The simplest approach for monitoring participation is to keep an attendance record or *participant log*. For community-wide interventions, this might involve having a staff member observe and document the number of different people (or families) who use a particular setting during a given period of time. For example, for 2 hours each day over the course of a week, project staff could document the number of people who use a community playground or attend a community center. It is also possible to count or make a list of the people who participate in a particular community activity. Another strategy is to randomly survey community members to ask whether they are familiar with the project, and whether they have participated in any of the project activities.

For smaller group activities, such as social support groups, it is relatively simple to keep an attendance log that documents who attends each meeting of the group. For projects that ask participants to engage in certain tasks between group meetings (e.g., visit other group members, practice certain new skills), a record can be kept at each meeting of each participant's between-session completed tasks.

Why is it important to keep track of who participates in an intervention? First, this allows us to assess whether we are reaching those people for whom the intervention was designed. Second, keeping a participant log allows us to keep track of how regularly people are participating in the various intervention activities. This will be important later on when we conduct outcome evaluations, as there is usually a strong relationship between the degree to which people participate in an intervention and the intervention's effectiveness. Stated differently, those people with the greatest degree of participation tend to experience the greatest benefit from a project.

Imagine a support group offered to distressed widows. Some of the women attend all 10 meetings of the group, whereas other women attend less regularly, some showing up every other week and others attending only one or two meetings. We can expect that those women who attend more of the meetings will experience a greater benefit from the intervention. *Only by keeping a participant log will we be able to keep track of each woman's level of participation in the program.* When evaluating the effectiveness of the support group, our primary aim is to show that it is effective for those women who actively participate in it. What constitutes "active" participation? There is no set rule, although generally participation below 50% (e.g., attending less than half of the meetings of a support group) is regarded as partial or nonattendance. It would, for example, be a valuable finding if we could show that women who attended at least half of the sessions showed a marked increase in psychological well-being, and those who attended all of the sessions experienced an even greater improvement.

Identifying Prospective Participants Who Are not Being Reached by the Intervention

It is relatively easy to keep track of who *is* participating in an intervention. It is somewhat more challenging to identify those individuals or families who might benefit from the program but are *not* participating in it. If we know the approximate size of the target group (e.g., the number of widows in the community), we can easily compare the number of people from the target group that *have* participated in the intervention with the total number of members of the group. This will give us a good idea of the number of potential participants who have not yet gotten involved in the project.

Often, however, we don't know the size of the target group. For example, we may not know how many individuals are struggling with depression or trauma in a community, and we may not have the time or resources to carry out a community-wide assessment. In such cases, how can we know whether we are reaching most of those people who might benefit from our intervention? One useful approach is to ask program staff (who are normally members of the local community), as well as program participants, to identify other community members whom they believe might benefit by participating in the intervention.

Identifying Obstacles to Participation

There are numerous reasons why community members might not participate in a mental health or psychosocial intervention. They might be concerned about a negative stigma associated with participating in the program; they might need to work during the time that program activities are offered; they might not be aware of the intervention or may have an inaccurate idea of what it involves; they may be concerned about issues of confidentiality; or they may not have anyone available to watch their children while they participate in the program. Most such obstacles to participation can be readily overcome with a bit of flexibility and creativity on the part of program staff.

There are a couple of simple strategies for identifying the specific obstacles that affect participation in the community you work in. One approach is to ask people who *are* participating to talk about why they think other community members are *not* participating. Another approach is to either informally or through formal interviews or focus groups ask *non-participants* about the reasons they have chosen not to take part in the intervention. Once the obstacles to participation have been identified, program staff can then work with community members to find ways of overcoming those obstacles, and thereby expand the reach (and thus the impact) of the program.

OUTCOME EVALUATION

Whereas process evaluations provide the information we need in order to know if our programs are being implemented—and implemented in the ways in which we have planned—we need to gather additional data to know if our programs are having their intended effect. Collecting information for the purpose of assessing the effectiveness of a program is referred to as *outcome evaluation*. Outcome evaluations can be difficult to conduct under the best of circumstances and may feel impossible to carry out under the fluid and often chaotic conditions of conflict zones and refugee camps. The authors do not portend to have solutions for all the complex challenges that arise when assessing the effectiveness of programs being carried out in these turbulent contexts; however, suggestions are offered that may help in designing and conducting more useful and informative outcome evaluations under these less than ideal conditions.

Outcome evaluations are designed to answer the questions:

- How well did the program achieve its goals and objectives?

- Who benefited most from the intervention or what components of the program had the greatest impact?

- Did the program have unintended consequences (positive or negative)?

- What was learned that would inform future interventions or other similar programs?

There are many ways of answering these questions and a variety of issues to consider when designing your outcome evaluation. The following sections highlight some of these issues and suggest strategies for handling challenges that can arise when designing the evaluation, choosing appropriate methods and measures or analyzing, interpreting, and reporting the results of an outcome evaluation.

Strategies for Evaluating the Effectiveness of Ecological Interventions

Outcome evaluation begins with a series of questions that need to be answered in order to know the degree to which a program has been effective in meeting its expectations. If the expectations for the program have not been clearly articulated, it will be very difficult to design a successful evaluation. This may sound self-evident but it is surprising how much difficulty many program staff have explaining exactly what their program's goals and objectives are. *Goals* are the general aspirations of a program and are often stated in fairly broad terms (e.g., to reduce post-conflict distress and increase feelings of well-being in a particular displaced population). Program *objectives* are the specific methods used to achieve the program's goals and need to be stated in more precise and *measurable* terms (e.g., organize 20 12-week adult therapy groups to reduce symptoms of depression and anxiety and increase social connectedness among participants). Objectives that are too broad or vague do not readily lend themselves to evaluation. Frequently programs have multiple objectives and there should be *outcome indicators* associated with each individual objective. Outcome indicators are the specific items that are used to judge the success of a program and should be directly tied to the goals and objectives. An example of program goals and objectives is found in Box 1 (next page), which comes from the intervention with Sierra Leonean refugees described in chapter 2 of this volume.

In general, the term *effects* refers to immediate program outcomes while *impacts* refers to the more enduring long-term outcomes (the usage differs by field). We use the terms somewhat interchangeably in this chapter as many of the strategies described are useful for both.

There are many good articles and books covering the basic principles for conducting outcome evaluations (e.g., Fetterman, Kaftarian, & Wandersman, 1996; Kazdin, 1992; Linney & Wandersman, 1991; Wholey, Hatry, & Newcomer, 1994); therefore we do not go into detail on 'the basics' here, but rather focus on applying some of these basic ideas to the evaluation of interventions in high adversity contexts like post-conflict zones.

Considerations in Designing an Outcome Evaluation

One of the fundamental reasons that many program evaluations fail is simply poor planning. Although significant efforts are made to develop detailed intervention plans, relatively little time and effort is put into designing the evaluation components. Outcome evaluation, like research, will produce much more meaningful results when it is well designed and conducted in as rigorous a manner as possible. While there may be limits on the rigor that can be achieved in the contexts in which

TABLE 10.1. Objectives and Goals From a Project With Sierra Leonean Refugees*

Goal	Objective	Outcome measure
1. To provide psycho-education and mental health services to Sierra Leonean adults living in Guinean refugee camps.	1. Implement eight, 12-week therapy groups (four male & four female) for 8 to 12 adults per group in each refugee camp in which the program is operating. Groups will be designed provide psychoeducation, reduce post-trauma symptoms and increase social functioning and ability to engage in the tasks of daily living.	1.1 Symptom checklists for depression, anxiety, somatic symptoms and PTSD administered at intake, & 1, 3, and 6 months (quantitative) 1.2 Measure of social connectedness and community involvement (quantitative) 1.3 Behavior checklist of indicators of involvement in daily activities (quantitative). 1.4 Participant and community focus groups organized four times per year (qualitative)
2. To create a cadre of peer counselors who are able to provide culturally appropriate mental health services to their fellow refugees	2. Professional expatriate psychotherapists will provide long-term applied training (topic-specific trainings, in-session modeling, pre- and post-therapy training and ongoing case supervision) to refugee peer counselors (ratio of approximately 10 trainees for each senior staff). Training will continue throughout employment with the program and be adapted to the changing needs and abilities of each staff.	2.1 Written examinations on basic counseling skills and the impact of war on individuals, families and communities. Conducted following initial month of training and then on a semi-annual basis (quantitative/qualitative) 2.2 Quarterly supervisor ratings on counseling skills, ability to incorporate training into practice and job performance (qualitative/quantitative)

*Note: These goals and objectives are taken from the project described in chapter 3. They are selected examples from a larger set and do not represent a complete evaluation design.

many ecological interventions operate, there are ways to improve the odds of ending up with useful results.

Begin by designing the outcome evaluation at the same time you develop the intervention plan for your program. Make it part of your proposal or implementation plan from the outset. All too often outcome evaluation is an afterthought for ecological mental health interventions and psychosocial programs that is added on after the program has been developed and is in operation or when additional funding is sought. It is much harder to develop and implement a successful evaluation post-hoc. As you go through the process of developing evaluation questions and selecting measures keep returning to the basic questions: What was the program designed to achieve? How will you know if it was effective?

Collecting Data

Determining that a program has had an impact requires several types of information: baseline data, follow-up data and, if possible, comparison or control group data. *Baseline data* is collected from the target population on all of the dimensions of interest prior to the start of the intervention. Baseline data can be collected as part of an overall needs assessment or as a specific evaluation activity. This is the data with which all future assessments will be compared, and as such, all questions of interest must be included.

At a minimum there needs to be at least one *follow-up assessment* in which the measures administered during the baseline assessment are given again. Usually, a follow-up assessment is conducted at the end of each specific program activity or intervention cycle. Sometimes, however, there are multiple assessment points during or following an intervention.

Finally, it is impossible to make any conclusive statements about the effectiveness of a program without collecting baseline and follow-up data from community members who did not participate in the intervention, but who are, in all other ways, similar to program participants. Even if your follow-up assessment indicates a significant positive effect among participants, for example a large drop in symptoms, you cannot, with any certainty, attribute the change to your intervention or interpret its meaning without a comparison or *control group*. It is possible that during the period of your intervention, symptoms dropped in the entire community and the effects seen among program participants were not due to your intervention but to more general phenomenon like the passage of time or reduced tension in the region. It is even possible that symptoms could have dropped to a greater degree in the entire community than among your program participants, in which case the program would actually be impeding recovery. Control group data is the standard against which program results are compared in order to judge their significance.

Control groups can be created in several ways. Once the target audience has been identified, participants can be randomly assigned into groups—those who will participate in the intervention and those who will not. For obvious reasons this approach can be difficult to use in many ecological mental health interventions. However, if the program can only serve part of the target audience at a time, people can be randomly placed into sequential cycles of the intervention. If you have several types of interventions within one program, you can randomize the order in which people receive the different interventions or have some people receive several interventions at once (e.g., group therapy and life skills training) and compare them to those who receive single interventions.

All of these methods can be very difficult to organize and manage in the contexts we are discussing and finding a method for including a random "non-intervention group" or control group in the evaluation design may not be possible. It can be enough of a challenge to gather evaluation data from program participants in these settings and the added burden of identifying and following an adequate comparison sample can overwhelm program resources. Yet there are other ways to try and build a case for program effectiveness. As previously noted, you can use internal indicators like attendance records to determine if people who participated more frequently received greater benefit from an intervention than those who attended less often. This method was used by one of the authors in a recent program evaluation and it could be shown that higher attendance was related to greater symptom reduction among refugees receiving group therapy. Examining the attendance records also indicated that those with the most severe psychological symptoms at the baseline assessment were the most likely to drop out. A preliminary follow-up with these drop-out cases indicated that they were not ready to address their problems in a group setting and some requested individual sessions where they could discuss their problems "in private."

Other methods for substantiating effectiveness include gathering follow-up data on clients for whom you have baseline information but who did not participate in the intervention at all (a zero attendance group). We have found people very willing to participate in follow-up assessments even when they have not attended any parts of the intervention. This strategy also provides information about why some people chose not to participate (process evaluation data) and provides a chance to re-engage these people in tne program. It is useful to collect data that allows for examination of possible differences between those who engage and those who don't (e.g., demographic information like age and gender or experiential data like higher rates of traumatic exposure). Another method is to conduct baseline assessments with a cohort of participants prior to their engaging in an intervention (e.g., 1 month prior) and then re-assessing them when the program is about to begin. This pre-intervention or 'wait period' data can be compared with data collected at a similar period into the intervention and/or with data from another similar cohort who were assessed at the beginning and one month into the program (this is a "waiting-list" type strategy).

Planning for the Unpredictable

Another important design consideration in these contexts is to be prepared for change. If you know you are working in a continually changing or fluid environment, which is frequently the case when intervening with displaced populations, build this into your evaluation design. Although you cannot plan for every unexpected turn of events you should design your outcome evaluation around the reality of the situation as you have come to know it. Some strategies include:

- Keep measures brief so that information can be collected quickly. Assessing a few key indicators for each of the domains of interest will be less cumbersome for staff and participants than lengthy all-inclusive assessments. Brief measures also lend themselves to more frequent assessments.

- Shorten the time between data collection points. This is helpful if your program is suddenly interrupted and it will also allow you to analyze more precisely when significant changes occurred.

- Evaluate the effectiveness of specific techniques or components of the program or intervention as well as the overall impact. Knowing how individual parts of the intervention are succeeding can often be more informative than measures of overall effectiveness. It allows you to compare interventions and to analyze which parts of the program are having the most (or least) impact. This strategy also protects against ending up with no evaluation data, if the whole program ends prematurely or parts of the program are terminated.

- Have a system in place for tracking participants. In highly mobile situations such as refugee camps, it is helpful to collect good contact information, such as a friend or relative who might know where to find a participant or information about where someone intends to go if the situation changes (e.g., the camp is closed down). We have found this data crucial in locating the "zero attendance comparison group" discussed earlier.

- Have a plan in place that describes how confidential information will be protected or destroyed if staff needs to quickly relocate. For example, who will be responsible for evaluation data in an emergency situation? It is always better to destroy sensitive or confidential data if you are forced to evacuate than to leave it behind or transport it in an unprotected or unregulated manner.

Including Community Members in the Evaluation Process

An outcome evaluation will produce more meaningful results if you find ways to involve people from the local community in the evaluation process. We believe that this is an extremely important part of developing an appropriate evaluation strategy, and one that is quite often over-looked. Outcome evaluation should be a participatory process with as much local input and involvement as possible (Dalton et al., 2001; Fetterman et al., 1996). It is becoming more common for program developers to elicit community input when designing new *interventions* (usually during the needs assessment phase); however, few programs appear to seek local participation and input when designing the evaluation components of their programs.

Community involvement can have a significant impact on the success or failure of an evaluation. When community members are engaged in developing an outcome evaluation from the beginning, they feel ownership of the process. It is easier to get the community to *participate* in the evaluation if they have been involved in designing it. Through a cooperative design process, program staff and community members have an opportunity to develop an outcome evaluation that holds meaning for everyone concerned. It creates an environment in which they can begin to see evaluation as an important and valuable part of the program and not an added burden carried out only as a requirement of funding agencies and management at the "home office."

In addition, local participation can aid in developing more meaningful assessment questions and provide valuable feedback as to whether questions brought in from the outside will be understood by participants. They can tell you if the methods you have chosen to gather information will be accepted by the community or provide information that can impact the timing of your evaluation. If you know, for example, that it is inappropriate for women to meet alone with a man for an interview or that few people will be able to participate in a follow-up assessment because it is scheduled during a local festival, you can alter your design accordingly.

But it is important to do more than simply elicit local input. We suggest, whenever possible, hiring local staff to implement the evaluation or, at a minimum, include people from the community as regular members of your evaluation team. In our own programs, we have trained local staff to conduct interviews, facilitate focus groups, administer checklists, analyze data, and write reports. This often requires more time and effort spent recruiting, training, and supervising; however, the benefits are well worth the investment. In part, this is another way of empowering the community you are serving. By creating local expertise in designing and carrying out program evaluation you are contributing to the sustainability of the program. There are direct benefits for the program as well. Along with being cultural resources, people are often more comfortable talking to someone from their culture who speaks their own language and understands the context for their answers.

That being said, it is also important to be aware of possible differences between the local staff you hire and the larger community. Often local staff are hired because they have more education, are multilingual or have worked previously for psychosocial programs. These differences in status or education may create barriers between local staff and program participants. We cannot assume that having someone from the community conduct an assessment will always result in more accurate information. A number of years ago, one of the authors was part of a longitudinal study examining the long-term psychological consequences for Khmer adolescents who lived through the horrors of the Pol Pot regime. He interviewed a young man who reported having had significantly high levels of post-trauma psychological symptoms since arriving in the United States several years earlier. When the interview was finished, the author briefly reviewed the assessment data reported by this young man from the previous summer and noticed that at that time he had indicated having had almost no symptoms. When questioned about this, the youth replied that during the previous assessment there had been an interpreter present, a Khmer man who was well respected in the community. He said he had not wanted to reveal his problems to someone from the local Khmer community but was willing to discuss them alone with the author, as he was "an American" and so it was alright.

We have found that it is not uncommon for people to be guarded with their comments when working through an interpreter due to concerns about confidentiality or underlying tensions created by differences in age, gender, religion, or culture. Common language does not necessarily translate into common beliefs or acceptance. The general point is that you cannot assume a specific intervention technique or methodology will work with any particular population or in any specific context until you do your homework and then try it out. You need to work with the community to understand how to adapt evaluation methods to local beliefs and conditions. Sometimes there are obstacles that you cannot do anything about and simply must live with but it is important to know what they are.

It is also helpful to keep in mind the skills of those who will be conducting the evaluation. What kind of training will they need to ensure that you get valid results? How much supervision will be required? It is best to keep the design and techniques within the ability of the staff carrying out the work. It is also good to avoid developing a plan that requires university trained researchers if local community members with minimal formal education will be responsible for overseeing and conducting the evaluation. It is also important to provide clear instructions for each step in the evaluation process with clearly defined responsibilities and lines of supervision. Manuals can be useful resources and are helpful for keeping the evaluation on track.

External Consultants

Finally, if you do not have the internal expertise to design your outcome evaluation, bringing in an outside consultant can be very helpful. Find someone who will take the time to understand your programs objectives as well as the population you are working with and the context in which the program will be operating. Outside experts who are called in for quick consultations sometimes bring along their own agenda (and sometimes their own measures) that may not be the best fit for answering your particular program's questions.

Choosing Measures of Program Success

Selecting appropriate measures for evaluating the effectiveness of an ecological mental health intervention can be challenging and there are a variety of issues that can influence the choices you make. It is important to begin with clear evaluation questions and then look for the methods and measures that will provide the answers—not the other way around: Do not let the measures dictate the evaluation. Some of the issues you will want to consider when selecting measures include:

- **Who does the evaluation need to inform?** You may want to start by considering the audience(s) that your evaluation must satisfy. These audiences, sometimes referred to as stakeholders, include your program staff (field staff responsible for implementing the program and staff from the home office), funding agencies, other groups who may want to replicate your program and the local community. Often these groups have different needs or agendas which may require collecting different information.

- **From whom should information be collected?** Many evaluations limit themselves to collecting data from program participants. However, evaluation results will be more informative and useful if you employ multiple measures and collect information from a variety of informants. For example, if you are trying to assess the effectiveness of a program for children, you will have a more complete picture if you can gather information from the children, their peers, caregivers, and other adults, such as teachers, who know the children in particular contexts. Program effects may be more evident in one setting than another (e.g., in a structured situation like school than in less structured situations like home or play settings). Important information can be missed when data are gathered in only one setting or from only one group of respondents.

- **Who are the targets of the intervention?** The methods you choose to evaluate the program will differ depending on the population(s) being targeted. For example, are you interested in the program's effect on individuals? families or systems? or community wide effects? Many programs are interested in measuring the program's impact on several (or all) of these levels.

Types of Information to Collect

There has been a tendency for ecological mental health interventions, and many psychosocial programs, to use measures of psychological symptoms as the sole method for establishing program success. Although measuring symptoms may be important and useful, there are other types of information that can also help establish program effectiveness. Types of data to consider collecting are:

- **Measures of psychological distress**: There are numerous standardized measures of psychopathology (many based on ICD or DSM taxonomies). The most frequently used by ecological mental health interventions and psychosocial programs assess depression, anxiety, somatic symptoms and post-traumatic stress disorder. Most often these measures will need to be translated, validated and adapted for use with new populations. The alternative is to develop new measures based on local problems and expressions of distress.

- **Process evaluation data**: Information gathered for the purpose of process evaluation can also be valuable when answering questions about program effectiveness. As described earlier, participation data and attendance logs can be useful for outcome evaluation as well.

- **Functional adaptation**: It can be useful to include measures that assess important areas of daily functioning, such as social adaptation, ability to parent children or engage in meaningful community activities in an outcome evaluation. Change that takes place in these domains can be as or more meaningful to participants than changes in psychological symptoms, and as such, they can be important indicators of program effectiveness. However, because there are no established measures of adaptive functioning, and because these behaviors are so culturally and situationally determined, you will need to develop your own measures (for an excellent approach to developing culturally appropriate measures of functioning, see Bolton & Tang, 2002).

- **Referral or service utilization data**: Gathering information on how well program participants are able to follow through on referrals made for them to other programs, or are able to utilize other services available to them, can be helpful when evaluating program success. For example, it may be useful to know if people who have participated in your mental health intervention are more likely to enroll in skills training or job placement programs than they were prior to the intervention (or more likely to enroll than a comparison sample).

- **Ongoing outside events**: It is important to gather information on significant events that impact the local environment. Conditions such as increasing levels of violence or changes in access to important resources such as food, water, and medicine, while possibly unrelated to your specific program, may have a significant influence on your program's effectiveness. A detailed log of events that have taken place concurrently with an intervention can often prove to be crucial when interpreting the evaluation results.

There is another set of considerations to be made concerning the *nature* of the data to be collected for the evaluation. Two common distinctions that can impact your measure selection are qualitative vs. quantitative and emic vs. etic.

Qualitative Versus Quantitative Measures

Evaluation methods are frequently categorized according to whether they provide us with numbers (quantitative data) or words (qualitative data) and there has been an ongoing debate over the relative usefulness of each type in evaluating program effectiveness. *Quantitative methods* provide numerical data that can be analyzed with statistical methods. The quantitative techniques most frequently used in psychosocial outcome evaluations are checklists, surveys, and structured interviews. The numerical data derived from these techniques can be used for hypothesis testing (e.g., we expect that people who attended more than 50% of the intervention activities will have significantly more social connections at the 3-month follow-up assessment than those who attend less than 50% of the activities) and summarizing results for reports (e.g., percentage and frequency data).

Qualitative methods, on the other hand, provide narrative data that are primarily descriptive and interpretative, and highlight the unique or individual characteristics of the target population in its natural context. Methods include unstructured interviews, focus groups, and observation, as well as techniques like video taping, group mapping, role plays, and drama. Qualitative techniques have traditionally been associated with attempts to understand program effects from a local perspective, whereas quantitative techniques have been associated with a more scientific or outsider's perspective.

Recently, these traditional distinctions have been breaking down. Programs are developing quantitative checklists and surveys that reflect local beliefs and concerns and are using qualitative methods to collect baseline and follow-up data to assess changes in understanding or knowledge. For example, one of the authors conducts numerous brief interviews during the needs assessment phase of program development to gather information on local concepts of well-being and individual problems that have resulted from living through the war (a qualitative technique). The data generated through these interviews is then used to create new baseline and follow-up measures for assessing program effectiveness. These new checklist style measures (a quantitative technique) will be based on local perceptions.

Traditional survey and interview style techniques for evaluating program effectiveness often combine qualitative and quantitative methods as well. Sometimes a specific quantitative question like, "Are you separated from your family?" (yes/no) are followed by a qualitative question like, "How has this affected you?" The reverse strategy is also used. A mental health intake assessment might ask, "Tell me why you came to our program today?" or "What kind of assistance do you hope to receive?" These open-ended qualitative questions can be followed with a variety of quantitative questions that are of specific interest to the program (e.g., a list of post-trauma symptoms or common reasons people give for participating in the program).

Both types of approaches have their strengths and when used together can provide richer results. Recently, one of the authors was analyzing symptom data from a community mental health intervention and found a consistent and statistically significant relationship between age, depression, and anxiety; while being young was related to higher anxiety scores, being older was associated with higher levels of depression. This quantitative finding was interesting, but it took qualitative data, gathered through interviews with program participants, to give meaning to the finding. Younger refugees described feeling as though life was passing them by while they sat in the camp; they should be going to school, starting a business and building a future for themselves. They expressed impatience with their situation, and were anxious to get on with their lives. Older refugees, on the other hand, expressed little hope of being able to start over again or rebuild their lives when they returned home from the camps and were more focused on the tremendous losses they had experienced.

Emic Versus Etic Measures

Another area of consideration when selecting evaluation measures is the degree to which program staff and/or other stakeholders are interested in understanding the intervention's effectiveness from an *emic* (insider or local) or *etic* (outsider or observer) perspective. Generally, when you use standardized measures or quantitative assessment tools that were originally developed for use with a different population than the one with which you are working, you are taking an etic approach. For example, assessing a construct such as depression among Filipinos or Vietnamese using a measure originally developed for use with middle class White Europeans would represent an emic approach. On the other hand, when you use measures or techniques that were locally derived, or methods that were designed to understand the impact of a program as community members perceive, experience, and understand it, you are taking a more emic evaluation approach. It is easy to see why qualitative techniques are often associated with emic approaches while quantitative techniques are linked with etic approaches. As demonstrated in the previous section, however, this generalization is not always valid.

As ecological mental health interventions have become more culturally sensitive, there has been a tendency to view emic methods as *good* assessment techniques while etic methods are characterized as *bad*, or at least less desirable techniques. As usual, the reality is more complicated than this and there are a variety of reasons why a particular program might choose to include one type or the other. For example, a program might choose to include etic measures out of a desire to compare their results with those from other programs—in which case it is helpful to use common measures. In fact, the desire to generalize the results of one program to other populations (and vice versa) is a common underlying reason why some evaluators prefer standardized measures. It is difficult to compare results across programs or populations when the data collected are by definition specific to the local community and context, which is the case with emic data.

Another commonly cited reason for using existing or standardized measures is pragmatics. It is simply much easier and efficient to use a measure that has already been developed and found to be useful with other populations. Many program staff feel that they just do not have the expertise or resources to create their own measures.

In addition, funding agencies sometimes ask programs to include particular measures of program success as a requirement for funding. Almost always these are quantitative, etic measures that have demonstrated their effectiveness in other settings. They may not, however, be a good fit for evaluating a particular population or program. If faced with this situation, we suggest countering with a well thought out alternative method. Based on the experience of colleagues, funding agencies are often willing to accept substitute methods when a sound alternative plan is proposed and are becoming more receptive to methods that incorporate emic perspectives.

Historically, the outcome measures used by most ecological mental health interventions and psychosocial programs have been etic in nature, but there appears to be a growing tendency to approach evaluation from a more emic perspective. More often in recent years, programs are interested in understanding and measuring their effects as they are experienced by the participants. There is an awareness that outcome evaluations are much more meaningful if they include local perspectives. Methods that have traditionally been used by anthropologists, such as social mapping and narrative techniques are being incorporated into outcome evaluations. Some of the techniques previously described, such as eliciting community input into the evaluation process and including community members on the evaluation team can help keep a program from becoming too "outsider focused."

Using Existing Measures or Creating Your Own

After you have developed your evaluation questions, identified the domains which need to be assessed, and considered the various measurement issues raised in the previous sections, you need to decide on the actual methods and measures you will use. There are basically three approaches available. You can choose to use existing measures, adapt existing measures for use with your specific population, or create new measures. Each of these approaches has its strengths, weaknesses, and challenges.

Some of the strengths of using existing measures were presented earlier: the knowledge that they have been useful in other settings, the ability to compare findings with other programs, and the efficiency of not having to create measures. But there are problems as well. It is important to remember that a measure developed and standardized on one population is not necessarily valid for use with another. There is no such thing as a measure being "somewhat valid"—it either is or it isn't. Rarely have traditional measures been validated for use with the populations being served by ecological psychosocial and mental health programs for refugees. Nonetheless, many programs, including our own, have gone ahead and used existing measures in these contexts (for the reasons stated earlier) and with the time-limited nature of many interventions and the lack of resources for evaluation, this will likely continue to be the case into the foreseeable future.

There are a number of things that can be done to make existing measures more useful in new settings. Begin by translating the measures into the local language. The most commonly used strategy for this involves translation and back-translation (Behling & Law, 2000; Brislin, 1970). The first step is to have one person, fluent in both the language of the original measure and the local language, translate the measure into the local language. A second person, with the same skills, is given the translated version only (they do not see the original measure) and they translate it back into the original language. This "back-translation" is then compared with the original measure and any discrepancies between the translated and original version are resolved by the two translators. It is important that the two translators fully comprehend *the meaning* of the items in the measure if they are to arrive at a meaningful final product. We recommend adding an additional step to the measure translation process by having a group of bilingual staff and community members read the back-translated measure (for language and meaning) with the task of achieving group consensus for the items. It is also helpful to then pilot the translated measures with a small group of community members to ensure that all items are readily understood as intended. A failure to take these precautionary steps can lead to unexpected (and problematic) results. For example, one of us was involved with the adaptation and translation of a conventional measure of children's behavioral problems, for use among indigenous Guatemalans living in refugee camps in southern Mexico. To our surprise, on an item assessing audio hallucinations most of the parents reported that their children *often* heard voices when no one was actually present. We had spent enough time in the camps to know that most children were *not* psychotic (none were, in fact). Upon further exploration, it became clear that children heard the voices of people not actually present because the houses were made of cornstalks or loosely bound boards through which the voices of neighbors could easily heard. Piloting the measure and closely examining the results allowed us to identify and correct a significant gap between the intended and actual understanding of an instrument item.

Interview style measures should also be translated into the local language—even if the staff administering them are bilingual and can translate on the spot. Unless there is a translation to go by, different interviewers will often ask questions in somewhat different ways. Even the same interviewer will translate questions differently on different administrations.

When intervening with populations of limited literacy, written measures can also be given interview style. Pictures or diagrams can be used in place of, or along with, typical rating scales to overcome literacy problems or comprehension issues related to cultural differences. For example, a card with a picture of four glasses with varying amounts of water has been used to help people rate symptoms on a *never* (empty glass) to *always* (full glass) Likert scale. In another instance, children used a card with a sketch of a person crying on the right and a person smiling on the left (connected with a line) to indicate how they felt over the previous week. A grid was laid over the card and the children's answers were coded depending on where in the grid their mark fell.

The third alternative, creating new measures, has two primary advantages: You can create measures that specifically address the evaluation questions of interest to your program, and you can collaborate with the local community and develop measures that capture their feelings, beliefs, and expressions of distress. If your program is interested in assessing areas for which there are few, if any existing measures, for example increased trust, social connectedness, or the ability to handle daily domestic responsibilities, there will be little choice but to create new measures. But even if the program is interested in evaluating post-traumatic psychological symptoms, like depression or anxiety, you may want to create new measures that reflect local post-traumatic feelings and experiences.

There are a variety of ways to create measures that reflect local feelings and beliefs. Focus groups can provide insight into the local perspective when creating new measures. Another method that is gaining popularity is to gather information from the community in a standardized way, for example through a series of brief interviews or surveys. The interview or survey data is then examined for common themes or high frequency responses and the results of this analyses are used to create the new measures, but ones that are based on local concepts (a method of this kind was described earlier in the 'qualitative vs. quantitative' section; see also Bolton & Tang, 2002). There are a variety of resources available to assist with the process of scale development (e.g., Dawis, 1993; DeVellis, 1991).

Analyzing, Interpreting, and Reporting the Results of an Outcome Evaluation

If an outcome evaluation has been well designed and implemented the analysis and reporting phase is often fairly straightforward and rewarding. But once again, the context and conditions can create added challenges which should be considered.

Data Management

The results of an outcome evaluation can only be as good as the data on which it is based. It is important to manage the data collection and data entry processes closely. We have known psychosocial projects that got to the analysis phase of their evaluation only to find that problems in the quality of the data precluded meaningful analyses or interpretation. Most of the time, if the problems had been identified earlier in the process, they could have been easily rectified. Some of the ways to avoid problems include meeting regularly with the evaluation team to ensure that everyone is conducting the assessment in the same manner. It can be useful to have evaluation team members sit in on each other's assessments. It is usually wise to enter evaluation data in an ongoing way (i.e., do not wait until all the data are collected to begin entering and examining them). In one of our own programs, assessments were left to accumulate with the intention of entering the data over a brief period (the assumption was that it would be easier to supervise and retain consistency). Without warning, there were a series of violent rebel attacks, the refugee camps were evacuated and, in the process, almost 9 months of evaluation data were either lost or destroyed. The only data that remained were those that had been already entered into the computer and stored on discs, which could be easily transported.

At times, the relatively unregulated conditions of field work can lead to a more casual approach to data management. It is important to use the same care in safeguarding confidential data that you would use if you were operating in a university or clinical setting. Set up clear rules surrounding access to, and handling and storage of sensitive information; and review these processes, and the reasoning behind them, with the entire evaluation team. The rights of program participants to privacy should always supercede the evaluation needs of the program.

Analyzing Data

Programs choose between having local staff analyze data in the field and sending the data off-site to have it analyzed. Frequently local program staff feel that they lack the expertise to analyze their own data onsite, thus they choose to send it on to more skilled program evaluation staff, either at their home office or to external consultants, who can use more sophisticated approaches in analyzing the data. The appeal of this approach is obvious. But there are advantages to conducting the outcome evaluation analyses locally. It keeps the program staff involved in the process and avoids the situation where the data they have worked hard to collect gets sent away with no further word; or the results are returned with no explanation of how they were generated. Analyzing data in the field helps take the mystery out of the process and contributes to building local capacity by giving community team members access to it.

When analyzing data in the field it can be helpful to keep the techniques simple, and, once again, staff will do better with step-by-step instructions and a how-to manual. Many basic summary statistics like averages, frequencies, and percentages, as well as impressive graphs and figures, can be generated with basic spreadsheet programs like Microsoft Excel. Local program staff are much more likely to have experience using these programs than statistical software packages. However, one of the authors has had great success recruiting and training refugee staff to use statistical software and now has research and evaluation staff capable of running many comparative and predictive statistics in the field.

Interpreting the Results

Sometimes program results are self-explanatory and do not require much interpretation. Other times, however, outcome evaluation results need context to give them meaning. Once you have analyzed your data and have the basic results, it is helpful to discuss them with your staff, program participants, and other members of the community. Ask them what they think about the findings. Do they reflect their experience of program impact? Were there additional program effects that were not captured by the evaluation results? This provides an opportunity to explore unintended effects of the program or to look for explanations for surprising or unexpected results. As previously mentioned, it can be enlightening to examine the results of the outcome evaluation in relation to other concurrent events that may have impacted the success of your program.

Finally, it is important to remember that there can always be at least three reasons for negative findings from a program evaluation. First, for a variety of reasons the program may not have been effective and negative results may reflect the unfortunate reality of a problematic program design. As difficult as this can be, it is one of the important reasons for conducting an outcome evaluation—to learn if our interventions are having their intended effects. Second, the program may have been well designed, implemented, and possibly effective under other circumstances but "outside factors" were undermining the program effectiveness. And finally, negative findings may be the result of a poorly designed or implemented outcome evaluation. That is, the evaluation itself may have been flawed, thus providing inaccurate results. It is always important to take time and explore the reasons behind any set of evaluation results.

Reporting Evaluation Results

Most of the time, outcome evaluation data and the reports generated from it, flow in one direction: from the program to the home office or management level staff, and then on to the funding agencies. Rarely, in our experience, do results get reported back to the local staff who provided the intervention (and often collected the data), the participants, or other community members. However, rapid feedback of results to these stakeholders is important. If the program is having positive effects, the reports can provide encouragement for local staff and build support for the program in the community. But regardless of the actual findings, these are the people who have been collecting the data or participating in the evaluation, and they need to know the results of their efforts.

Take the time to adapt the reports for each audience so that the information is meaningful for them. Pictures and graphs can be useful where literacy is a consideration. One of the authors recently sat in on a community presentation by a program where many summary statistics were presented orally. In a follow-up discussion we learned that only one person in the audience knew what a percentage was, and that while everyone had smiled and nodded politely during the talk, very little of it had been understood.

Although report formats and styles vary considerably, there is some basic information that should be included in the evaluation section of a report.

- The outcome evaluation section of a report frequently begins with a summary of the findings from the process evaluation: was the program implemented as planned; did the activities take place; was the target audience reached, etc. Too often, however, process evaluation data are *all* that is reported for ecological mental health and psychosocial interventions working in adverse contexts. Although process evaluation data can tell us a great deal that is useful about how an intervention was implemented and who it did and did not reach, process data, by themselves, cannot tell whether an intervention was or was not effective.

- It is helpful to provide a brief summary of the methods that were used to assess program effectiveness. This will save the person reviewing the report from having to refer back to the original proposal to make sense of the results.

- Provide a complete summary of your findings. Highlight and elaborating them specifically for each audience.

- Describe any problems that were encountered in the evaluation process and how you intend to address these concerns.

- Finally, state your plans for any ongoing or future evaluations of the program (e.g., post-intervention follow-up assessments or community impact evaluations).

CONCLUSION

For the sake of presentation, program evaluation has been presented in this chapter in a somewhat linear fashion. In reality, the processes that were described are interrelated and iterative, both informing and dictating each other as the evaluation is designed and implemented. Good outcome evaluation is not static but should be an active process that is constantly re-examined and adapted to meet changing needs of a program. We have an obligation to our programs, our funders, and the participants in our interventions, to do a better job of evaluation and to pass what we learn on to others. There is increasing attention to the sustainability of interventions in post-conflict regions. Ecological mental health projects and psychosocial programs have often focused on empowering local staff with training and intervention skills; however, local staff also need the skills necessary to effectively evaluate their work. We hope that the suggestions considered in this chapter are helpful for those individuals and organizations who desire a better understanding of the effectiveness of their programs. Success begins by making evaluation a priority.

REFERENCES

Bolton, P., & Tang, A. (2002). An alternative approach to cross-cultural function assessment. *Social Psychiatry and Psychiatric Epidemiology, 37,* 537-543.

Dalton, J., Elias, M., & Wandersman, A. (2001). *Community psychology: Linking individuals and communities.* Belmont, CA: Wadsworth/Thompson Learning.

Dawes, R. (1994). *House of cards: Psychology and psychotherapy built on myth.* New York: Free Press.

Dawis, R. (1993). Scale construction. In A. Kazdin (Ed.), Methodological issues and strategies in clinical research (pp. 193-213). Washington, DC: American Psychological Association.

Dean (focus groups), D. (1994). How to use focus groups. In J. Wholey, H. Hatry, & K. Newcomer (Eds.), *Handbook of practical program evaluation* (pp. 338-349). San Francisco: Jossey-Bass.

De Jong, J. (2002). Public mental health, traumatic stress and human rights violations in low income countries. In J. de Jong (Ed.), *Trauma, war, and violence: Public mental health in socio-cultural context* (pp. 1-92). New York: Kluwer Academic/Plenum Publishers.

DeVellis, R. (1991) *Scale development.* Newbury Park, CA: Sage.

Enett, S., Rosenbaum, D., Flewelling, R., Bieler, G., Ringwalt, C., & Baily, S. (1994). Long-term evaluation of drug abuse resistance education. *Addictive behaviors, 19,* 113-125.

Fetterman, D., Kaftarian, S., & Wandersman, A. (Eds.). (1996). Empowerment evaluation. Thousand Oaks, CA: Sage.

Kazdin, A. (Ed.). (1993). *Methodological issues and strategies in clinical research.* Washington, DC: American Psychological Association.

Kruger, R. (1994). *Focus groups.* Thousand Oaks, CA: Sage.

Linney, J., & Wandersman, A. (1991). *Prevention plus III: Assessing alcohol and other drug prevention programs at the school and community level: A 4 step guide to useful program assessment.* Rockville, MD: US Department of Health and Human Services, Office for Substance Abuse Prevention.

Miller, K. (1999). *Program evaluation for HIV/AIDS prevention.* Chicago: Midwest Hispanic AIDS Coalition.

Miller, K. (Co-producer), Billings, D. (Co-producer), & Farias, P. (Co-producer). (1995). *Playing to grow: Creative education programs for children* [Instructional video]. (Available from K. Miller, Psychology Department, SFSU, 1600 Holloway Avenue, San Francisco, CA 94132)

Miller, K., & Billings, D. (1994). Playing to grow: A primary mental health intervention with Guatemalan refugee children. *American Journal of Orthopsychiatry, 64,* 346-356.

Wholey, J., Hatry, H., & Newcomer, K. (Eds.), (1994). *Handbook of practical program evaluation.* San Francisco: Jossey-Bass.

11

Innovations, Challenges, and Critical Issues in the Development of Ecological Mental Health Interventions With Refugees

Lisa M. Rasco and Kenneth E. Miller

The projects outlined in this volume represent some of the most creative and challenging mental health and psychosocial intervention work with refugees today. The contributing authors describe a wide range of ecological interventions designed to promote the psychological well-being of refugees in a diversity of settings—from refugee camps within or along the tenuous borders of developing countries to more permanent resettlement communities in nations such as the United States. Although the methodologies and theoretical underpinnings of the interventions vary, all of the projects are guided by a community-based, ecological model, which emphasizes drawing on community strengths and resources and involving community members as stakeholders and active collaborators in the development and implementation of psychosocial interventions.

Box 11.1
Summary of Ecological Principles

(For expanded description, see chapter 1, pp. 35-48)

1. Psychological problems often reflect a *poor fit* between the demands of people's settings and the adaptive resources to which they have access. Ecological interventions should seek to alter problematic settings, create alternative settings better suited to people's needs and capacities, or enhance people's capacity to adapt to existing settings.

2. Ecological interventions should prioritize and address problems that are of concern to community members.

3. Whenever possible, prevention should be prioritized over treatment, as preventive interventions are generally more effective, cost-efficient, and humane than an exclusive reliance on the treatment of problems once they have developed.

4. Local values and beliefs about psychological well-being and distress should be incorporated the into the design, implementation, and evaluation of community-based interventions.

5. Whenever possible, ecological interventions should be integrated into existing community settings and activities to enhance community participation and long-term sustainability.

6. Capacity building, rather than direct service provision by mental health professionals, should be an intervention priority—especially in communities that underutilize or have limited access to professional mental health services. Capacity building reflects the ecological focus on empowerment (i.e., helping people achieve greater control over the resources that affect their lives).

In this chapter, we step back and offer reflections on a number of critical issues that arose as common themes across this body of work. We first note the innovations, strengths, and ways the various projects exemplify the principles of ecological interventions discussed in chapter 1 (see summary in Box 11.1). Yet, even as we look to the work of the contributors for inspiration and guidance, their candid discussions of obstacles they've encountered make it clear that the field is not without challenges. Therefore, we next outline some common difficulties researchers and practitioners face when conducting ecologically oriented intervention work with refugees. We hope that highlighting these critical issues will help lay the groundwork for the development and sharing of constructive solutions. Toward these ends, we discuss the importance of developing well-elaborated models of risk and protection to guide intervention work, and offer a broad organizational frame to aid this endeavor. Next, we discuss the need for better conceptualizations of distress and well-being at the family and community levels, as well as the need for a clear articulation of intervention goals and the difficulties involved in choosing these goals when a wide range of material and psychosocial needs exist. We also consider the importance of clearly articulating linkages between models of risk and the design of psychosocial interventions, as well as the challenges involved in program evaluation. Finally, we discuss conceptual and practical impediments to creating culturally sensitive interventions that blend Western and local approaches to healing, and offer ideas about how to address these obstacles.

Although this chapter is not meant to cover all of the critical issues facing the field of ecological approaches to refugee mental health and well-being, our intention is to organize and frame a number of key issues as important foci for ongoing discussion and to stimulate critical reflection on how these challenges might be addressed in the diverse settings in which they arise.

STRENGTHS AND INNOVATIONS

Although the theoretical foundations and methodologies of the projects in this volume vary, all of the interventions adhere in important ways to the basic tenets of an ecological approach to intervention (see Box 11.1). For example, in accordance with the first ecological principle, a number of the interventions involve the creation or alteration of community settings to support and build local capacity and enhance people's ability to adapt to existing settings. Goodkind, Hang, and Yang (chap. 9) describe how their "learning circles" intervention for Hmong refugees built local capacity by bringing together resources from the University and Hmong communities to strengthen the skills of, and empower, all community participants. Tribe and colleagues (chap. 5) describe the training of women, all of whom had participated in empowerment programs for war widows in Sri Lanka, to work at local extension offices and become "be-frienders" to other women in their communities— thereby extending the reach of their psychosocial intervention. Weine and colleagues (chap. 8) describe the success of a family-oriented, psychosocial support and resource intervention, which helped ease the transition of Bosnian and Kosovar refugees to their new lives in the United States. These projects not only created settings for group learning, empowerment, and psychological support, but also enhanced participants' ability to adapt to their new settings by providing crucial information and education about services, resources, and rights in their communities.

In addition, true to the second ecological principle, all of the projects involved active collaboration between project developers, staff, and community members in intervention design and implementation. Rather than imposing a ready-made agenda on refugee communities, a number of project teams drew on methods that prioritized communities' self-identified needs. For example, Tribe and colleagues (chap. 5) conducted "fact-finding missions", during which each community's specific needs were identified by local community members and service organizations working in various Sri Lankan refugee camps, prior to the development of empowerment groups for war widows living in those camps. The results of these inquiries significantly shaped the agendas for the various women's empowerment groups. Similarly, other chapter authors describe the employment of needs assessments, focus groups, meetings with community elders, and so forth to establish the needs of communities and elicit the support of key community members to help design and implement mental health interventions to address those needs.

As Ecological Principle 3 states, an ecological approach to intervention prioritizes prevention over treatment, and accordingly, the projects in this volume aimed to build local capacity to address difficulties and decrease the probability of long-term, chronic suffering among community members impacted by the stresses of forced displacement. Rather than primarily directing resources to set up Western-style, expert run clinics for the treatment of psychopathology, many projects promoted the reestablishment of local healing and psychosocial support networks, as well as community activities and meeting places to provide safe, supportive, and predictable environments to promote community healing. However, it is clear that many refugees and displaced persons *do* experience high levels of war-related and displacement-related distress, and contributors such as Hubbard and Pearson (chap. 3) and van de Put and Eisenbruch (chap. 4) illustrate innovative ways in which treatment-focused interventions can be culturally appropriate, utilize community resources, and strive to empower communities by helping them develop greater capacity to address their own mental health needs. Stated otherwise, while the ecological model prioritizes prevention over treatment, it in no way negates the importance of treatment for individuals experiencing significant distress. The challenge is to develop treatment-focused interventions that are contextually grounded, empowering in nature, and that utilize local resources rather than rely on scarce outside professionals.

Along these lines, several projects incorporated local approaches to healing (Ecological Principle 4), a topic we discuss in some detail in the final section of this chapter. Also, to increase the likelihood of program utilization and sustainability, many projects were integrated into familiar and nonstigmatized community settings (Ecological Principle 5), such as schools (Kostelny and Wessells, chap. 6), homes (van de Put and Eisenbruch, chap. 4) neighborhood community centers (Weine et al., chap. 8) and various community meeting places within or adjacent to refugee camps or zones of conflict (Buitrago Cuéllar, chap. 7; Hubbard and Pearson, chap. 3; Tribe and colleagues, chap. 5; and Wessells and Monteiro, chap. 2).

Finally, the interventions in this volume focused on strengthening the capacity of communities to cope with and heal from displacement-related stressors, as well as the effects of violence and war-related loss (Ecological Principle 6). For example, Hubbard and Pearson (chap. 3) described the training of local psychosocial agents to address the mental health needs of psychologically distressed Sierra Leonean refugees unable to take advantage of relief services, and Wessells and Monteiro (chap. 2) described how community members and local service providers were trained to facilitate normalizing and healing activities for thousands of internally displaced children and youth in Angola, and how a mobile unit of intensively trained local staff traveled to various communities to provide ongoing supervision and support for psychosocial interventions. In a similar vein, the staff of Corporación AVRE (chap. 7) trained local community members to work as Popular Therapists and Multipliers of Psychosocial Actions with a broad range of distressed communities affected by violent conflict and displacement in Columbia. While initially providing on-going supervision to the local staff doing the front-line work, the goal of these projects has been to train local staff who do not rely heavily on outside mental health experts, thereby building local capacity to manage necessary psychosocial intervention work. Indeed, Hubbard and Pearson describe how local psychosocial agents (PSAs) continued to provide assistance to distressed Sierra Leonean refugees even after a rebel attack forced them to relocate and necessitated the temporary withdrawal of expatriate project staff providing supervision and training. They also note that the PSAs began to train other community members to provide psychosocial assistance (spontaneously "training trainers") and were eager to continue a new phase of their work during the process of repatriation. These chapters provide promising examples of how trained community members can provide ongoing, dependable psychosocial support to their communities even under very difficult circumstances.

Clearly, the field is rich with dedicated and creative individuals coordinating innovative programs true to the principles of an ecological approach to mental health intervention. Yet, it is also clear from the contributors' descriptions of their projects that there remain notable challenges facing the field—and in the following sections, we elaborate a number of these critical issues in the hopes of stimulating discussion and ideas about how to address some of the challenges involved in designing, implementing, and evaluating ecological interventions for and with refugee communities.

CHALLENGES AND FUTURE DIRECTIONS

The Need for Elaborated Risk Models

An important endeavor in the field of refugee mental health, as in any field of health-related research and intervention, is the development and elaboration of risk models[1] that guide the design, implementation, and evaluation of psychosocial interventions. As Kostelny and Wessells (chap. 6) suggest, we can look to risk and resilience theory from the fields of public health and developmental psychopathology to inform the development of risk models, which organize our understanding of how risk factors[2]—such as the multiple stressors commonly associated with the refugee experience—in the presence or absence of protective factors, translate into psychosocial outcomes at the individual, family, and

---

[1]Throughout the remainder of this chapter, we use the term *risk* rather than *causal* model because we do not have the appropriate studies to indicate a causal or etiologic relationship between common elements of the refugee experience (e.g., exposure to political violence and displacement) and indicators of psychosocial distress among refugees. However, a number of correlational studies indicate important associations among various refugee experiences and psychosocial outcomes, and therefore help us identify risk and protective factors (e.g., see recent review by de Jong, 2002; and chapter 1, this volume). Moving from models of risk to causality requires studies that establish criteria such as longitudinal time sequence, ruling out of alternative explanations, etc. (Freedman, 1999). However, meeting these criteria is particularly difficult in this field because we rarely have "pre-conflict or displacement" measures (other than retrospective accounts). Yet, with more large-scale intervention research and evaluation studies, we may begin to establish more of these criteria and move in the direction of building causal models to better understand these relationships.

[2]As Rutter (1987) explained, risk factors should not be thought of as static events—but, rather, as sets of circumstances that set in motion a series of events or mechanisms that, in certain contexts, increase the likelihood of particular negative outcomes.

community levels. A number of pre- and post-migration risk factors—
such as loss of or separation from family members, lack of shelter,
torture, imprisonment, poverty, discrimination, exposure to combat,
sexual assault, and so forth—have been associated empirically with
increased psychosocial distress in a range of refugee populations (de
Jong, 2002; Steel & Silove, 2000). Research and theory indicate that the
greater the number, severity, and chronicity of risk factors experienced
by individuals or communities, the greater the probability of the
expression and severity of adverse psychosocial outcomes associated
with those risk factors (Coie et al., 1993; Garbarino & Kostelny, 1996;
Rutter, 1979; Rutter & Garmezy, 1983).

A well-articulated risk model, based on empirical data or sound
theory, offers a theoretical "roadmap" outlining paths between risks and
psychosocial outcomes of interest, and, ideally, delineating specific
mechanisms (including mediating or moderating variables) linking risk
to outcome. In the design of interventions, these models help us make
predictions, visualize potential intervention points along the path from
risk to outcome, and—during the evaluation phase—allow us to
pinpoint what is or is not working in our interventions by drawing
attention to discrepancies between predictions from the model and
actual outcome data. Well-elaborated risk models, therefore, advance the
science of prevention and intervention by helping us continually hone
and correct our guiding models, improve the design of interventions,
and even design models to guide the extension of successful
interventions to new populations. In a nutshell, risk models identify
clearly which problems need to be addressed; specify the factors that
increase the likelihood of people developing particular problems; specify
the pathways by which risk factors impact people's well-being; and
ideally, specify variables that either increase or reduce people's
vulnerability to developing the target problems in the face of the risk
factors.

A comprehensive risk model for understanding the impact of
trauma, loss, and displacement-related stressors on refugee mental
health and well-being would account for the mental health and
psychosocial difficulties—ranging from symptoms of PTSD and
depression to broad social problems, such as the breakdown of support
networks—that are commonly observed and documented in refugee

populations. Well-elaborated risk models take into consideration both (1) risk factors, associated with various negative outcomes, that might be prevented or ameliorated and (2) protective factors[3] that moderate the impact of risk and might be harnessed to foster well-being and decrease the likelihood of maladaptive psychosocial outcomes in the presence of unavoidable stressors (e.g., de Jong, 2002). For our specific purposes, a risk model relevant to refugee mental health would outline how exposure to political violence, migration, social upheaval, and displacement-related stressors are thought to place refugees at risk for a number of adverse psychosocial outcomes—including symptoms of trauma, anxiety, and/or depression in individuals, distress and tension among families, and social disruptions in communities.

A Broad Framework for the Development of Risk Models

The authors in this volume have drawn on a range of theoretical models—from theories of trauma to theories of political and social empowerment—to ground and guide their intervention work with refugees and displaced persons. In reflecting on these theoretical foundations and on the empirical literature summarized in chapter 1, we have constructed a general, global risk model that may be useful across the diverse settings in which refugees are found (Fig. 11.1). The model we have sketched is not meant to represent all of the underlying mechanisms involved in the translation of risk to psychosocial and mental health outcomes—but is meant to offer a guiding framework for mapping the potential impact of common war and displacement-related stressors (i.e., risk factors) on the psychosocial well-being of refugees.

---

[3]Although it is an understandable tendency—when dealing with situations of human suffering and psychosocial distress—to emphasize the abundant stressors, refugee communities are equally remarkable for their resilience and adaptability. For this reason, protective factors, such as relocating with an intact family or gaining meaningful employment upon resettlement, should be considered in the construction of risk models, as they are thought to buffer or mitigate the negative psychosocial impact of various risks in ways that should be more carefully studied and understood.

Figure 11.1. The Adverse Effects of Political Violence and Displacement on Individuals, Families, and Communities

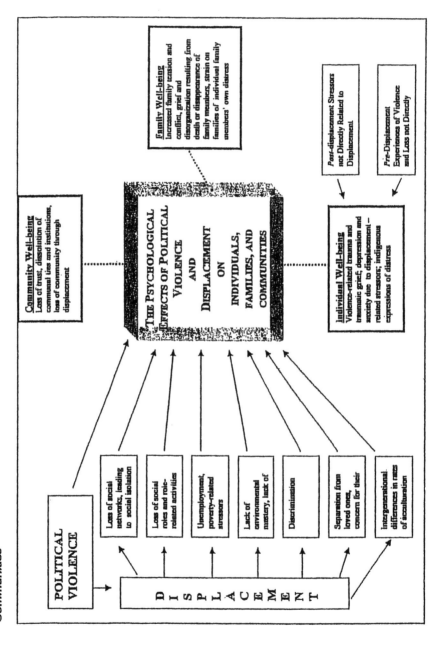

A number of risk factors associated with the refugee experience are outlined on the left-hand side of Figure 11.1. Although risk factors associated with negative psychosocial outcomes are often conceptualized as occurring either within *individuals* (physiologic vulnerability to stress, poor coping skills), *families* (single-parent household, marital discord), or *communities* (high poverty, few mental health resources), risk also might be viewed as the result of a *poor fit* between individuals, families, or communities and their environments. For instance, a particular coping style may only be "poor" or "maladaptive" in a particular setting. From this perspective, we would not speak of at-risk individuals or groups, but consider at-risk contexts or person–environment transactions. In our model, most of the displacement related stressors—such as discrimination, lack of environmental mastery, loss of familiar social roles and support networks—might be conceptualized as person–environment *mismatches* that lead to adverse psychosocial outcomes. When risk is viewed in this ecologically contextualized manner, we would argue that risk factors are best targeted with ecologically grounded interventions that take into account person–environment transactions (Barrera, 2000; Felner, Felner, & Silverman, 2000; Kelly, 1987; Vincent & Trickett, 1983). For example, although it might be difficult to alter an individual's physiological reactivity or previous exposure to stress, it *is* possible to develop community resources and adapt current environments to support resilience and protect or buffer individuals— who may be highly reactive to stress or who have experienced high levels of trauma exposure—from negative psychosocial outcomes.

It is important to note that risk factors for various forms of psychosocial distress often *vary* across populations (Coie et al., 1993; de Jong, 2002; Steel & Silove, 2000), and the risk factors included in Fig. 11.1 should not be assumed to be exhaustive or relevant for all refugee groups, or linked to psychosocial distress in the exact same manner across populations. However, the model provides a general schema outlining the *types* of stressors that commonly impact the lives of refugees in adverse ways—and provides an illustrative list of factors to take into consideration when building and testing risk models for the populations with whom we work.

Although we have stressed the importance of protective factors when creating models of risk and resilience, we did not include them in the general risk model pictured in Figure 11.1. However, the *inverse* of any of the risk factors outlined on the right of the diagram could be considered a protective factor. For example, the stress of losing supportive social networks in its inverse would be the maintenance or development of crucial social ties—an important protective factor thought to mitigate the stress of displacement for refugees (e.g., Gorst-Unsworth & Goldenberg, 1998; Kinzie et al., 1986; Miller et al., 2002). Other important protective factors not specifically implied by our model, but that might be harnessed and fostered in community-based interventions, include involvement in recreational activities (sports, dances, concerts) and empowering organizations such as workers unions and human rights groups, living in safe neighborhoods or smaller sized camps, access to good schools and jobs, and the maintenance of religious or political ties and activities that provide comfort and meaning in trying circumstances (de Jong, 2002; Steele & Silove, 2000). From an ecological perspective, effective interventions are likely to be those that identify and strengthen protective factors—such as the often overlooked resources present in refugee communities—while minimizing the salience of risk factors that may compromise people's well-being.

The stressors related to political violence and displacement, shown on the left-hand side of Fig. 11.1, impact the psychosocial well-being of refugees at multiple, interrelated levels including: individual health and psychological functioning; the structure and functioning of families; and community well-being. These multilevel psychosocial outcomes are represented by the box on the right hand side of Fig. 11.1. Depending on which level is targeted by a particular intervention or intervention component, the model can be re-organized so that individual, family, or community level outcome is at the far right, while the other levels might then represent mediating or moderating variables.[4] For example, one component of an intervention may entail the development of a women's

---

[4]As described by Baron and Kenny (1986), a mediating variable helps account for the relationship between two factors. For instance, feelings of profound guilt may help explain (i.e., mediate) the positive association between witnessing the violent death of a family member and the development of severe depression. A moderating variable, on the other hand, affects the direction or strength of the relationship between two variables (see example in text about the women's weaving collective).

weaving collective, designed to ameliorate depression in *individual* participants and enhance their financial well-being by creating a socially supportive setting in which their crafts can be produced and marketed. It may be that a *family* level variable, such as whether or not women have spouses who support their working, is an important moderating variable. Perhaps only those women with supportive spouses will benefit from participation in the collective, given that women with unsupportive spouses may experience increased distress because their participation in the intervention increases tensions at home. Community level variables—such as attitudes about women working in the community (e.g., women's access to loans)—might also moderate the outcomes of this type of intervention. This is simply to illustrate that the general framework of risk outlined in Fig. 11.1 can be "reorganized," depending on the outcome(s) of interest (i.e., individual, family, or community-level), and can include important mediating and moderating variables at the individual, family, and community level(s) that might influence specified outcomes in important ways.

Intervention Foci: Multiple Levels of Interest

As noted, the psychosocial outcomes in Fig. 11.1 represent the multiple levels of distress often associated with the risk factors commonly experienced by refugees and displaced persons. Although numerous mental health interventions for these populations focus primarily on *individual level* distress as the primary intervention target and outcome of interest, the broad theoretical model that guides the work of ecologically minded researchers and practitioners acknowledges that trauma, loss, and displacement impact the psychosocial well-being and functioning of target populations at multiple, interconnected levels, including those of the individual, the family, and the community.

Although each of these multiple, interacting levels of psychosocial well-being is clearly important, in the psychological sciences, formulations of well-being and distress have rarely been articulated or operationalized beyond the individual level. Mental health workers are trained to assess symptoms of distress in individuals, and accordingly, most mental-health oriented research and intervention work with refugees targets individual level symptoms and functioning as the outcomes of interest. As summarized in chapter 1, research clearly indicates that exposure to violence is correlated with symptoms of trauma (nightmares, flashbacks, avoidance, hyperarousal, numbing, dissociation) among refugees (Arroyo & Eth, 1986; Fox & Tang, 2000; Kinzie, Sack, Angell, Clark, & Ben, 1989; Kinzie, Sack, Angell, Manson, & Rath, 1986; Miller et al., 2002; Mitchulka, Blanchard, & Kalous, 1998; Mollica et al., 1993; Mollica et al., 1998; Thabet & Vostanis, 2000; Weine et al., 1998), and displacement related stressors are associated with symptoms of depression and anxiety (Gorst-Unsworth & Goldenberg, 1998; Miller et al., 2002; Pernice & Brook, 1996; Thabet & Vostainis, 2000). And although it is of great importance to understand how political violence and displacement-related stressors impact individuals, it is equally important to understand how larger systems, such as families and communities, are affected by violence and displacement. It is also essential to examine the ways that family and community-level distress and well-being impact individuals, and to understand the dynamic interactions among these interrelated levels of functioning. In order to clarify these relationships, we need conceptual models and assessment methodologies that allow us to operationalize and evaluate forms of well-being and distress at the family and community levels. To capture distress and well-being at these levels, we must draw on methodologies from such fields as family systems research, sociology, anthropology, and public health.

Family Well-Being and Distress

Many researchers and practitioners in the field of refugee mental health point to the primary importance of the family in refugee communities with whom they work (see Weine et al., chap. 8, and Wessells and Monteiro, chap. 2). As Weine and colleagues note, for refugees—who have experienced the dissolution of familiar social networks and institutions—the family, however intact, is often the only remaining social group to whom refugees can turn for support and a sense of belonging; thus, it is important to understand how refugee families are functioning. Family-level outcomes of interest might include the level of family cohesion or tension, the functioning of marital or parent–child relationships, and the integrity of extended family networks after displacement. However, better articulated models of optimal versus compromised family functioning that are *specific to different refugee groups*[5] are needed to help illuminate the impact of stressors at the level of the family and to operationalize notions of "distress and well-being" at the level of the family.

In family research, familial distress and well-being have been conceptualized in a number of ways, including: (1) the aggregation of the self-reported distress or well-being of individual family members, (2) the assessment of the integrity of various relational subsystems (e.g., the marital dyad, siblings, parent–child relationships, intergenerational relationship among extended family) through observational coding and/or self-report of members of the subsystem (e.g., Cowan, Powell, & Cowan, 1998), or (3) the assessment of more global, "emergent" functioning — such as family cohesiveness and tension (Moos & Moos, 1986). These approaches to family assessment could be employed to collect information about family functioning in refugee populations.

Drawing on work from family researchers such as Philip and Carolyn Cowan (e.g., Cowan, Powell, & Cowan, 1998), one potentially fruitful direction for future research on refugee families would be to use a model of family functioning that outlines how multiple relationship domains (or subsystems) may be affected by exposure to violence and displacement related stressors. For example, it would be reasonable to predict that the marital relationship is affected by stressors associated with the refugee experience (e.g., the impact of trauma and unresolved grief on marital intimacy, the effects of prolonged separation due to

---

[5]Ethnographic information regarding indigenous notions of "well functioning" versus "poorly functioning" families could be collected from focus groups or interviews with key informants from refugee populations, and would highlight important dimensions of family functioning to consider in family-focused interventions with refugee groups. Drawing on methods described by Hubbard and Miller (chap. 10, this volume) — individuals could be asked to describe the qualities that families who are doing well (before *and* after political violence or resettlement) and families who are not doing well. With this type of information, it would be possible to develop models of family functioning relevant and specific to different refugee groups that could guide and inform family-focused theory, research, and intervention with refugees.

violence and displacement on marital relationships, and the relation of war trauma and exile-related stressors to the increased rates of domestic violence that have been reported in some refugee groups). In addition, parent-child relationships are likely to be affected by displacement related stressors such as differing rates of acculturation between parents and children, and the concomitant pressures on children to assume "adult" roles, such as translators and culture brokers for their parents (Berry, 1997; Camino & Krulfield, 1994; Cornille, 1993; Farver, Narang, & Bhadha, 2002). Other family relationships likely to be affected by the stressors associated with being a refugee are sibling relationships and intergenerational ties with grandparents and extended family, who are often split up during flight and resettlement (Alley, 1982; Beiser, 1988; Ganesan, Fine, & Yilin, 1989).[6] Finally, the nested ecology of the family (e.g., Bronfenbrenner, 1986)—their interactions with wider social systems such as the neighborhood, social and peer groups, school, work, religious groups, and service systems (see Weine et al., chap. 8)—is likely to be adversely impacted by displacement, which grossly disrupts the familiar social ties and connections to resources that families rely on in their communities.

In conclusion, we have much to learn about the ways in which refugee families are impacted by the stressors associated with the refugee experience, what types of protective factors might work to buffer these risks at the level of the family, and what types of interventions work best to support or improve family functioning. Developing culturally specific models of optimal and distressed family functioning for different refugee groups, and drawing on assessment methods from family researchers to capture this important dimension of psychosocial well-being, will help us deepen our understanding of risk and resilience among refugee families and improve family-oriented intervention work with refugees.

---

[6]Indeed, extended family relationships are considered more important in many refugee communities than they are in most Western societies, where the nuclear family is often of primary importance. Therefore, the loss of extended family ties and supports might be especially detrimental to the family functioning of many refugee groups (Barudy, 1989; Gilad, 1990; Stein, 1985).

Community Well-Being and Distress

Many ecologically minded researchers and practitioners are interested in how communities function and how the "social fabric" may be impacted by violence and stress (see Buitrago Cuéllar, chap. 7). For instance, political violence and displacement often lead to the loss of key community members, the breakdown of social institutions and helping networks (such as links with religious and traditional healers and community elders), loss of trust in neighbors and in important social institutions (such as police and judicial systems) due to deceit and corruption, loss of access to basic necessities (clean water, food, health care), and loss of basic protection, safety, and justice (Martin-Baró, 1989; Summerfield, 1995; Wessells & Monteiro, 2001). Seminal thinkers such as Martin-Baró (1985, 1989) have eloquently described how this kind of social breakdown increases suspicion, hostility, and anxiety among individuals, families, and larger (ethnic or political) groups, and how violent approaches to conflict resolution can become normalized and routine under conditions of prolonged conflict (Martín Baró, 1989; Wessells and Monteiro, chap. 2, this volume). In addition, as noted in chapter 1, community violence often involves the conscription of whole segments of a community's youth into the horrors of armed conflict (Boothby, 1994; Machel, 1996), as well as sexual violence against women and girls (Aron, Corne, Fursland, & Zelwer, 1991; Landesman, 2002), creating massive obstacles to community rebuilding after conflict due to the stigmatization of former child soldiers, unmarriageable rape victims, and the creation of a generation of "children of rape" (Landesman, 2002).

Although ecologically minded interventionists are usually quick to acknowledge that community-level functioning is an important dimension of psychosocial well-being, it is not entirely clear how to operationalize and assess community-level well-being, distress, or dysfunction. Here we might turn to fields such as sociology and public health to provide us with assessment methodologies to capture indicators of community distress and disruption, as well as optimal community functioning. As ecologically minded mental health workers, it is imperative that we continue to struggle to better capture this level of psychosocial functioning, to better understand how healthy and unhealthy communities function, as well as the impact of community functioning on the individuals and families.

Clarifying Intervention Rationales

In addition to developing well-elaborated risk models to guide interventions with refugee communities, we also should strive to be as transparent and reflective as possible in providing a theoretical rationale for our intervention designs. In our own work, and in reading the work of others who develop interventions, we have found that this seemingly straightforward task can be a challenge; and yet, when developing interventions, it is crucial that the targeted psychosocial outcomes or problems to be addressed be clearly specified, and that risk models—based on sound conceptual models or empirical work—guide the design of interventions. Journal articles, grant applications, and even theoretical pieces related to intervention often fail to link applied intervention work with relevant theoretical and empirical literatures. Too often, in fact, there exist completely separate bodies of theoretical or empirical literature, on the one hand, and applied (often unevaluated) intervention work and practice, on the other—with very little overlap between the two. There is a need for more theory-driven, evaluated intervention studies across diverse refugee populations to help bridge these divides between research, theory, and practice. When intervention targets and underlying theory are laid out clearly and interventions evaluated, interventions themselves can become tests of our guiding models of psychosocial risk, protective factors, and of modes of healing in various populations. These critical topics are elaborated in the following sections.

Choosing and Specifying Intervention Goals

It is important to remember that there can be no discussion of risk without a particular outcome, or set of outcomes, in mind (i.e., individuals, families, and communities must be at risk *for* something), and it is crucial that the mental health or psychosocial difficulties that an intervention is designed to address be clearly conceptualized and articulated at the outset. It has become commonplace in mental health-related fields to speak of at-risk populations; however, it is imperative when designing interventions, and certainly evaluation research, that we are as clear and specific as possible about intervention targets—whether they be individual distress (symptoms of trauma, depression, or anxiety) or well-being (feelings of hope, empowerment), or specific family or community markers of distress or well-being. In fact, the specification of intervention targets and goals should be the *first step* in the design of an intervention. Having clearly articulated intervention goals allows us to focus on addressing *specific* difficulties and helps clarify the evaluation design—specifying which outcomes to follow and assess—so that we know whether our interventions are working as intended. However, when working with refugee populations experiencing a multitude of stressors that impact their psychosocial functioning at multiple levels—it is often difficult to decide *which* psychosocial difficulties to target and *at what level* to intervene.

Recall the multiple stressors experienced by the former child soldiers described in chapter 2 by Wessells and Monteiro. These youth commonly experience a range of psychosocial difficulties, including profound social stigma, lack of job skills and opportunities, poverty, physical injury, loss of family members, as well as symptoms of trauma, anxiety, and depression. As Wessells and Monteiro note, a mental health intervention designed to ameliorate symptoms of trauma and depression in this population (e.g., through individual or group therapy), without attention to broader social issues—such as the reintegration of these youth into their communities and basic job training—would probably not be very successful in relieving their symptoms of psychological distress. Very real social conditions maintain their symptoms of distress, and it is crucial, therefore, that these social conditions be addressed in psychosocial interventions designed to improve their psychological well-being. As this example illustrates, psychosocial interventions for populations experiencing broad psychosocial difficulties should ideally address multiple levels of distress—or, at least, be part of coordinated services that work to improve health and well-being at the individual, family, and community levels. Yet, even for such broad-based interventions, it is important to specify particular psychosocial intervention targets at these various levels.

When deciding upon the foci of psychosocial interventions, it is important to work collaboratively with community members to identify and prioritize intervention goals. As described by numerous authors in this volume, this process includes collecting information through needs assessments, focus groups, key informant interviews, and so forth—to determine a community's self-identified psychosocial needs. However, as several of the authors note, the types of problems identified by community members do not always match up with the interventionist's training, agenda, or understanding of the psychosocial needs of that community. Yet, it is crucial that intervention goals reflect the concerns of the community, or at the very least, be the product of a collaborative defining of priorities. Clearly, there will be instances when conflicting ideas arise around the identification of intervention goals, such as whether to focus on mental health (e.g., resolving symptoms of trauma), psychosocial well-being (e.g., creating settings that facilitate social support and the rearticulation of valued social roles), or economic security (e.g., developing micro-enterprise programs that increase family income, thereby increasing self-sufficiency, lowering the risk of malnutrition, and reducing poverty-related stress). In such cases, some collaborative negotiation of goals—based on mutual sharing of sometimes conflicting theories and beliefs about distress and healing, and a reciprocal recognition of the community's priorities and the organization's capacities and areas of expertise—is essential. It is imperative that time be allotted to this process of sharing and negotiation of goals, which will help ensure community support for and appropriateness of the intervention.

Based on the discussions of numerous authors in this volume (see, e.g., Tribe & colleagues; Hubbard & Pearson) it is understandably the case that community members often prioritize basic material and socioeconomic needs over mental health and psychosocial concerns. Clearly, a community's most basic needs, such as food and shelter, should be addressed first and foremost, and an ecological model leads naturally in the direction of coordinated program design and implementation to address multiple levels of need, with mental health and psychosocial services being an integrated part of a broad infrastructure that includes attention to basic health care, material assistance, and social services. However, it is important to stress that an ecological perspective also underscores capacity building in all forms of intervention, so that refugee communities move toward ever greater degrees of self-sufficiency to meet their own basic material, physical, mental health, and psychosocial needs.

Linking Models of Risk and Intervention To Intervention Design

Once the problems[7] to be addressed are identified, it is important to look to empirical work and conceptually sound theories of risk and protection to inform the design of interventions. Models of risk and protection can provide ideas about what stressors might be ameliorated and what resources or supports developed in refugee communities to encourage health and well-being. For example, if the goal of an intervention is to decrease feelings of depression and increase feelings of empowerment within a refugee community, an interventionist could draw on empirically supported or theoretically grounded risk and intervention models to decide where and how to intervene.[8] For instance, social isolation has been identified as a risk factor for depression (Miller et al., 2002), and lack of access to resources is theoretically linked to feelings of disempowerment (Goodkind, Hang, & Yang, chap. 9). Therefore, an intervention designed to address these psychosocial difficulties among members of a refugee community might seek to build social support among participants (through the creation of a support circle or collective) to alleviate depression, and facilitate access to community resources (through the provision of information or improving the accessibility of service provision) to increase feelings of empowerment among community members.

Given that risk and protective factors may vary across and even within different refugee populations (de Jong, 2002; Steele & Silove, 2000), it is ideal to draw on risk models empirically derived from the

---

[7]Many ecological interventionists choose to take a strengths-based approach, in which case it may be resources or protective factors (rather than problems) that are identified as the intervention focus.

[8]Theoretically grounded models may include non-Western theories of healing that may be quite effective in local contexts.

refugee population of interest and to collect locally relevant information about risk and protective factors during the groundwork phase of an intervention. If information specific to a population of interest is unavailable and time does not permit the gathering of new data, then it may be reasonable to refer to risk models developed from information on similar groups (e.g., culturally similar groups or those facing similar stressors).

Just as locally informed risk models help inform the development of sound interventions, the selection of intervention methods should incorporate local beliefs and practices (see Ecological Principle 4). For example, one might identify depression as an intervention goal and link depression to the loss of loved ones through violence or the loss of valued social roles; however, at the actual intervention level, methods of reducing depression may involve a combination of tested (e.g., increased social support) and untested strategies, such religious prayer or ceremony. In culturally sensitive interventions, some elements of a risk or intervention model may include non-empirically supported relations among variables (e.g., the relation between traumatic events, soul loss, and "*susto*" among Guatemalans and Salvadorans; Marsella, Bornemann, Ekblad, & Orley, 1994). To Guatemalan or Salvadorian refugees, frightening events represent risk factors for *susto* because the soul is thought to flee the body when frightened, leading to vulnerability and illness. Although no empirical data are available to either support or refute the proposed mechanism (soul loss) by which *susto* results, traditional healers work to restore the soul and are often claimed to be effective at restoring a sense of well-being by doing so (Farias, 1994).

Therefore, although we emphasize the use of empirically supported or theoretically sound risk and intervention models, this is not to imply that all such methods must have been tested in Western, randomized and controlled intervention trials. The conceptual "soundness" of a model may be based on empirical data, theory, and/or coherent and well-established local belief systems, the effectiveness of which can be tested in evaluations of community-based, ecological interventions.

In sum, whatever the ultimate design of an intervention, it is crucial that there be a clear and explicit linking of intervention components to conceptually sound underlying models of risk and intervention. We have found that it is not always clear *why* interventions are designed as they are—and, if interventions are designed to address multiple problems, it is not always clear which components of those intervention are meant to address which problems (and how). If the links between the design and the guiding theoretical frame of an intervention are not made explicit, it is difficult to evaluate whether an intervention has an impact on the outcomes of interest, and which component of the intervention is having an impact on which targeted problems. Drawing on empirical work or sound theory to provide a clear rationale for interventions also helps to ensure that, with often limited resources, we develop interventions that are both testable and grounded in fairly strong evidence or theory supporting the likelihood of their efficacy.

Building a Knowledge Base of Effective Community-Based Approaches

Many of the interventions in this field incorporate common elements such as social support, utilization of paraprofessionals, and the integration indigenous and Western methods of healing. However, it is important to consider what empirical or theoretical knowledge base we have to support these intervention methods. For example, the importance of social support in helping to ameliorate the impact of various stressors has been well-established across diverse groups (see review by Barrera, 2000), and the efficacy of paraprofessionals in administering psychotherapeutic interventions has also received some support (although it is not entirely clear over what range of treatments; see review by Christensen & Jacobson, 1994). However, fewer studies have examined the efficacy of integrating Western and indigenous approaches to healing, and as Wessells (1999) cautions, it is necessary to evaluate the efficacy of indigenous healing methods (as well as their efficacy in combination with Western approaches) in ameliorating distress and promoting well-being among refugees in various contexts.

At this point, ecological interventions with refugees are built on a fairly limited empirical knowledge base about what is and is not effective. However, this is equally true of clinic-based treatment approaches to refugee mental health, where intervention strategies have been guided by findings from research with non-refugee populations, or more commonly, have not been guided by empirically supported approaches at all.

Therefore, it would be extremely useful to the field for those who are implementing ecological mental health interventions to evaluate their efforts and to begin creating a knowledge base regarding the efficacy of various intervention approaches commonly employed by ecologically oriented interventionists. By clearly laying out the foci, design, and theoretical grounding of our interventions, by evaluating their efficacy, and by continuing to share our successes and failures in applying and adapting ecological approaches to intervention in different contexts—we can begin to build just such a foundation—helping to define the scope of and lend increased legitimacy to ecological intervention approaches to refugee mental health and well-being.

Program Evaluation

The design and implementation of innovative, ecological interventions for refugees is an incomplete endeavor without the inclusion of an evaluation component to determine whether or not interventions are working as intended. Unfortunately, program evaluations are often overlooked or added on as afterthoughts in many fields of intervention. Evaluations are particularly challenging in the types of settings (i.e., in or near zones of conflict) described in many of the preceding chapters, particularly when intervention projects are not designed or conceived of as research-oriented projects. Some of the notable obstacles encountered by contributors to this volume include: a lack of culturally appropriate assessment materials (and little time or resources to create them), assessment fatigue among community members, difficulties with consistent participant involvement and follow up, and even having to destroy assessment records when forced to relocate from one camp to another.

It is also clear from the preceding chapters that interventions designed for refugees living in the relative safety of developed host countries such as the United States are more likely to integrate a systematic evaluation component as part of their intervention design than those designed as part of an emergency response to a crisis in a developing country. In this volume, projects in developed resettlement countries were often linked with university (e.g., Goodkind, Hang, & Yang, chap. 9) or academic/medical settings (e.g., Weine et al., chap. 8) with ample resources to support evaluation efforts, whereas interventions conducted in unstable and often dangerous refugee camps settings rarely had access to such resources.

However, despite the numerous challenges involved, all of the chapter authors emphasized the importance of evaluating their intervention work to help identify what was and was not effective so that they might improve upon their projects. Some of the projects attempted to overcome limitations of time and resources through evaluation strategies that included informal qualitative feedback and follow-up with program participants and staff. Yet it is clear that the field is in need of structured evaluation methods that will work for interventions implemented in the shifting and often dangerous contexts in which most refugees live. Toward this goal, Hubbard and Miller (chap. 10) provide conceptual insights and practical suggestions toward designing and conducting evaluations that work in these challenging contexts, and the reader is referred to that chapter for a more extensive discussion of this topic.

In short, we advocate making the evaluation an integral part of the original design for any intervention project, no matter how rapidly it needs to be implemented. The evaluation for a pilot project may be a less formal, process-oriented evaluation that allows for flexible feedback-driven improvements in the program; while a more rigorously designed intervention study might include both process and outcome evaluation components, as well as qualitative and quantitative methods, which enhance the ability to track implementation fidelity, who is (and is not) participating and why, and whether the intervention outcome goals are being achieved at various follow-up points. Having an evaluation team — working on measurement design, interviews, observations, data management, and analyses — that includes local community members is imperative if we are to work within the ecological frame of community empowerment and true collaboration and instill a sense of ownership in and dedication to the success of community-based interventions. Community members are ideal observers, interpreters of qualitative data, linguistic interpreters, interviewers, etc. (Wandersman, 1999).

Many basic process and outcome evaluation methods can be taught to and utilized by community members with some basic supervision (see Hubbard & Miller, this volume). For some of the more complex evaluation questions that involve tracking multilevel change across time, one promising future direction might include collaboration between those in the field (whether it be a community center or refugee camp) and university or research settings where some of the data could be sent and analyzed with sophisticated statistical methods and resources. Yet, Hubbard and Miller caution that that a sole reliance on outside consultants that takes the evaluation process completely out of the hands of local community members can have the unintended consequence of making the evaluation process more mysterious than necessary and of decreasing community investment and interest in the success of the program. Therefore, they conclude that just as an ecological approach emphasizes the training and supervision of local paraprofessionals in techniques of mental health intervention, so too should this approach include the training of local staff in basic research evaluation techniques. Indeed, Hubbard reports considerable success in training local refugee staff to run comparative and predictive statistics in the field (Hubbard & Miller, chap. 10).

Integrating Western and Culturally Indigenous Approaches to Healing

All of the contributors to this volume, along with numerous practitioners in the field of refugee mental health, are engaged in the challenging practice of integrating Western and local approaches to healing and restoring a sense of well-being in refugee communities. Indeed, a central theme appearing across this volume is the need to better understand ethnocultural variations in conceptualizations of distress, well-being, and healing, and to use this knowledge to create culturally meaningful interventions with refugees. The researchers and practitioners who engage in this integrative practice are essentially creative pioneers drawing on methods from diverse fields such as anthropology, sociology, psychology, religion, and medicine. Unfortunately, there is no well-elaborated guiding model for this endeavor, and little sharing of practical strategies, successes, and failures among those engaged in this work.

Need for Methodologies

It is increasingly recognized that it is of primary importance to ground any mental-health or psychosocial intervention for refugees in a thorough understanding of local cosmologies and world-views, especially in relation to topics such as health, well-being, suffering, and healing.[9] However, it is not always clear *how* to go about doing this — and, until fairly recently, there have been few sources of guidance for the collection and use of ethnographic information in psychosocial interventions with refugees.

Fortunately, a number of researchers and practitioners from fields such as psychiatry, psychology, and anthropology have provided some basic suggestions and guidelines for others doing applied, health-related cross-cultural work. Arthur Kleinman, a medical anthropologist and cross-cultural psychiatrist at Harvard, suggests a standard series of eight questions to guide the collection of ethnographic information about medical and psychiatric disorders (Kleinman, 1983; Kleinman, Eisenberg, & Good, 1978). These types of questions (see Box 11.2) — designed to reveal culture-specific understandings of the etiology, the course, and mechanics of an illness, as well as ideas about treatment and healing — can be used to build a general understanding of "explanatory models" and local idioms of distress from various refugee communities.

---

[9]Particularly when working with children and families of different ethnocultural groups, it is useful to understand culturally indigenous notions of psychosocial well-being and distress against a backdrop of local notions of child development and expectations about social roles and relations (such as parenting and gender roles). An understanding of local views related to human development and social expectations provides an important context for understanding psychosocial distress and well-being and can help to prevent serious misunderstandings when developing interventions with culturally diverse populations.

Box 11.2
Kleinman's Eight Questions

1. *What do you call the problem?*

2. *What do you think has caused the problem?*

3. *Why do you think it started when it did?*

4. *What do you think the sickness does? How does it work?*

5. *How severe is the sickness? Will it have a short or long course?*

6. *What kind of treatment do you think the patient should receive? What are the most important results you hope he/she receives from this treatment?*

7. *What are the chief problems the sickness has caused?*

8. *What do you fear most about the sickness?*

In addition, there are a growing number of resources that researchers and practitioners can draw on to familiarize themselves with culture-bound syndromes and local expressions of distress relevant to their work with various refugee populations. Descriptions of culture specific disorders can be found in a range of sources including anthropological literatures, the appendix of the *DSM-IV*, and chapters in edited compilations such as *Beyond Trauma: Cultural and Societal Dynamics* (Kleber, Figley, & Gerson, 1995), *Ethnocultural Aspects of Posttraumatic Stress Disorder* (Marsella, Friedman, Gerrity, & Scurfield, 1996), and *Honoring Differences: Cultural Issues in the Treatment of Trauma and Loss* (Nader, Dubrow, & Stamm, 1999). A number of web-based resources, such as the website for the Refugee Studies Centre at Oxford University (http://www.rsc.ox.ac.uk/), contain information on culture specific descriptions of distress in a variety of refugee populations. Although the availability of these resources reflects a growing appreciation of the need to understand ethnocultural variations in symptoms and experiences of distress, it is not always easy to access sufficiently detailed, relevant, and up-to-date information about cross-cultural expressions of distress specific to refugee populations of interest.

Therefore, it remains imperative for those of us working in the field to take the time to collect basic ethnographic information from refugee groups with whom we work.

It is also essential to balance our understanding of how different ethnocultural groups understand illness and distress with an understanding of how these groups conceptualize health, healing, and well-being, and how Western notions of health, which implicitly guide many interventions, compare with local beliefs and practices (Prilleltensky & Nelson, 2000). An elaborated understanding of local concepts of health and well-being provides an important background and context for understanding distress and deviation from health. In addition, developing locally grounded understandings of well-being can help practitioners formulate intervention goals that are congruent with local ideals of health and well-being. Toward these ends, a number of strategies are available for gathering information about local beliefs and practices related to well-being, as well as distress. For example, Prilleltensky and Nelson (2000) have described the use of focus groups to develop an understanding not only of how different Australian immigrant groups conceptualize well-being, but also—to highlight potential impediments to service provision—how these notions contrast with those of Australian social service providers. Prilleltensky, Nelson, and Peirson (in press) developed a useful set of questions to guide the collection of information about culture-specific notions of well-being (see Box 11.3) that can help identify important protective factors that can be supported and developed in interventions. Each of these questions is repeated to probe understandings of general well-being, as well as personal, relational, and collective well-being.

Similarly, it is possible to collect qualitative information about local notions of well-being and distress by conducting focus groups in which community members are asked to identify characteristics of individuals who are doing well (emotionally, behaviorally, cognitively, and spiritually) and those who are not. Information can be gathered through interviews with key informants, ideally representing diverse sectors of the community—such as teachers, parents, health workers, traditional healers, the elderly, and youth. In their work with refugees from Sierra Leone, Hubbard and his colleagues at the Center for Victims of Torture in Minnesota (see chaps. 3 and 10, this volume) have used this approach, asking Sierra Leoneans to identify the qualities of both children and adults who were, and were not, doing well after surviving the conflict in their homeland.

Box 11.3
Prilleltensky's Questions*

1. *What is the meaning of well-being for you?*

2. *What contributes to it?*

3. *What interferes with its attainment?*

4. *How can it be maintained?*

5. *How can it be restored when it is absent?*

* Each of these questions is repeated to probe understandings of general well-being, as well as personal, relational, and collective well-being.

The qualitative data that is collected from these types of interviews and focus groups can be used in a variety of ways. For example, from the lists of indicators of wellness and distress that are generated, one can calculate which indicators are mentioned most frequently in a given population, or ask participants to sort the indicators into clusters to create culturally relevant dimensions of wellness or distress (which can then be factor analyzed to identify empirically derived clusters). In addition, questionnaires for the collection of quantitative data can be developed using the most frequently occurring indicators, and then either a simple total scale score could be derived indicating people's relative degree of wellness or distress, or people's responses to the various items on the questionnaire could be factor analyzed to generate empirically sound dimensions or factors that represent locally relevant syndromes of distress. This approach to creating grounded, culture-specific understandings of wellness and distress can be used by researchers and practitioners working with a variety of refugee populations and has been used effectively by not only Hubbard's group, but also by MacMullin and Laughry (2002) in their work with formerly abducted child soldiers in Northern Uganda, by Bolton and his colleagues in their work with survivors of violence in Rwanda and

Uganda (Bolton, 2001; Bolton & Tang, 2002), and by Kinzie, Manson, Vinh, Tolan, Anh, and Pho (1982) in their work with Vietnamese refugees.

It would be of great benefit to have these innovative methods for collecting culturally relevant information about distress and well-being organized and easily available to others working in the field. Ethnographic data collection should be standard practice when developing interventions with refugees, and it should be made less mysterious and intimidating for program staff without training in anthropological field methods. Clearly, more work needs to be done on the development of data gathering methodologies that are accessible, standardized, and yet flexible enough for use across diverse contexts.

A final note on this matter is that although there exists a growing number of resources and methodologies to guide the collection of ethnographic information relevant to psychosocial distress and well-being, numerous contributors to this volume raise the issue of practical impediments to their employment. As many authors made clear, the pressing immediacy of emergency situations, limited resources (translators, interviewers), and assessment fatigue in communities bombarded with humanitarian aid and relief workers pose very real obstacles to the collection of thorough ethnographic information prior to the development and implementation of interventions with refugee communities. For these reasons, many practitioners understandably feel the urgency to move ahead without thorough knowledge of how their own conceptions of mental health and well-being match up with those of local populations, and attempt to clarify misunderstandings as they go along. However, urgently implemented interventions that are not built upon local understandings of psychosocial distress and well-being run the risk of alienating participants and can lead to frustrating clashes between program staff and local community members who are the intended beneficiaries of the intervention. For these reasons, despite the challenges involved, it is crucial to allow sufficient time for the collection of ethnographic data and for mutually educative interaction (about worldviews and cosmologies) with community members.

Putting Integrative Approaches
Into Practice

Although there are resources to turn to for guidance in collecting ethnographic data relevant to mental health in different ethnocultural groups, knowing how to use this information to inform interventions and putting these culturally grounded understandings into practice remains very much an art and challenge. Mental health professionals and consultants often enter settings as "outside experts," carrying their own worldviews and agendas. However, it is important to recognize that local beliefs systems and meanings represent powerful substrates for healing (Kleinman, 1980; Kleinman & Sung, 1979). Working within local frameworks of understanding to relieve symptoms of distress (e.g., helping people re-balance their chi or honor their deceased ancestors through traditional burial rituals) may contribute more to the healing process than relying solely or primarily on modes of healing that are commonplace in the developed nations (e.g., individual psychotherapy) but may be unfamiliar, and even suspect, in many regions of the world (Kleinman, 1980).

On the other hand, although it is important to avoid cultural and psychological imperialism (Dawes, 1997), we must be careful not to go to the opposite extreme and romanticize all things indigenous (Wessells, 1999). After all, some medicine men still use arsenic and lead in their healing ceremonies (Fadiman, 1997, p. 267). Indigenous beliefs and healing practices are rarely subjected to systematic evaluation and should not be assumed automatically to be helpful for all members of a particular community, or for all manifestations of psychosocial and health problems (Wessells, 1999). In addition, there is no reason to assume *a priori* that belief systems and practices related to healing psychological, psychosocial, or spiritual distress that have been shown to be effective in one cultural context (such as Western cultures) will not be effective elsewhere. Similar mechanisms of healing, such as the use of groups as sources of instrumental and social support, may be found in widely diverse settings; whereas other processes, such as formalized ceremonies for grieving the death of loved ones, may be nearly universal, although the specific expression of grief and the rituals that accompany it may vary cross-culturally (Kleinman, 1988). Therefore, in our desire to be culturally sensitive, we should not assume that Western intervention theories and techniques are never transferable in our work with indigenous groups.

In light of these dilemmas, it has been argued (e.g., Wessells, 1999) that the most effective approach to designing psychosocial interventions for culturally diverse groups involves an *integration* of indigenous understandings and healing practices with Western concepts and approaches. Indeed, this is the approach illustrated by many of the contributors to this volume. Examples of such integrative approaches include the intervention for internally displaced Angolans described by Wessells and Monteiro (chap. 2) which involved the reconstruction of traditional meeting huts (*jangos*) for community gatherings, and combined psychoeducation of project staff (about, e.g., Western notions of child development and the effects of war on children) with the support and instigation of culturally familiar activities—such as cleansing ceremonies, traditional singing, and normalizing activities for children—thought to promote healing. The Cambodian project described by van de Put and Eisenbruch (chap. 4), rooted in rich ethnographic research, aimed to strengthen and rebuild age-old networks (that had been seriously weakened by the social upheaval in Cambodia) between community members and traditional healers while setting up complimentary psychoeducation and Western clinical services alongside traditional help-seeking networks.

Along these lines, in chapter 3, Hubbard and Pearson describe how ritual was incorporated into group psychotherapy for Sierra Leonean refugees and illustrate how this integrative work is not always straightforward. They describe how early attempts to incorporate traditional Sierra Leonean ceremony into the project's therapy groups were met with resistance by some of the Christian group members who found the ceremonies—which involved ritualistic appeasement of deceased ancestors—sacrilegious. This led to a shift in the practice of incorporating traditional Sierra Leonean ceremony to a model that involved group members creating their own unique group ritual (with meaning specific to that group) to initiate and deepen their therapeutic work together. Hubbard and Pearson concluded that the use of ritual was important to the groups, but where it came from was less so. This highlights the important point that cultures are neither homogenous nor static, and trying to figure out which local traditions to support and incorporate into interventions (as well as who subscribes to them and who doesn't) is never a simple endeavor, but critical to consider when creating interventions that interweave Western and local approaches to healing.

As these examples illustrate, open-minded, respectful negotiation and collaboration among consultants, local and expatriate program staff, and a diversity of community members concerning how to put integrative, culturally sensitive interventions into practice is imperative. Through a process of ongoing program evaluation (see chap. 10) of both Western and local approaches to healing, it becomes possible to identify which intervention methods are effective, which need to be modified, and which ought to be dropped. This process is by no means simple, as anyone who has attempted to collaborative work with numerous stakeholders knows. However, taking the time to contextually ground our interventions greatly enhances the likelihood of their having a positive impact.

Negotiating Culture Clashes

There is also a clear need for sharing among practitioners and consultants in the field regarding how they have negotiated the inevitable culture clashes that arise when attempting this integrative work. We are, for example, greatly interested in Hubbard and Pearson's (chap. 3) ethnographic findings that both Sierra Leonean refugee men and women identified Sierra Leonean women who were functioning "well" after the war as obedient. It is intriguing to consider what to *do* with this information (i.e., how might it inform intervention goals?). No matter how culturally sensitive they would like to be, many practitioners or consultants would be reluctant to design an intervention to help Sierra Leonean women become more obedient, so as to return to a culturally sanctioned "more optimal" state of functioning. As careful ethnographic work is conducted, it is likely that a number of ethnocultural conceptions of well-being will be revealed that conflict notably with notions of well-being held by researchers and practitioners developing interventions with different refugee populations, and we will have to figure out how to negotiate and respect these differences.

In a similar vein, it is not uncommon for conflicts to arise among program consultants, staff, and community members concerning beliefs and practices that are not related to concepts of healing per se, but to broad, ideological cultural beliefs and practices. For example, program consultants and local staff may have different ideas about the promotion of healthy child development or appropriate social roles and practices that may relate directly to intervention implementation and goals (e.g., whether girls should be allowed to play sports; see chap. 6; or even more sensitive and fraught, whether domestic abuse or the physical punishment of children should ever be regarded as acceptable).

Along these lines, a number of authors in this volume share how they have negotiated these types of cultural and ideological differences during the implementation of their interventions. For example, Kostelny and Wessells (chap. 6) relate their experience of working with front-line, local staff in East Timor whose ideas about physically disciplining children were at odds with those of the Christian Children's Fund consultants. Program consultants approached this dilemma through the use of guided questions to explore with the staff how they felt as children when they were physically punished. Kostelny and Wessells note that this process worked to shift some of the perceptions held by local staff, and that together they were able to collaboratively and creatively come up with mutually satisfactory ideas for disciplining children. In the TAFES groups discussed by Weine and colleagues (chap. 8), project staff found that they needed permission from Kosovar men to involve families in the intervention (and to even talk to Kosovar women), and although they were careful not to confront patriarchal practices in a manner that would lead to a backlash among Kosovar men or hinder participation in the intervention, they did find ways to encourage Kosovar women to speak up in the context and safety of the tea groups. In this way, they were able to help the Kosovar women's voices to be heard. Finally, Tribe and colleagues (chap. 5) had to do some careful and diplomatic negotiation with a male community leader who felt that the best way to help Sri Lankan war widows was not to provide them with empowering information and access to resources, but to find them all husbands. All of these situations illustrate the need for creative and sensitive negotiation of goals and agendas among program consultants, local and expatriate staff, and local community members if interventions are to be successful.

In sum, as the field moves forward, it is vital that we continue to share with one another the complex clashes and struggles that often arise when attempting to integrate Western and indigenous approaches to psychosocial intervention and healing. As we work to create a dialogue (and even debate) about the issues raised in the various chapters in this volume, we will have the opportunity to learn from one another's strategies, successes, and failures. This is an exciting time to be engaged in applied, integrative, cross-cultural intervention work. As the world becomes an ever more interconnected, global community, we have the opportunity to learn from and to build upon a wide range of wisdom and healing traditions that can broaden and deepen psychosocial approaches to healing and restoring well-being in refugee communities.

CONCLUSIONS

Although we have only just begun to touch upon some of the critical issues facing those engaged in developing ecological interventions for refugees, we hope that we have provided a useful, if preliminary, framework of some key topics and suggestions for future directions. As elaborated in chapter 1 of this volume, due to a severe dearth of clinic-based resources and services, as well as notable linguistic and cultural barriers to their use, there is a need for an alternative approach to addressing the mental health needs of refugees—one that does not rely on the traditional clinical model as its cornerstone. The goal of this volume has been to highlight the work of individuals who are committed to staking out an alternative path for addressing the mental health and psychosocial needs of refugees. This path, based on an ecological model of intervention, offers a promising direction for the future of refugee mental health interventions. Clearly, this path is not without some significant challenges, but the contributors to this volume illustrate how researchers and practitioners working in collaboration with community members are finding innovative and creative ways to address these challenges. We hope that this volume instigates sharing and discussion among those participating in or thinking about conducting similar work in the field, and hope it provides helpful ideas and strategies to those who strive to put into practice ecologically grounded interventions to restore health and well-being to refugee communities across the globe.

REFERENCES

Alley, J. C. (1982). Life-threatening indicators among the Indochinese refugees. *Suicide and life threatening behavior, 12*(1), 13-20.

Aron, A., Corne, S., Fursland, A., & Zelwer, B. (1991). The gender-specific terror of El Salvador and Guatemala: Post-traumatic stress disorder in Central American women. *Women's Studies International Forum, 14,* 37-47.

Arroyo, W., & Eth, S. (1986). Children traumatized by Central American Warfare. In R. Pynoos & S. Eth (Eds.), *Post-traumatic stress disorder in children* (pp. 101-120). Washington, DC: American Psychiatric Press.

Baron, R. M., & Kenny, D. A. (1986). The moderator mediator variable distinction in social psychological research: Conceptual, strategic, and statistical considerations. *Journal of Personality and Social Psychology, 51*(6), 1173-1182.

Barrera, M. (2000). Social support research in community psychology. In J. Rappaport & E. Seidman (Eds.), *Handbook of community psychology* (pp. 187-214). New York: Kluwer Academic/Plenum.

Barudy, J. A. (1989). A programme of mental health for political refugees: Dealing with the invisible pain of political exile. *Social Science & Medicine, 28*(7), 715-727.

Beiser, M. (1988). Influences of time, ethnicity and attachment on depression in Southeast Asian refugees. *American Journal of Psychiatry, 145*(1), 46-51.

Berry, J. W. (1997). Immigration, acculturation, and adaptation. *Applied Psychology: An International Review, 46*(1), 5-34.

Boothby, N. (1994). Trauma and violence among refugee children. In A. J. Marsella, T. Bornemann, S. Ekblad, & J. Orley (Eds.), *Amidst peril and pain: The mental health and well-being of the world's refugees* (pp. 239-259). Washington, DC: American Psychological Association.

Bolton, P. (2001). Local perceptions of the mental health effects of the Rwandan genocide. *Journal of Nervous and Mental Disease, 189,* 243-248.

Bolton, P., & Tang, (2002). An alternative approach to cross-cultural function assessment. *Social Psychiatry and Psychiatric Epidemiology, 37,* 537-543.

Bronfenbrenner, U. (1986). Ecology of the family as a context of human development. *American Psychologist, 32,* 513-531.

Camino, L. A., & Krulfield, R. M. (1994). *Reconstucting lives, recapturing meaning: Refugee identity, gender, and culture change*. London: Gordon and Breach.

Christensen, A., & Jacobson, N. (1994). Who (or what) can do psychotherapy. The status and challenge of non-professional therapies. *Psychological Science, 5*, 8-14.

Coie, J. D., Watt, N. F., West, S. G., Hawkins, J. D., Asarnow, J. R., Markman, H. J., et al. (1993). The science of prevention: A conceptual framework and some directions for a national research program. *American Psychologist, 48*(10), 1013-1022.

Cornille, T. A. (1993). Support systems and the relocation process for children and families. In B. Settles, D. Hanks, & M. Sassman (Eds.), *Families on the move: Migration, immigration, emigration, and mobility* (pp. 281-298). New York: Haworth Press.

Cowan, P., Powell, D., & Cowan, C. P. (1998). Parenting interventions: A family systems perspective. In W. Damon (Ed.), *Handbook of child psychology* (5th ed., Vol. 4). New York: Wiley.

Dawes, A. (1997, July). *Cultural imperialism in the treatment of children fol-lowing political violence and war: A Southern African perspective*. Paper presented at the Fifth International Symposium on the Contributions of Psychology to Peace, Melbourne, Australia.

de Jong, J. T. V. M. (2002). Public mental health, traumatic stress and human rights violations in low-income countries: A culturally appropriate model of times of conflict, disaster and peace. In J. T. V. M. de Jong (Ed.), *Trauma, war, and violence: Public mental health in socio-cultural context* (pp. 1-93). New York: Kluwer Academic/Plenum.

Fadiman, A. (1997). *The spirit catches you and you fall down: A Hmong child, her American doctors, and the collision of two cultures* (1st ed.). New York: Farrar Straus and Giroux.

Farias, P. (1994). Central and South American refugees: Some mental health challenges. In A. Marsella, T. Bornemann, S. Ekblad, & J. Orley (Eds.), *Amidst peril and pain: The mental health and well-being of the world's refugees* (pp. 101-114). Washington DC: American Psychological Association.

Farver, J. A. M., Narang, S. K., & Bhadha, B. R. (2002). East meets West: Ethnic identity, acculturation, and conflict in Asian Indian families. *Journal of Family Psychology, 16*(3), 338-350.

Felner, R. D., Felner, T. Y., & Silverman, M. M. (2000). Prevention in mental health and social intervention: Conceptual and methodological issues in the evolution of the science and practice of prevention. In J. Rappaport & E. Seidman (Eds.), *Handbook of community psychology* (pp. 9-42). New York: Kluwer Academic/Plenum.

Fox, S., & Tang, S. (2000). The Sierra Leonean refugee experience: Traumatic events and psychiatric sequelae. *Journal of Nervous and Mental Disease, 188,* 490-495.

Freedman, D. (1999). From association to causation: Some remarks on the history of statistics. *Statistical Science, 14,* 243-258.

Ganesan, S., Fine, S., & Yilin, T. (1989). Psychiatric symptoms in refugee families from Southeast Asian: Therapeutic challenges. *American Journal of Psychotherapy, 43*(2), 218-228.

Garbarino, J., & Kostelny, K. (1996). The effects of political violence on Palestinian children's behavior problems: A risk accumulation model. *Child Development, 67*(1), 33-45.

Gilad, L. (1990). Refugees in Newfoundland: Families after flight. *Journal of Comparative Family Studies, 21,* 379-396.

Gorst-Unsworth, C., & Goldenberg, E. (1998). Psychological sequelae of torture and organised violence suffered by refugees from Iraq: Trauma-related factors compared with social factors in exile. *British Journal of Psychiatry, 172,* 90-94.

Kelly, J. G. (1987). Swampscott anniversary symposium. *American Journal of Community Psychology, 15*(5), 511-561.

Kinzie, J., Manson, S., Vinh, D., Tolan, N., Anh, B., & Pho, T. (1982). Development and validation of a Vietnamese language depression rating scale. *American Journal of Psychiatry, 10,* 1276-1281.

Kinzie, J., Sack, W., Angell, R., Clark, G., & Ben, R. (1989). A three year fol-low-up of Cambodian young people traumatized as children. *Journal of the American Academy of Child and Adolescent Psychiatry, 28,* 501-504.

Kinzie, J., Sack, W., Angell, R., Manson, S., & Rath, B. (1986). The psychiatric effects of massive trauma on Cambodian children: I. The children. *Journal of the American Academy of Child and Adolescent Psychiatry, 25,* 370-376.

Kleber, R., Figley, C., & Gersons, B. (1995). *Beyond trauma: Cultural and societal dynamics.* New York: Plenum Press.

Kleinman, A. (1980). *Patients and healers in the context of culture: An exploration of the borderland between anthropology, medicine, and psychiatry.* Berkeley: University of California Press.

Kleinman, A. (1983). Culture, mind and therapy: An introduction to cultural psychiatry, *American Journal of Psychiatry, 140*(2), 252-253.

Kleinman, A. (1988). *The illness narratives: Suffering, healing, and the human condition.* New York: Basic Books.

Kleinman, A., Eisenberg, L., & Good, B. (1978). Culture, illness, and care: Clinical lessons from anthropologic and cross-cultural research. *Annals of Internal Medicine, 88*(2), 251-258.

Kleinman, A., & Sung, L. H. (1979). Why do indigenous practitioners successfully heal? *Social Science & Medicine Part B--Medical Anthropology, 13*(1B), 7-26.

Landesman, P. (2002, September 15). A woman's work. *New York Times, Sunday Magazine,* p. 82.

Machel, G. (1996). *The impact of armed conflict on children.* Report of the Expert of the Secretary General Cape. New York: United Nations.

MacMullin, C., & Loughry, M. (2002). *The psychosocial adjustment of formerly abducted child soldiers in Northern Uganda.* Manuscript submitted for publication.

Marsella, A. J., Bornemann, T., Ekblad, S., & Orley, J. (1994). *Amidst peril and pain: The mental health and well-being of the world's refugees.* Washington, DC: American Psychological Association.

Marsella, A., Friedman, M. J., Gerrity, E., & Scurfield, R. M. (Eds.) (1996). *Ethnocultural aspects of post-traumatic stress disorders: Issues, research and applications.* Washington, DC: American Psychological Association.

Martin-Baró, I. (1985). *Accion e ideologia: Psicologia social desde Centroamerica.* San Salvadore: UCA Editores.

Martin-Baró, I. (1989). Political violence and war as causes of psychosocial trauma in El Salvador. *International Journal of Mental Health, 18,* 3-20.

Miller, K. E., Weine, S. M., Ramic, A., Brkic, N., Bjedic, Z. D., Smajkic, A., et al. (2002). The relative contribution of war experiences and exile-related stressors to levels of psychological distress among Bosnian refugees. *Journal of Traumatic Stress, 15*(5), 377-387.

Mitchulka, D., Blanchard, E., & Kalous, T. (1998). Responses to civilian war experiences: Predictors of psychological functioning and coping. *Journal of Traumatic Stress, 11,* 571-577.

Mollica, R., Donelan, K., Svang, T., Lavelle, J., Elias, C., Frankel, M., et al. (1993). The effect of trauma and confinement on functional health and mental health status of Cambodians living in Thailand-Cambodia border camps. *Journal of the American Medical Association, 27,* 581-586.

Mollica, R., McInnes, K., Pham, T., Fawzi, M., Smith, C., Murphy, E., et al. (1998). The dose-effect relationships between torture and psychiatric symptoms in Vietnamese ex-political detainees and a comparison group. *Journal of Nervous & Mental Disease, 186,* 543-553.

Moos, H. R., & Moos, S. B. (1986). *Family environment scale manual (2nd ed.).* Palo Alto, CA: Consulting Psychologist Press.

Nader, K., Dubrow, K., & Stamm, B. H. (1999). *Honoring differences: Cultural issues in the treatment of trauma and loss.* Philadelphia, PA: Brunner Mazel.

Pernice, R., & Brook, J. (1996). Refugees' and immigrants' mental health: Associations of demographic and post-migration factors. *Journal of Social Psychology, 136,* 511-519.

Prilleltensky, I., & Nelson, G. (2000). Promoting child and family wellness: Priorities for psychological and social interventions. *Journal of Community and Applied Social Psychology, 10,* 85-105.

Prilleltensky, I., Nelson, G., & Peirson, L. (Eds.). (in press). *Promoting family wellness and preventing child maltreatment.* Canada: University of Toronto Press.

Rutter, M. (1979). *Changing youth in a changing society: Patterns of adolescent development and disorder.* London: The Nuffield Provincial Hospitals Trust.

Rutter, M. (1987). Psychosocial resilience and protective mechanisms. *American Journal of Orthopsychiatry, 57*(3), 316-331.

Rutter, M., & Garmezy, N. (1983). Developmental psychopathology. In P. Mussen (Ed.), *Handbook of child psychology* (Vol. 4). New York: Wiley.

Steel, Z., & Silove, D. (2000). The psychosocial cost of seeking and granting asylum. In A. Y. Shalev, R. Yehuda, & A. C. McFarlane (Eds.), *International handbook of human response to trauma* (pp. 421-438). New York: Kluwer Academic/Plenum.

Stein, B. N. (1985). The experience of being a refugee: Insight from the research literature. In C. L. Williams & J. Westermeyer (Eds.), *Refugee mental health in resettlement countries* (pp. 5-23). New York: Hemisphere.

Summerfield, D. (1995). Addressing human response to war and atrocity: Major challenges in research and practices and the limitations of Western psychiatric models. In R. Kleber, C. Figley, & B. Gersons (Eds.), *Beyond trauma: Cultural and societal dynamics* (pp. 9-37). New York: Plenum Press.

Thabet, A., & Vostanis, P. (2000). Post-traumatic stress disorder reactions in children of war: A longitudinal study. *Child Abuse and Neglect, 24,* 291-298.

Vincent, T. A., & Trickett, E. J. (1983). Preventative interventions and the human context: Ecological approaches to environmental assessment and change. In R. D. Felner (Ed.), *Preventive psychology: Theory, research, and practice* (pp. 67-81). New York: Pergamon.

Wandersman, A. (1999). Framing the evaluation of health and human service programs in community settings: Assessing progress. *New Directions for Evaluation, 83,* 95-102.

Weine, S., Vojvoda, D., Becker, D., McGlashan, T., Hodzic, E., Laub, D., et al. (1998). PTSD symptoms in Bosnian refugees 1 year after resettlement in the United States. *American Journal of Psychiatry, 155,* 562-564.

Wessells, M. G. (1999). Culture, power, and community: Intercultural approaches to psychosocial assistance and healing. In K. Nader, N. Dubrow, & H. Stamm (Eds.), *Honoring differences: Cultural issues in the treatment of trauma and loss* (pp. 267-280). Ann Arbor, MI: Edwards Brothers.

Wessells, M. G., & Monteiro, C. (2001). Psychosocial interventions and post-war reconstruction in Angola: Interweaving Western and traditional approaches.

In D. Christie, W. V. Wagner, & D. Winter (Eds.), *Peace, conflict, and violence: Peace psychology for the 21st century* (pp. 262-275). Upper Saddle River, NJ: Prentice-Hall.

Author Index

Subject Index

Subject Index